Transbronchial and Endobronchial Biopsies

Transbronchial and Endobronchial Biopsies

Philip T. Cagle, MD
Professor of Pathology and Laboratory Medicine
Weill Medical College of Cornell University
New York, New York
Director, Pulmonary Pathology
The Methodist Hospital
Houston, Texas

Timothy C. Allen, MD, JD
Chairman
Department of Pathology
The University of Texas Health Science Center at Tyler
Tyler, Texas

Keith M. Kerr, FRCPath, FRCPEd
Consultant Pathologist
Department of Pathology
Aberdeen Royal Infirmary
Professor of Pulmonary Pathology
Aberdeen University Medical School
Aberdeen, United Kingdom

Wolters Kluwer | Lippincott Williams & Wilkins
Health
Philadelphia · Baltimore · New York · London
Buenos Aires · Hong Kong · Sydney · Tokyo

Senior Executive Editor: Jonathan W. Pine, Jr.
Managing Editor: Jean McGough
Project Manager: Jennifer Harper
Manufacturing Coordinator: Kathleen Brown
Marketing Manager: Angela Panetta
Design Coordinator: Stephen Druding
Production Services: International Typesetting & Composition

© 2009 by LIPPINCOTT WILLIAMS & WILKINS, a Wolters Kluwer business

530 Walnut Street
Philadelphia, PA 19106 USA
LWW.com

All rights reserved. This book is protected by copyright. No part of this book may be reproduced in any form by any means, including photocopying, or utilized by any information storage and retrieval system without written permission from the copyright owner, except for brief quotations embodied in critical articles and reviews. Materials appearing in this book prepared by individuals as part of their official duties as U.S. government employees are not covered by the above-mentioned copyright.

Printed in China

Library of Congress Cataloging-in-Publication Data

Cagle, Philip T.
  Transbronchial and endobronchial biopsies/Philip T. Cagle, Timothy C. Allen, and Keith M. Kerr
    p. ; cm.
  Companion book to: Color atlas and text of pulmonary pathology/editor-in-chief, Philip C. Cagle ; associate editors, Timothy C. Allen . . . [et al.]. 2nd ed. 2008.
  Includes bibliographical references and index.
  ISBN-13: 978-0-7817-8517-4
  ISBN-10: 0-7817-8517-0
  1. Lungs—Biopsy. 2. Lungs—Diseases—Cytodiagnosis. 3. Lungs—Cancer—Cytodiagnosis.
 I. Allen, Timothy C. II. Kerr, Keith M. III. Color atlas and text of pulmonary pathology. IV. Title.
    [DNLM: 1. Lung Diseases—pathology. 2. Biopsy—methods. 3. Bronchi—pathology.
 4. Bronchial Diseases—pathology. 5. Lung—pathology. WF 600 C131t 2009]
    RC734.B56C34 2009
    616.2'400223—dc22

2008008246

DISCLAIMER

Care has been taken to confirm the accuracy of the information presented and to describe generally accepted practices. However, the authors, editors, and publisher are not responsible for errors or omissions or for any consequences from application of the information in this book and make no warranty, expressed or implied, with respect to the currency, completeness, or accuracy of the contents of the publication. Application of the information in a particular situation remains the professional responsibility of the practitioner.

The authors, editors, and publisher have exerted every effort to ensure that drug selection and dosage set forth in this text are in accordance with current recommendations and practice at the time of publication. However, in view of ongoing research, changes in government regulations, and the constant flow of information relating to drug therapy and drug reactions, the reader is urged to check the package insert for each drug for any change in indications and dosage and for added warnings and precautions. This is particularly important when the recommended agent is a new or infrequently employed drug.

Some drugs and medical devices presented in the publication have Food and Drug Administration (FDA) clearance for limited use in restricted research settings. It is the responsibility of the health care provider to ascertain the FDA status of each drug or device planned for use in their clinical practice.

To purchase additional copies of this book, call our customer service department at (800) 638-3030 or fax orders to (301) 223-2320. International customers should call (301) 223-2300. Visit Lippincott Williams & Wilkins on the Internet: at LWW.com. Lippincott Williams & Wilkins customer service representatives are available from 8:30 am to 6 pm, EST.

10 9 8 7 6 5 4 3 2

The editors wish to dedicate *Transbronchial and Endobronchial Biopsies* to two legendary figures who made the Texas Medical Center in Houston a great international center for pulmonary pathology: Claire Langston, now retired, and the late S. Donald Greenberg. For decades, these two individuals made tremendous contributions to knowledge in the field of pulmonary pathology, but they are perhaps best known and beloved for their immense personal influence as mentors and teachers of numerous academic progeny, several of whom are represented among the editors of this book.

Preface

It has been a number of years since a textbook dedicated specifically to the histopathology of transbronchial and endobronchial biopsies has been published. Because the diagnostic approach to transbronchial and endobronchial biopsies differs from that of larger surgical specimens, we were asked to provide a companion to the *Color Atlas and Text of Pulmonary Pathology* with specific descriptions and illustrations to assist pathologists with these smaller biopsies.

Transbronchial and Endobronchial Biopsies is intended to provide rapid answers in daily practice, including a fully searchable online text and image bank that are not usually readily available in standard textbooks. *Transbronchial and Endobronchial Biopsies* offers a succinct, user-friendly approach to the diagnosis of both neoplastic and nonneoplastic lung diseases for transbronchial and endobronchial biopsies, including malignant and benign neoplasms, infections, intra-alveolar infiltrates, diffuse interstitial diseases, transplant-related pathology, nonneoplastic large airways pathology, and pediatric pulmonary pathology. Unlike any other current lung pathology textbook, all figures are from transbronchial or endobronchial biopsies, thus accurately representing the limitations, artifacts, and diagnostic approach to these small tissue samples. To honestly reflect the experience of the practicing pathologist, each of the diagnoses is first illustrated with a low power overview of the biopsy for orientation. Subsequent higher power figures from the same biopsies document the specific diagnostic features. Artifacts, pitfalls, and special clues that point to a diagnosis on a tiny tissue sample are discussed and illustrated. The text is confined to specific points for accurate diagnosis on a small tissue sample.

Similar to its companion book, the *Color Atlas and Text of Pulmonary Pathology*, *Transbronchial and Endobronchial Biopsies* is dedicated to the memory of one of the early pioneers in the interpretation of biopsies from the flexible bronchoscope in the late 1960s and early 1970s, the late Dr. S. Donald Greenberg. Dr. Greenberg was a mentor to many of the editors of this book. We also dedicate this book to Dr. Claire Langston, who also has been a mentor to many of the editors and recently retired.

Philip T. Cagle, MD
Timothy C. Allen, MD, JD
Keith M. Kerr, FRCPath

Associate Editors

Roberto Barrios, MD
Professor of Pathology and Laboratory Medicine
Weill Medical College of Cornell University
New York, New York
Active Physician
Pathology and Laboratory Medicine
The Methodist Hospital
Houston, Texas

Megan K. Dishop, MD
Assistant Professor
Department of Pathology
Baylor College of Medicine
Pathologist
Department of Pathology
Texas Children's Hospital
Houston, Texas

Armando E. Fraire, MD
Professor
University of Massachusetts Medical School
Attending Pathologist
UMass Memorial Health Care
Worcester, Massachusetts

Jaishree Jagirdar, MD
Professor of Pathology
Department of Pathology
University of Texas
Director of Anatomic Pathology
Department of Pathology
University Hospital
San Antonio, Texas

Abida Haque, MD
Professor of Pathology and Laboratory Medicine
Weill Medical College of Cornell University
New York, New York
Attending Pathologist
The Methodist Hospital
Houston, Texas

Kun Y. Kwon, MD, PhD
Professor and Associate Superintendent
Department of Pathology
Keimyung University Dongsan
    Medical Center
Daegu, South Korea

Jae Y. Ro, MD, PhD
Professor of Pathology
Weill Medical College of Cornell University
New York, New York
Director of Surgical Pathology
The Methodist Hospital
Houston, Texas

Anna Sienko, MD, FRCP(C)
Associate Professor
Department of Pathology and Laboratory
    Medicine
Weill Medical College of Cornell University
New York, New York
Attending Pathologist
The Methodist Hospital
Houston, Texas

Contributing Author
Clifford G. Risk, MD, PhD
Pulmonologist
UMass Marlboro Hospital
Marlboro, Massachusetts

Contents

Preface   vii
Associate Editors   ix

1   Overview of Transbronchial and Endobronchial Biopsies   1
    Timothy C. Allen and Philip T. Cagle

2   Artifacts and Nonspecific Changes   3
    Timothy C. Allen and Philip T. Cagle

3   Non–Small Cell Carcinomas   7
    Kun Y. Kwon, Keith M. Kerr, and Jae Y. Ro

4   Neuroendocrine Tumors   21
    Keith M. Kerr, Kun Y. Kwon, and Jae Y. Ro

5   Metastatic Cancers   29
    Keith M. Kerr

6   Preinvasive Lesions   35
    Keith M. Kerr

7   Hematolymphoid Malignancies   39
    Timothy C. Allen, Keith M. Kerr, and Jaishree Jagirdar

8   Benign Neoplasms   43
    Keith M. Kerr

9   Viruses   47
    Abida Haque and Philip T. Cagle

10 Bacterial Pneumonia   51
    Armando E. Fraire, Abida Haque, and Clifford G. Risk

11 Mycoplasma Pneumonia   55
    Armando E. Fraire

12 *Pneumocystis jiroveci*   57
    Abida Haque, Anna Sienko, and Philip T. Cagle

13 Mycobacteria 59
Abida Haque, Anna Sienko, and Philip T. Cagle

14 Fungus 61
Abida Haque, Anna Sienko, and Philip T. Cagle

15 Other Infections 65
Timothy C. Allen and Philip T. Cagle

16 Diffuse Alveolar Damage 67
Anna Sienko and Timothy C. Allen

17 Pulmonary Edema 71
Timothy C. Allen and Roberto Barrios

18 Organizing Pneumonia 73
Philip T. Cagle and Timothy C. Allen

19 Acute Fibrinous and Organizing Pneumonia 77
Anna Sienko

20 Aspiration Pneumonia 79
Timothy C. Allen, Roberto Barrios, Abida Haque, and Philip T. Cagle

21 Intra-alveolar Hemorrhage 83
Timothy C. Allen, Jaishree Jagirdar, and Philip T. Cagle

22 Eosinophilic Pneumonia 89
Roberto Barrios and Keith M. Kerr

23 Lipid Pneumonia 91
Timothy C. Allen and Roberto Barrios

24 Pulmonary Alveolar Proteinosis 93
Anna Sienko and Philip T. Cagle

25 Sarcoidosis 95
Armando E. Fraire

26 Hypersensitivity Pneumonitis 97
Armando E. Fraire and Philip T. Cagle

27 Collagen Vascular Diseases 101
Timothy C. Allen, Jaishree Jagirdar, and Philip T. Cagle

28 Drug Reactions 105
Timothy C. Allen, Jaishree Jagirdar, and Philip T. Cagle

Contents

29 Inflammatory Bowel Disease   109
Anna Sienko

30 Pneumoconioses   111
Timothy C. Allen and Philip T. Cagle

31 Idiopathic Interstitial Pneumonias   115
Timothy C. Allen and Philip T. Cagle

32 Lymphangioleiomyomatosis   121
Timothy C. Allen

33 Intravenous Drug Abuse   125
Timothy C. Allen

34 Langerhans Cell Histiocytosis   127
Timothy C. Allen and Philip T. Cagle

35 Acute Transplant Rejection   131
Anna Sienko

36 Other Transplant Associated Pathology   135
Anna Sienko and Philip T. Cagle

37 Nonneoplastic Large Airways Pathology   139
Timothy C. Allen, Jaishree Jagirdar, and Keith M. Kerr

38 Role of Transbronchial and Endobronchial Biopsies in Children   145
Megan K. Dishop

39 Bronchial Masses in the Pediatric Population   151
Megan K. Dishop

40 Tracheobronchial Biopsy for Primary Ciliary Dyskinesia   157
Megan K. Dishop

41 Legal Aspects of Endobronchial and Transbronchial Biopsy   161
Timothy C. Allen

Index   163

Transbronchial and Endobronchial Biopsies

Overview of Transbronchial and Endobronchial Biopsies

▶ Timothy C. Allen, MD, JD
▶ Philip T. Cagle, MD

Transbronchial and endobronchial biopsies are procedures of limited invasiveness performed by bronchoscopy, typically aided by fluoroscopy, with less morbidity and mortality than wedge lung biopsy, which is performed by thoracoscopy or by open surgery; however, they provide a limited amount of tissue from a restricted sampling area. Specimens typically are no more than 2 to 3 mm in size. Endobronchial biopsies may contain bronchial epithelium and underlying bronchial wall, including subepithelial tissue, bronchial glands, muscle, and cartilage. Peribronchial lymphatic and vascular structures may also be present. Successful transbronchial biopsies also include lung parenchyma.

The decision to attempt a transbronchial biopsy as opposed to a thoracoscopic or open wedge biopsy is based on (1) whether histopathologic diagnosis of the suspected disease is possible by small sample, (2) the probability of sampling diagnostic tissue by transbronchial biopsy, and (3) the risk/benefit ratio for the patient. Therefore, diagnosis by endobronchial or transbronchial biopsy depends on the type of disease and the distribution of the disease. Neoplasms, infections, and some interstitial lung diseases are diagnosable by endobronchial or transbronchial biopsy. The diagnostic yield for a focal endobronchial lesion is 90% to 100%, whereas the diagnostic yield for a more peripheral focal lesion, using guidance with fluoroscopy and by obtaining additional cytology samples, is 40% to 80%. Obviously, some lesions are too peripheral for bronchoscopic sampling and require transthoracic needle biopsy or other procedure for diagnosis. The overall diagnostic yield for diffuse lung diseases by transbronchial biopsy is 37%.

Diffuse lung diseases with a peribronchial distribution are particularly amenable to diagnosis by transbronchial biopsy. For example, the diagnostic yield for sarcoidosis by transbronchial biopsy ranges from 85% to 97%. In the case of certain other diffuse interstitial lung diseases, for example, usual interstitial pneumonia, transbronchial biopsy potentially provides a supportive role to the clinical/radiologic diagnosis but, by itself, does not provide sufficient tissue for a definitive histopathologic diagnosis.

In addition to the type and distribution of the diseases, diagnosis by transbronchial biopsy also depends on the number of samples taken, the skill of the bronchoscopist, the type of forceps used, and complications that may cut short the procedure. Transbronchial biopsies are associated with minor bleeding that may cause the inexperienced bronchoscopist to overreact and stop the procedure prematurely. More significant bleeding and pneumothorax may occur as major complications in <3% of transbronchial biopsy procedures.

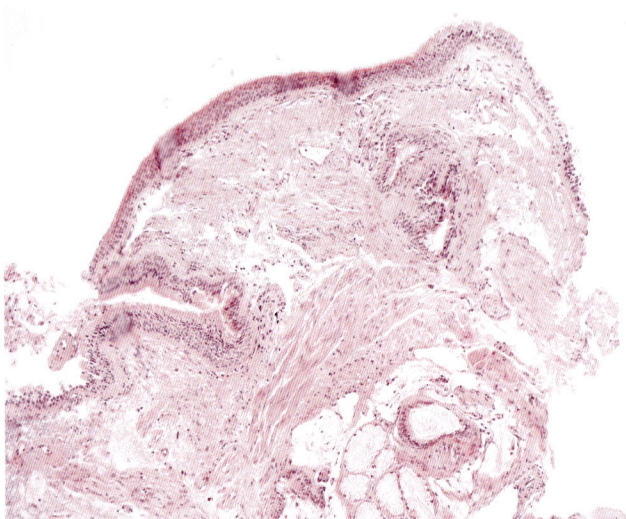

Figure 1.1: Low power of endobronchial biopsy shows normal bronchial mucosa and bronchial wall.

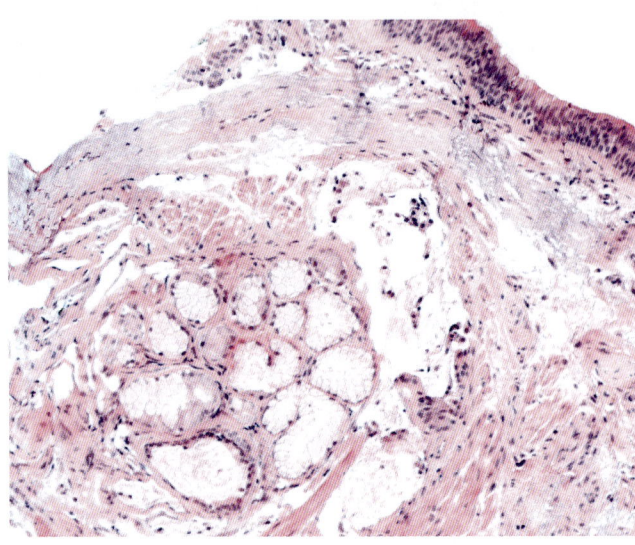

Figure 1.2: High power shows bronchial mucosa and underlying bronchial glands.

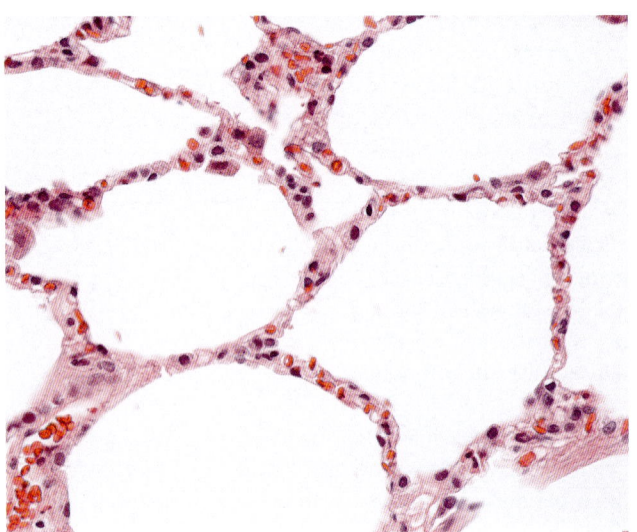

Figure 1.3: High power of transbronchial biopsy shows alveolar septa of lung parenchyma underlying bronchial wall.

Suggested Readings

Cagle PT. Endobronchial and transbronchial biopsies. In: Cagle PT, ed. *Diagnostic Pulmonary Pathology.* New York: Marcel Dekker; 2000.

Frost AE. Transbronchial biopsies: clinical perspective. In: Cagle PT, ed. *Diagnostic Pulmonary Pathology.* New York: Marcel Dekker; 2000.

Artifacts and Nonspecific Changes

▶ Timothy C. Allen, MD, JD
▶ Philip T. Cagle, MD

The pathologist should be aware of the artifacts and nonspecific changes that may be seen in a transbronchial biopsy in order to avoid misinterpretation of these as pathologic changes.

Tissue compression by transbronchial biopsy forceps causes collapse of lung parenchyma and, to a lesser extent, the bronchial wall. Lung parenchymal compression may appear on examination as rounded spaces or holes mimicking fungal organisms or lipid vacuolization. Collapsed lung parenchyma may be misinterpreted as fibrosis or increased cellularity within the interstitium. Bronchial wall compression, with collapse of blood vessels and loss of normal architecture, might mimic scarring within the bronchial wall. Bleeding is a normal result of the biopsy procedure and may occasionally mimic pathologic hemorrhage. When bleeding is associated with a pathologic condition, the biopsy generally contains associated fibrin and hemosiderin-laden macrophages. The adherence to strict criteria for the diagnosis of various conditions characterized by hemorrhage will help the pathologist avoid overdiagnosis of these conditions. Biopsy fixation in 10% formalin minimizes artifactual changes, whereas the use of alcohol-based non-aldehyde fixatives may increase the incidence of artifact, as may the use of saline to transport the biopsy to the laboratory.

Lymphocytes and other inflammatory cells may exhibit crush artifact. That crush artifact may occasionally be substantial enough to mimic small cell carcinoma. The diagnosis of small cell carcinoma must be made based only on the examination of intact (not crushed) small cell lung cancer cells.

Deep transbronchial biopsies may include pleura. Reactive mesothelial cells from the pleural surface should be recognized as such and not misinterpreted as a neoplasm.

A variety of endogenous structures may be found on transbronchial biopsy. Blue bodies may be present, occasionally in increased numbers that incorrectly suggest inorganic dust exposure. Blue bodies are intra-alveolar basophilic, laminated, calcified, frequently multiple concretions that range from 15 to 40 μm. Alcian blue and periodic acid-Schiff (PAS) stains highlight blue bodies. They are formed within macrophages and giant cells.

Calcium oxalate crystals occur within giant cells and may be seen along with blue bodies. They are found in association with granulomatous inflammation and are birefringent, identifiable with polarized light. The crystals are irregular, glassy sheets with sharply angled edges, ranging from 1 to 20 μm. Calcium oxalate crystals may mimic foreign material. Charcot-Leyden crystals, needle-shaped crystals seen within macrophages, form due to the collection of eosinophilic debris within macrophages and may be found in biopsies from patients with asthma, hypersensitivity pneumonitis, and eosinophilic pneumonia, among other diseases. Other endogenous structures, such as cholesterol clefts, psammoma bodies (calcospherites), dystrophic ossification, and Schaumann bodies may occasionally be found on transbronchial biopsy.

Exogenous structures such as ferruginous bodies, including asbestos bodies, may be found in transbronchial biopsies and are apparent both on hematoxylin and eosin (H&E) stain and iron stain. Although ferruginous bodies, including asbestos bodies, are not diagnostic of any disease state, it is important to differentiate them from other foreign material.

Reactive type II pneumocytes may be found in transbronchial biopsies in response to a variety of conditions including diffuse alveolar damage, infarct, and infections, among many other etiologies. They can also be seen adjacent to neoplasms, and care must be taken to recognize their reactive, benign nature and not to overdiagnose them as malignant cells.

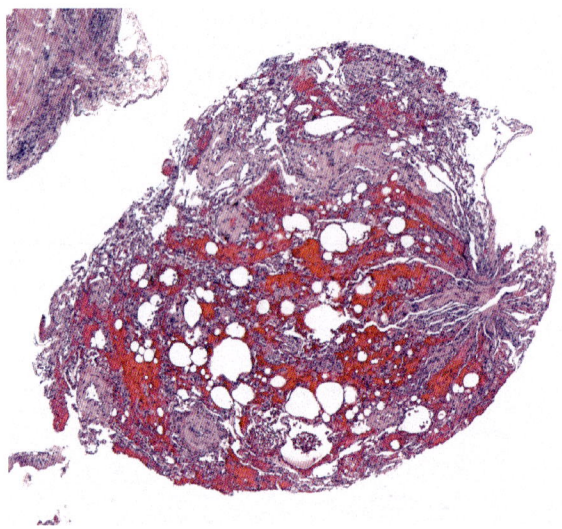

Figure 2.1: Low power of transbronchial biopsy shows fresh procedural hemorrhage within alveolar spaces and artifactual rounded spaces due to compression.

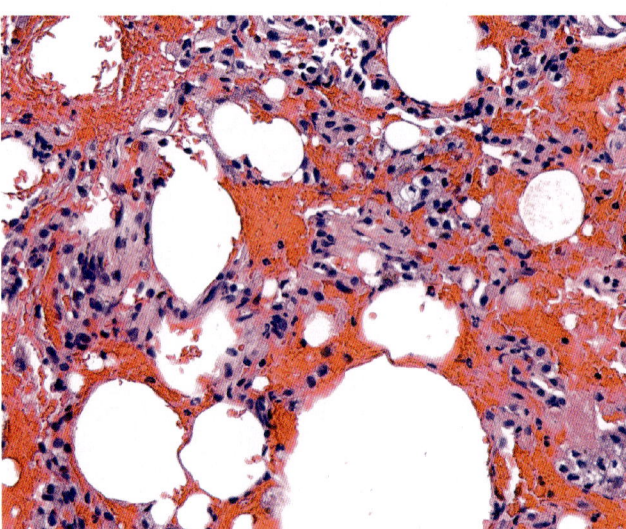

Figure 2.2: High power provides closer view of fresh procedural hemorrhage consisting of red blood cells within alveolar spaces and artifactual rounded spaces.

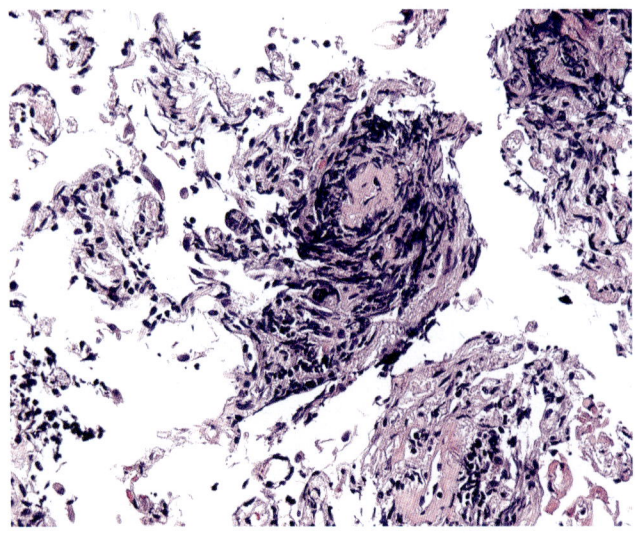

Figure 2.3: High power shows lymphocytes with crush artifact surrounding a parenchymal blood vessel.

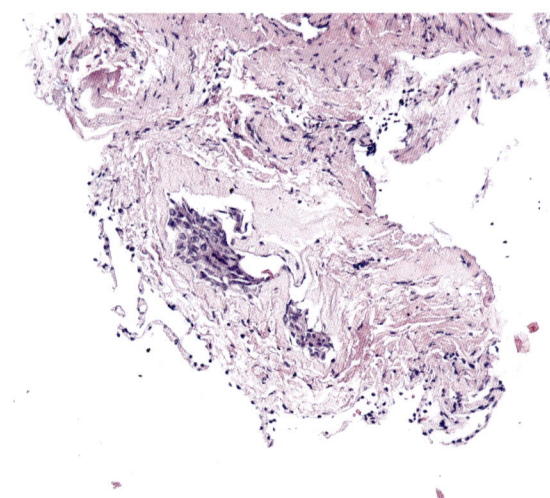

Figure 2.4: Low power shows epithelial cells within an apparent space in a transbronchial biopsy suggesting possible vascular spread of a neoplasm.

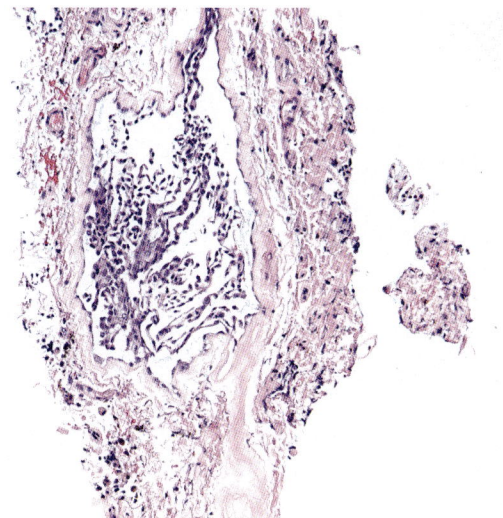

Figure 2.5: Higher power shows epithelial cells within a "space" that appears "lined" by cuboidal cells.

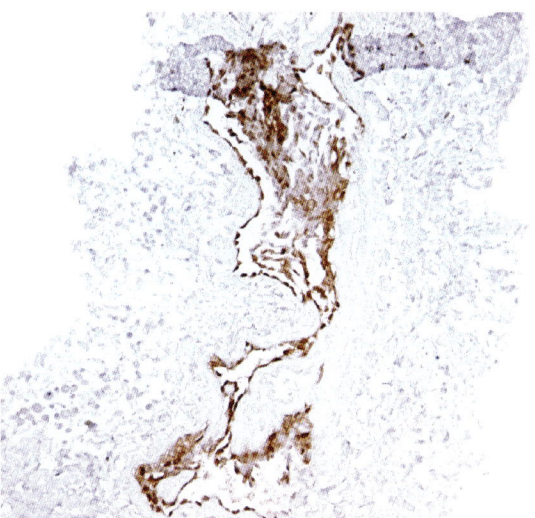

Figure 2.6: Calretinin immunostain demonstrates that the epithelial cells are consistent with mesothelial cells. This artifact is the result of *en face* embedding of a transbronchial biopsy that included pleura.

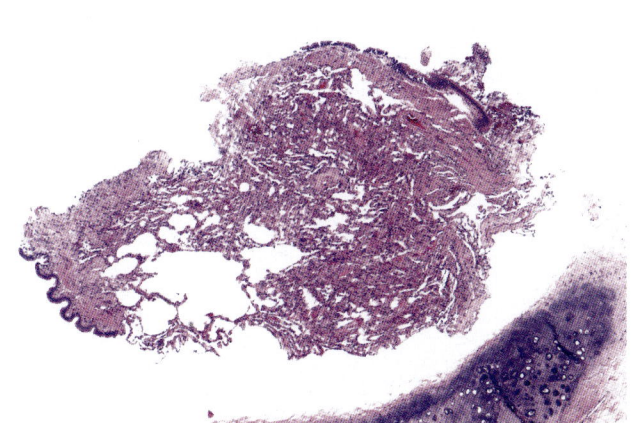

Figure 2.7: Transbronchial biopsy at low power appears to have parenchymal fibrosis. Biopsy of bronchial cartilage is present in the lower part of the field.

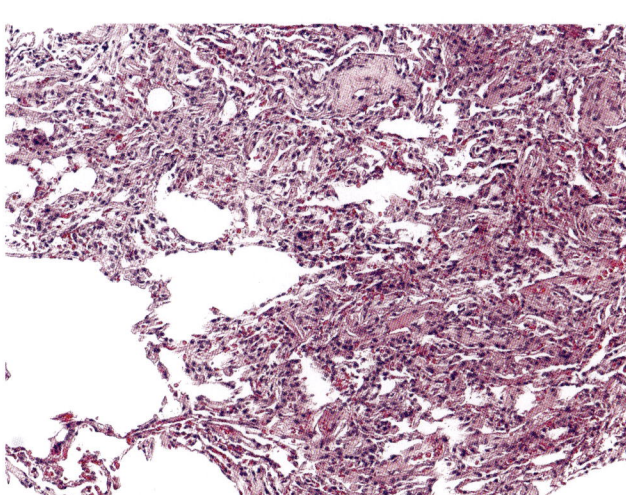

Figure 2.8: Higher power of tissue in Figure 2.7 shows that the apparent fibrosis is actually collapsed lung parenchyma. Attention to the individual alveolar septa at high power allows one to see that they are of normal thickness and it is their close proximity that gives the illusion of fibrosis at lower power.

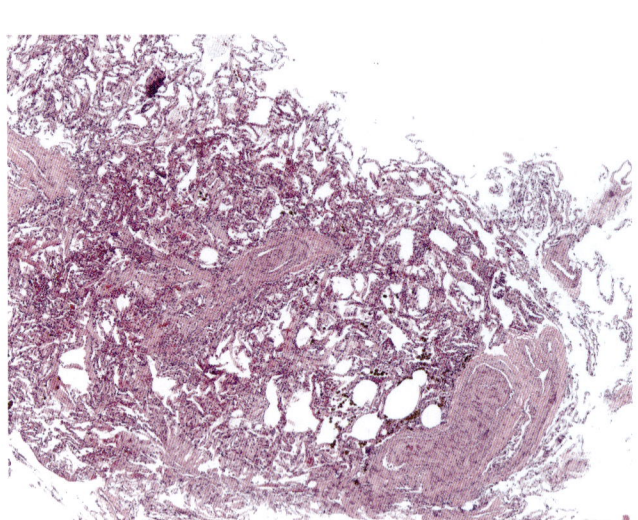

Figure 2.9: Low power of transbronchial biopsy shows large blood vessels cut longitudinally and tangentially. These vessels should not be mistaken for fibrotic tissue. Although the bronchus is not seen in this field, the large blood vessels probably accompany the bronchus through which the biopsy was taken.

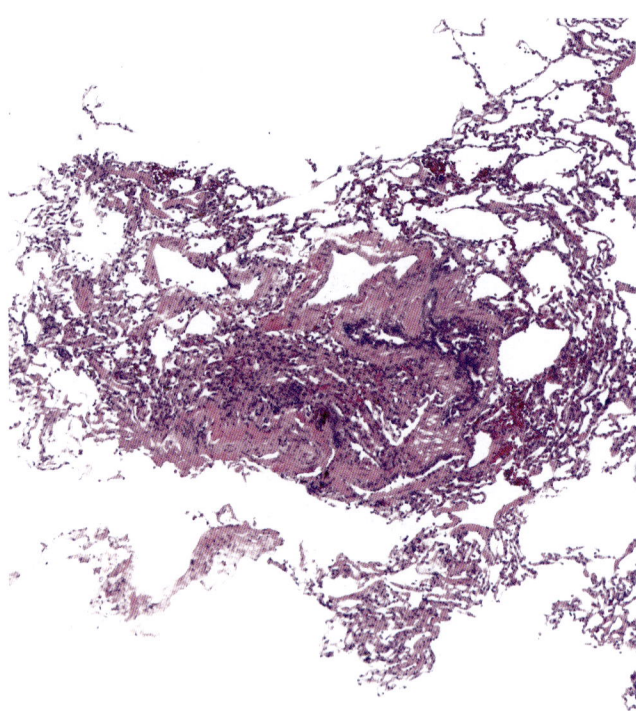

Figure 2.10: Low power of transbronchial biopsy shows bronchus and accompanying blood vessel cut *en face*. These structures should not be misinterpreted as fibrosis or other lesion.

Suggested Readings

Anton RC, Cagle PT. Intra- and extracellular structures. In: Cagle PT, ed. *Diagnostic Pulmonary Pathology.* New York: Marcel Dekker; 2000.

Cagle PT. Endobronchial and transbronchial biopsies. In: Cagle PT, ed. *Diagnostic Pulmonary Pathology.* New York: Marcel Dekker; 2000.

Non–Small Cell Carcinomas

▶ Kun Y. Kwon, MD
▶ Keith M. Kerr, FRCPath
▶ Jae Y. Ro, MD

Histologically, and largely through an imperative of patient management, lung carcinomas are divided into two major types: non–small cell lung carcinoma and small cell lung carcinoma. About 75% to 80% of lung carcinomas diagnosed on bronchial and transbronchial biopsy fall into the non–small cell carcinoma category. The diagnostic process involves a number of steps: identification of neoplastic conditions and, in particular, malignancy, recognizing the tumor is carcinoma, separation of small cell carcinoma from other (non–small cell) carcinomas, and, where possible, making a specific histologic subtype diagnosis of a non–small cell carcinoma.

Small tissue biopsies from endoscopy may contain only tiny fragments of atypical epithelium or small numbers of atypical cells. The biopsy procedure may also cause substantial crush artifact and there may be intense inflammation associated with any neoplastic process. Thus there will be situations in reporting endoscopic biopsies when a confident diagnosis of carcinoma is not possible. Cytological atypia insufficient to diagnose carcinoma may require a "suspicious" report with recommendation for further biopsy. It may be difficult to confirm an atypical squamous epithelium that is invasive, and thus a differential diagnosis with squamous dysplasia/carcinoma in situ (see later and Chapter 6) is appropriate. Immunostaining for cytokeratins may, in some situations, confirm an apparently infiltrating cell population as epithelial and thus assist a diagnosis of carcinoma, provided the cells in question are neither from the nonneoplastic bronchial epithelium nor mucous glands.

The World Health Organization (WHO) lung tumor classification of non–small cell carcinoma (Table 3-1) is based on examination of the whole or a substantial part of the tumor. Limited material in small samples sometimes makes a definitive diagnosis of non–small cell lung carcinoma subtype impossible to render. For many of the categories in Table 3-1, this would always be the case. Thus it is important to realize it is sometimes inappropriate to subclassify non–small cell lung carcinoma on small biopsy material, and we often only make a diagnosis of non–small cell carcinoma, not otherwise specified.

Squamous cell carcinoma is the most frequently diagnosed cancer in endobronchial biopsy material. Specific diagnosis requires recognition of either intercellular bridges or keratinization in the tumor. Sometimes either of these features will be present only focally, and a careful search of all tumor foci is required to identify it. Tumor cells are frequently large with irregular nuclei and coarse chromatin, nucleoli may be present but are not usually prominent, and cytoplasm is often dense and eosinophilic. The tumor usually invades the bronchial mucosa in irregular but well-defined sheets and nests of tumor cells. A basaloid variant of squamous cell carcinoma shows smaller cells and less cytoplasm and, potentially, it may be confused with small cell carcinoma. In the basaloid variant, tumor cells may show palisading at the margin of tumor cell nests. Some squamous cell carcinomas show clear cell areas, and an endobronchial tumor in particular may exhibit a papillary architecture. Distinction between in situ and invasive squamous cell carcinoma in the bronchus may be difficult, especially when subepithelial stroma is scant or absent. In situ carcinoma tends

Table 3-1	WHO Classification of Non–Small Cell Lung Carcinomas
Squamous cell carcinoma	8070/3
Squamous cell carcinoma variants	
Papillary	8052/3
Clear cell	8084/3
Small cell	8073/3
Basaloid	8083/3
Adenocarcinoma	8140/3
Adenocarcinoma variants	
Fetal adenocarcinoma	8333/3
Mucinous (colloid) adenocarcinoma	8480/3
Mucinous cystadenocarcinoma	8470/3
Signet-ring cell adenocarcinoma	8490/3
Clear cell adenocarcinoma	8310/3
Large cell carcinoma	8012/3
Large cell neuroendocrine carcinoma	8013/3
Basaloid	8123/3
Lymphoepithelioma-like carcinoma	8082/3
Clear cell	8310/3
Large cell with rhabdoid phenotype	8014/3
Sarcomatoid carcinoma	8033/3
Others	
Salivary-type carcinomas	

to exist in strips, whereas invasive tumor may demonstrate a more irregular pattern, comprising small islands or groups of cells, and a fibroblastic stromal reaction may be present. One further pitfall is the replacement of bronchial glands by extension of carcinoma in situ from the bronchial surface, mimicking invasive carcinoma and leading to misdiagnosis if the lobular architecture and occasional residual glandular cells are not recognized. Clinicopathologic correlation may help solve any problem, but repeat biopsy may also be necessary. In transbronchial lung biopsy, where more peripherally located squamous cell carcinoma invades lung parenchyma, nests of tumor cells may fill alveoli while the alveolar architecture remains intact. Squamous metaplasia with inflammatory reactive atypia in the lung periphery, occurring, for example, in the context of usual interstitial pneumonia or organizing diffuse alveolar damage may be misinterpreted as squamous cell carcinoma. As is always the case, knowledge of the clinical context, radiologic, and endoscopic findings should prevent misdiagnosis.

The peripheral location of adenocarcinomas makes them less often diagnosed in endoscopic biopsy material. Nonetheless, larger, more advanced adenocarcinomas may lie close to or involve an airway large enough to allow biopsy. A minority of adenocarcinomas probably originate in the proximal airways. The different patterns of invasive adenocarcinoma (acinar, papillary, micropapillary, and solid with mucin) may be appreciated in bronchial biopsies, although in practice acinar and papillary/micropapillary tumors are less common in such samples. In practice, given the tendency for many of these tumors to be relatively advanced and poorly differentiated, the solid pattern is most frequently found; occasionally the tumor has a cribriform architecture. Adenocarcinomas comprise a range of cell types depending on the architectural pattern present. Cells may be cuboidal, columnar, round, or oval. Cytoplasm may be eosinophilic, basophilic, or clear. A mucin stain may be extremely valuable in many instances, allowing identification of intracellular or extracellular mucin. Thyroid transcription factor-1 (TTF-1) and carcinoembryonic antigen (CEA) immunostaining also help to make a diagnosis of adenocarcinomas. Although the WHO classification of solid adenocarcinoma with mucin requires an arbitrary five cells with intracytoplasmic mucin vacuoles in each of two high-power fields, a more pragmatic approach is reasonable in bronchial or transbronchial biopsy specimens. The presence of mucin is sufficient for a presumptive diagnosis of adenocarcinoma, provided no other features are present to suggest an alternative. Mucin may be present in small vacuoles, finely divided granules, or in goblet-type cells. Extracellular mucin in gland lumina may be seen, and care must be taken not to confuse mucin in the tumor with mucin from the nonneoplastic bronchial epithelium or bronchial glands also present in the sample. Lymphatic invasion within the bronchial mucosa is not uncommon and may be associated with nodal metastases; occasionally this lymphatic carcinoma may be the only tumor present in the biopsy specimen, so careful searching for such tumor is always worthwhile.

Bronchioloalveolar carcinoma (BAC) may be detected in transbronchial biopsy when alveolated lung is sampled. This is characterized by the growth of tumor cells, often columnar with apical snouts (Clara cells), around alveolar walls. Given that the WHO definition of BAC is of a tumor composed entirely of this pattern, with no evidence of stromal, vascular, or pleural invasion, it is clear that this diagnosis can *never* be made on bronchial or transbronchial biopsy samples. If tumor showing this so-called lepidic growth is found, a diagnosis of adenocarcinoma showing a BAC pattern in the sampled tissue should be made and efforts made to correlate pathology with radiology and clinical findings. It is important to mention the BAC pattern, if identified, because this is associated, at least in some cases, with a greater chance of response to epidermal growth factor receptor (EGFR)-targeted tyrosine kinase inhibitors (Erlotinib, Gefitinib). Mucinous tumors, sometimes with mucin-filled goblet cells, may also exhibit this growth pattern (so-called mucinous BAC). In this instance the tumor cells may be present in small, sharply defined groups, lining only part of an alveolus. The presence of mucin, possibly in goblet cells, and the absence of ciliated cells helps distinguish this pattern of tumor from small reactive foci, for example foci of peribronchiolar metaplasia. In some cases of mucinous BAC, alveoli may contain either free mucin or many macrophages (muciphages) with foamy cytoplasm. Either of these features may appear in a transbronchial biopsy sample without any tumor cells. Clearly, carcinoma cannot be diagnosed in such an instance, but appropriate suspicion should be conveyed in the report.

Large cell carcinoma is another tumor type that cannot be diagnosed on bronchial or transbronchial biopsy. The pathologist has no way of knowing whether elements of undifferentiated carcinoma, comprising large cells, often prominent nucleoli, and abundant cytoplasm, are representative of the whole tumor or have been sampled from a lesion that shows definite differentiation, perhaps squamous cell or adenocarcinoma, elsewhere in the mass. In such circumstances the appropriate diagnosis to give is "non–small cell carcinoma, not otherwise specified." In practice, about 30% to 35% of carcinomas diagnosed on endoscopic biopsy fall into this category. Opting for the less specific diagnosis in the absence of definite differentiation features such as keratinization, intercellular bridges, or mucin, or even somewhat so-called softer features such as glands or papillae, will result in 80% to 90% accuracy in the diagnosis of squamous cell or adenocarcinoma. Otherwise, accuracy of squamous cell carcinoma diagnosis is around 70%, whereas adenocarcinomas are correctly classified in around 50% of cases when compared to the resected tumors. Cellular stratification and squamoid features are not reliable indicators of squamous cell carcinoma. In practice, a majority of cases classified as "non–small cell carcinoma, not otherwise specified" prove to be adenocarcinomas when resected. It follows that the variants of large cell carcinoma are also diagnoses that may be inappropriate to make in this context. Clear cells or basaloid tumor may be recognized, but these should be added as descriptors to a diagnosis of non–small cell carcinoma, rather than a specific variant diagnosis being offered. Large cell neuroendocrine carcinoma is discussed in Chapter 4.

Sarcomatoid carcinomas are defined in the WHO classification of lung tumors as lesions in which >10% of the lesion shows pleomorphic, giant cell, or spindle cell tumor. Once again, the limited sample of tissue in the endoscopic biopsy precludes such a definitive diagnosis. If tumor showing such features is encountered and definite differentiation is lacking, the best approach is to classify the tumor as non–small cell carcinoma and mention the sarcomatoid features. In this situation, care should, of course, be taken to exclude, as appropriate, true sarcomas or even diffuse malignant mesothelioma; clinicopathologic correlation is vital.

Many lung tumors are heterogeneous in appearance; approximately half show (usually small) areas of differentiation of other than the dominant type, and when the minority type exceeds 10% of the tumor, a mixed carcinoma may be diagnosed. Adenosquamous carcinoma is the best known mixed-type lung carcinoma. Yet again, this 10% rule dictates that these are tumors that cannot be correctly classified on endoscopic biopsy. Best practice is to diagnose carcinoma and describe what is present. Salivary-type carcinomas are rare in the bronchi and lung but have features identical to their better known counterparts arising in the salivary glands. Mucoepidermoid and adenoid cystic carcinomas are the most frequent and tend to predominate in the trachea and main bronchi.

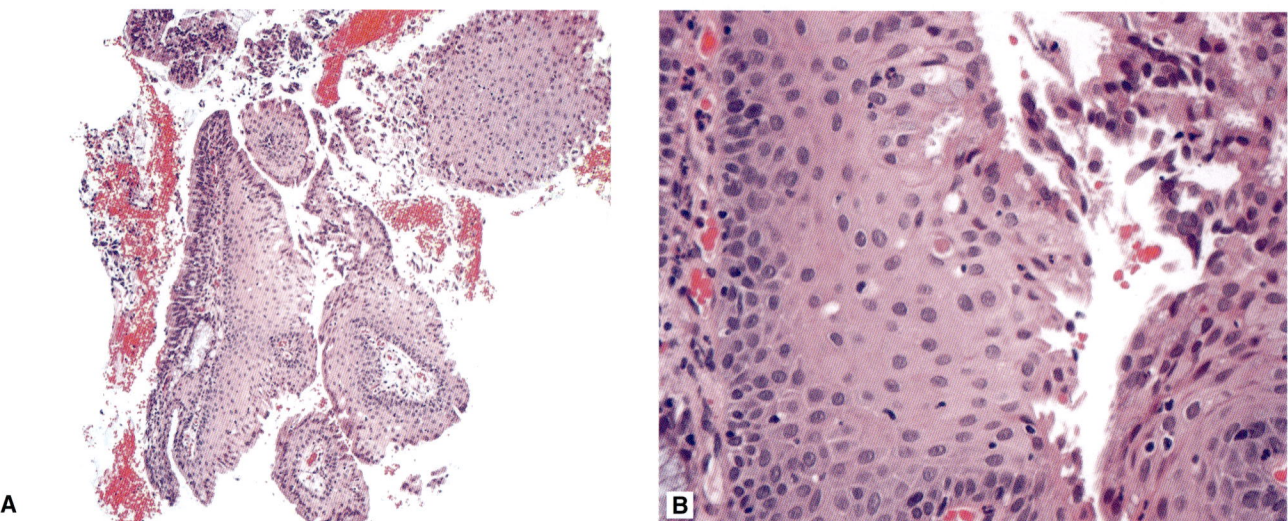

Figure 3.1: This bronchial biopsy shows respiratory epithelium but also metaplastic squamous epithelium that is focally atypical. The effects of fragmentation and malorientation can make distinction between squamous dysplasia/carcinoma in situ (see Chapter 6) and invasive disease difficult. In this case the lack of clear stromal invasion, mild atypia, and subtle residual columnar cells on the surface of some of the squamous epithelial islands helps rule out malignancy.

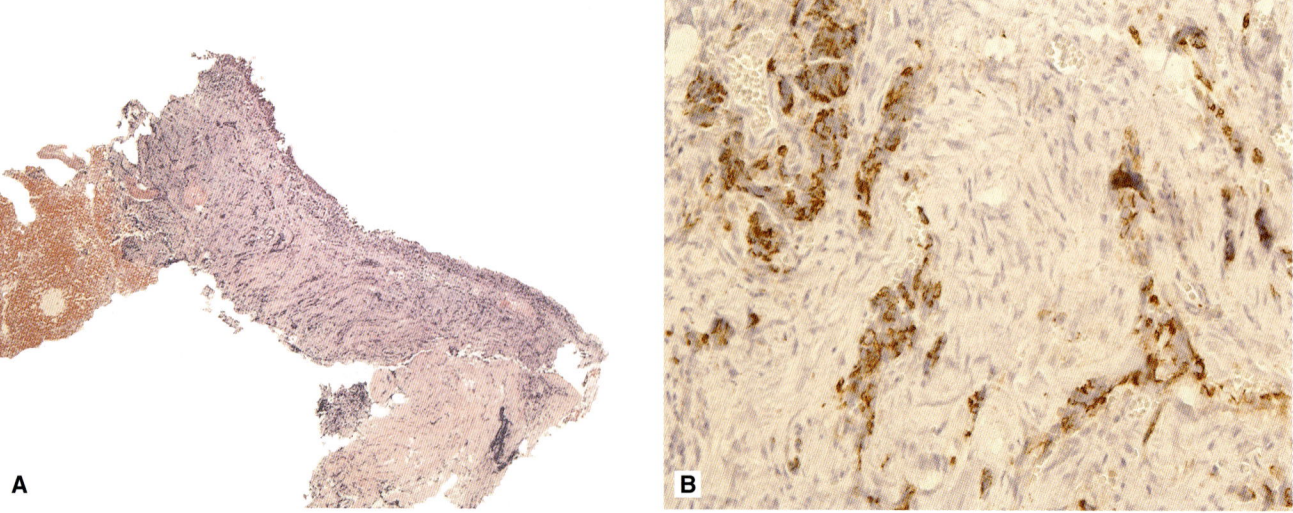

Figure 3.2: (A) Crushed specimens and intensely inflamed tissue can create diagnostic difficulty. (B) Sometimes immunostaining with cytokeratin may be useful in reaching a more definitive diagnosis of malignancy, although in this case it would be difficult to go much beyond a diagnosis of "carcinoma." The pattern distribution of crushed "infiltrating" epithelial cells, confirmed by the cytokeratin stain and the apparent fibroblastic stromal response, help secure a malignant diagnosis.

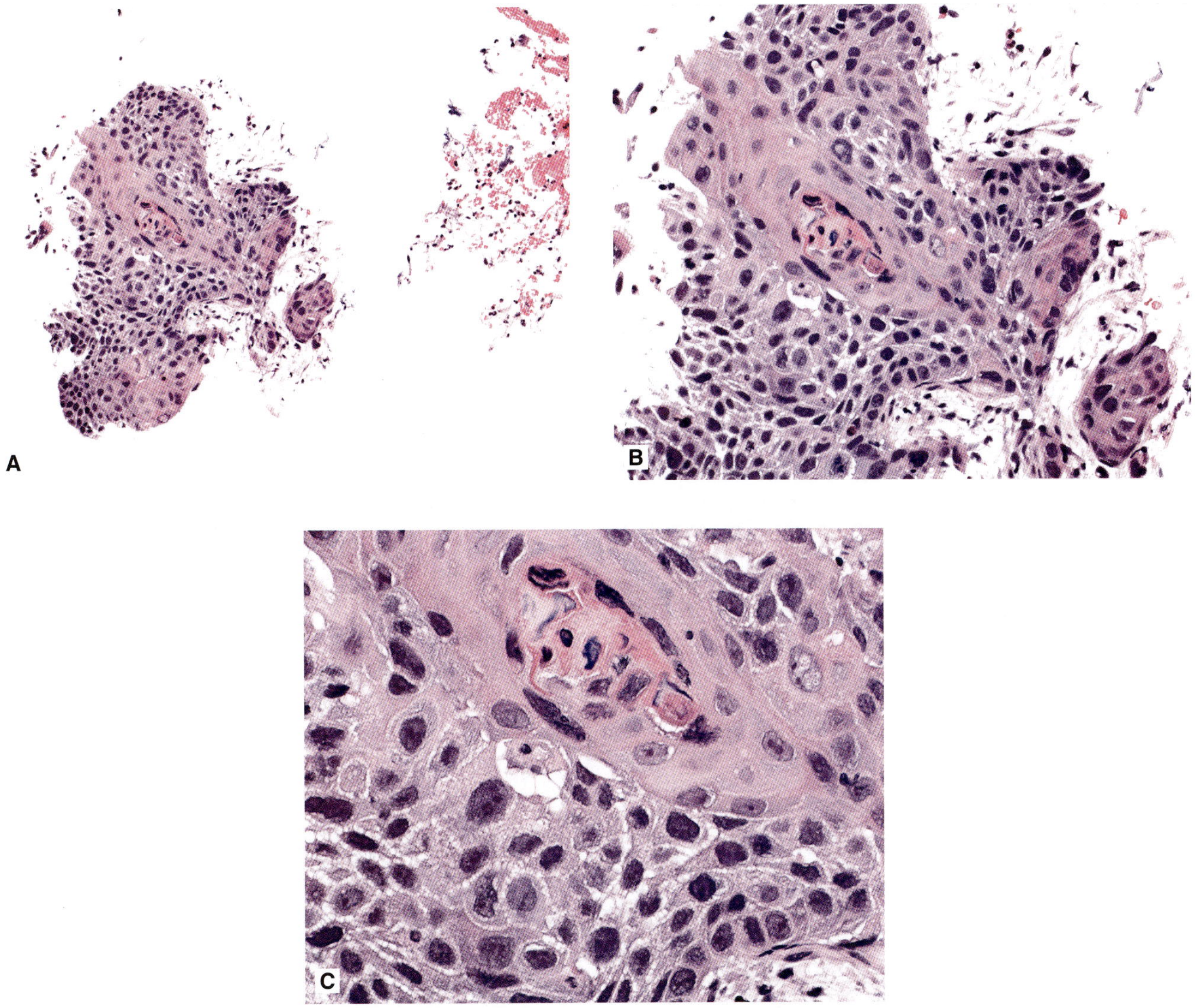

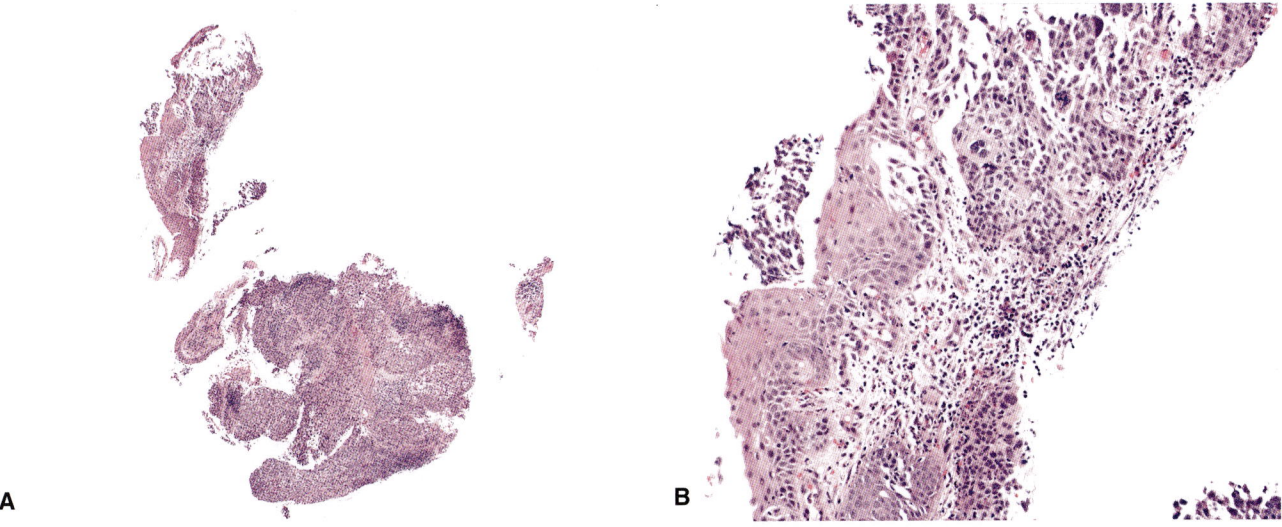

Figure 3.3: (A) This small bronchial biopsy fragment consists entirely of tumor. (B) This is squamous cell carcinoma. Although there is almost no stroma present in the sample to give a perspective of invasion, the topography of this zone of tumor is too irregular to consider carcinoma in situ. (C) This squamous cell carcinoma shows both keratinization with the formation of a keratin "pearl" and intercellular bridges. These are the two features that allow definitive diagnosis of squamous cell carcinoma. Note the irregular nuclear morphology and the coarse clumped chromatin.

Figure 3.4: (A) Two bronchial biopsies, the lower one infiltrated by tumor, the upper showing squamous epithelium on the surface and tumor beneath. (B) A higher power view of the upper fragment shows a squamous metaplastic surface epithelium with mild atypia on the left, deep to which there is invasive non–small cell carcinoma. (*Continued*)

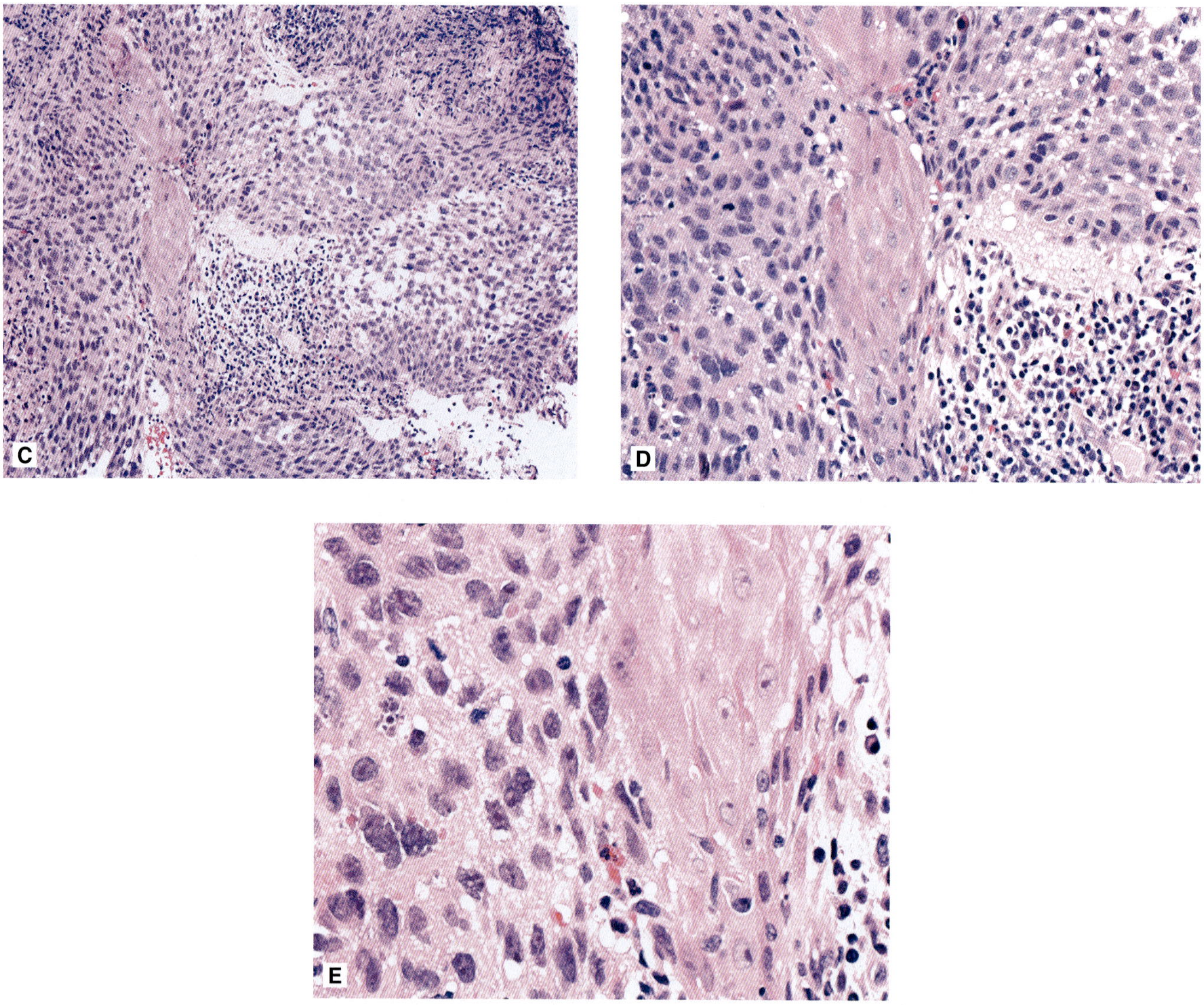

Figure 3.4: (*continued*) (C) The invasive tumor in the lower fragment shows sheets of cohesive non–small cell carcinoma with chronic inflammation in the intervening stroma. (D) Much of the tumor in this field shows poorly differentiated non–small cell carcinoma (left and top right) but in the center is a strip of more differentiated tumor with more abundant eosinophilic cytoplasm and more regular nuclei. The appearances suggest squamous differentiation. (E) Squamous differentiation is confirmed by the identification of intercellular bridges between those cells with eosinophilic cytoplasm. Note the difference in nuclear morphology between the differentiated and poorly differentiated areas.

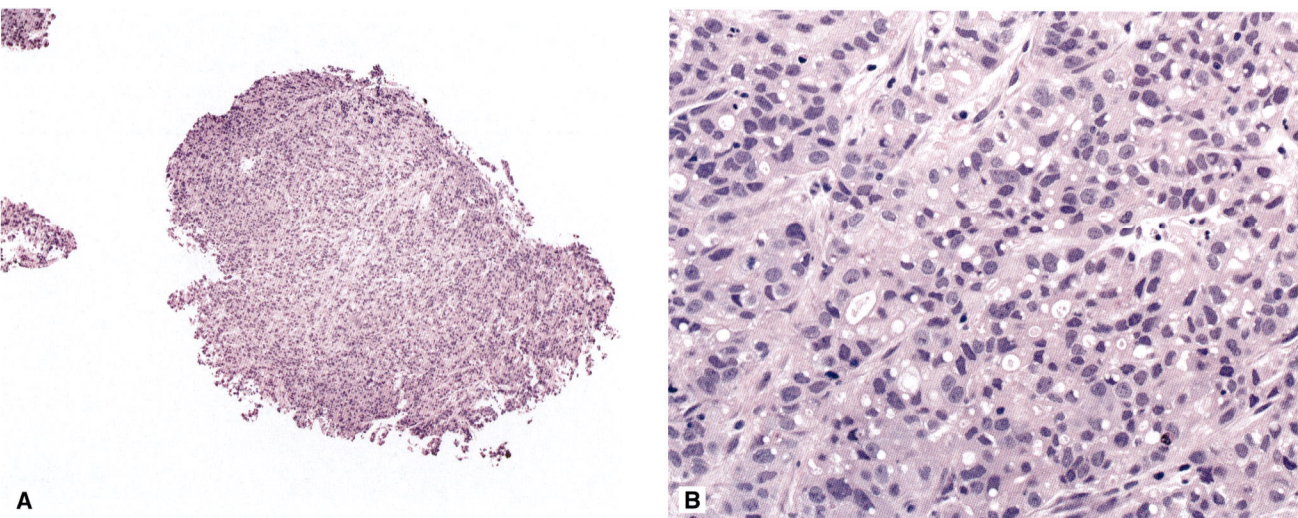

Figure 3.5: (A) This bronchial biopsy is almost completely replaced by a poorly differentiated adenocarcinoma. Such a large amount of tumor in a sample of adenocarcinoma is unusual. (B) This adenocarcinoma shows a rather cribriform architecture with occasional glands and many intracellular vacuoles. (*Continued*)

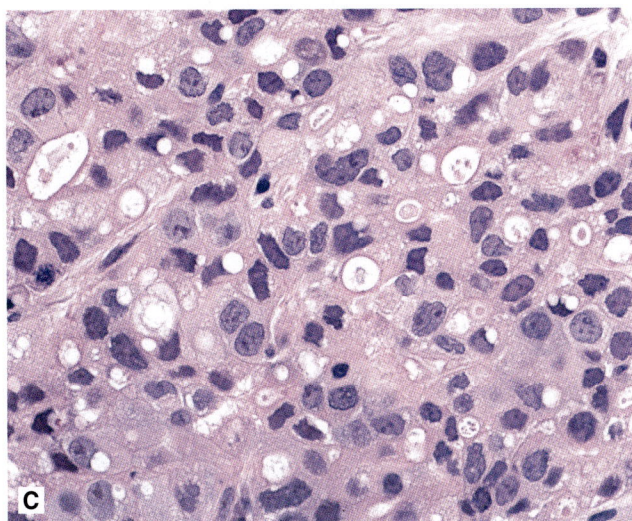

Figure 3.5: (*continued*) (C) There is nuclear pleomorphism and nucleoli are visible. Many intracellular mucin vacuoles are evident.

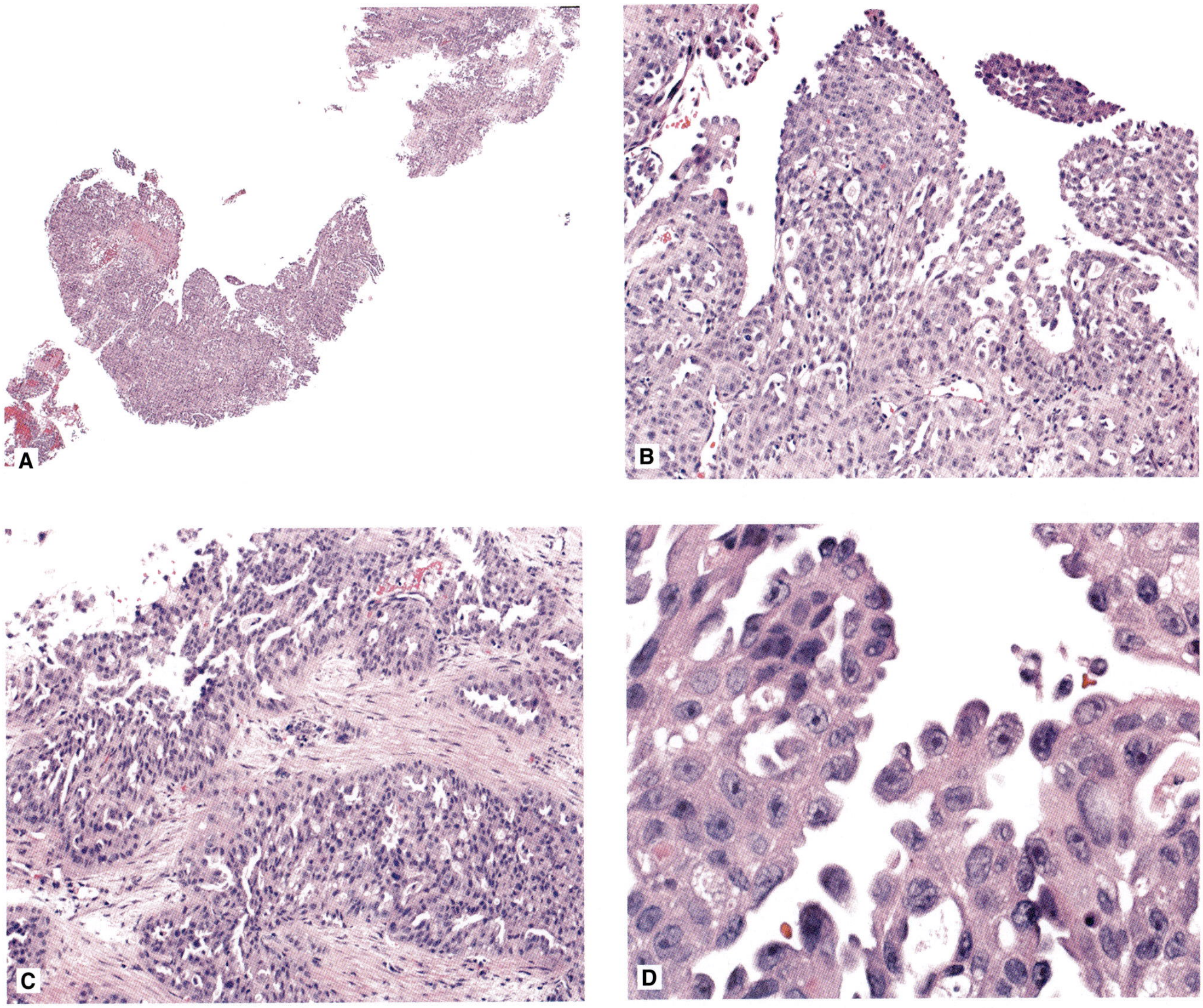

Figure 3.6: (A) Several fragments of bronchial biopsy infiltrated by adenocarcinoma. (B) This adenocarcinoma shows a papillary architecture in places, some solid foci and prominent vascularity. Note the Clara-like peg cells on the surface of the papillary tumor. (C) In other parts of this tumor, an acinar pattern is evident. Even in a bronchial biopsy the frequent mixture of adenocarcinoma patterns may be appreciated. (D) Papillary adenocarcinoma on the surface of the biopsy. The tumor cells have prominent nucleoli, oval nuclei, and sharp cell membranes, typical of adenocarcinoma. (*Continued*)

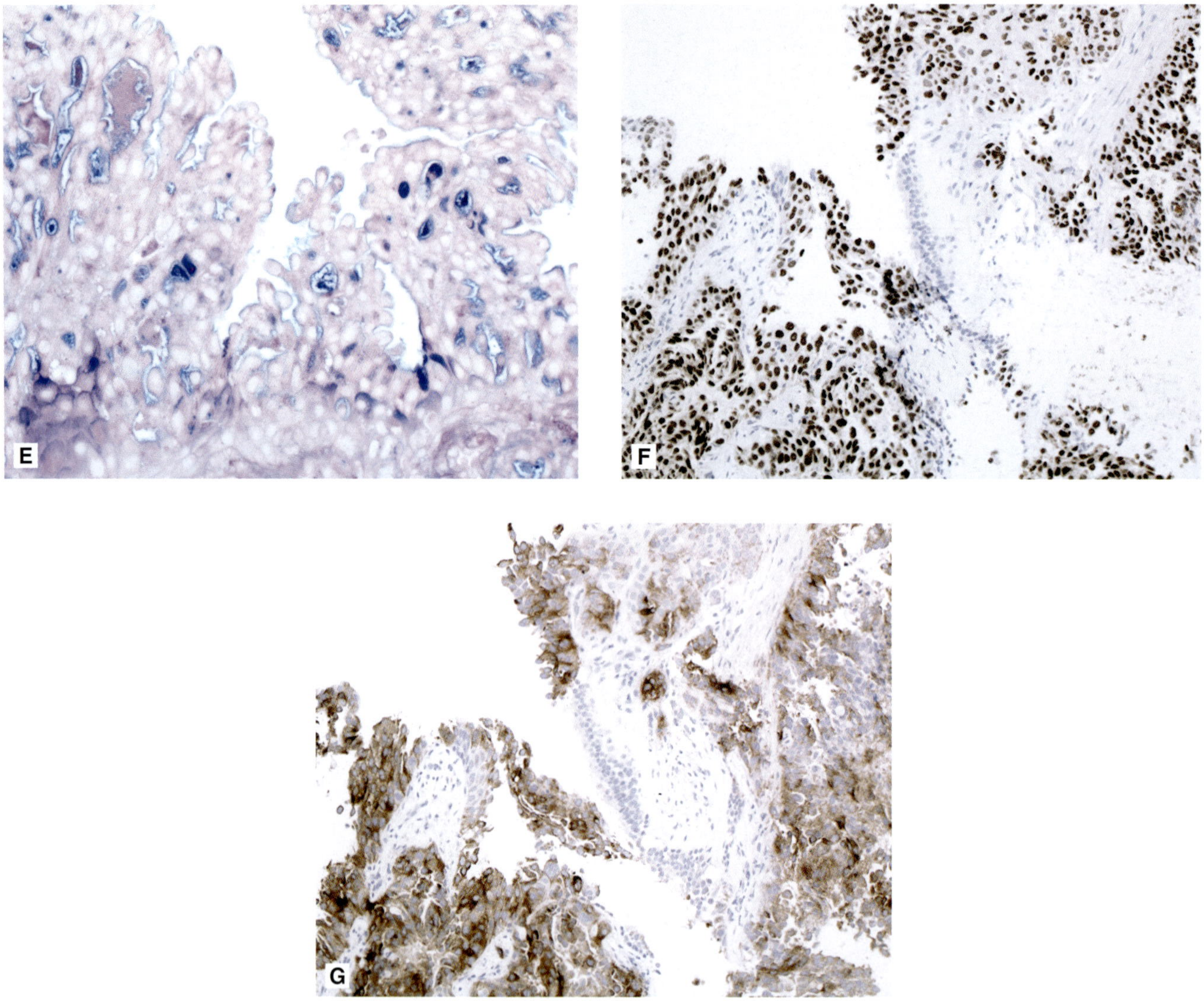

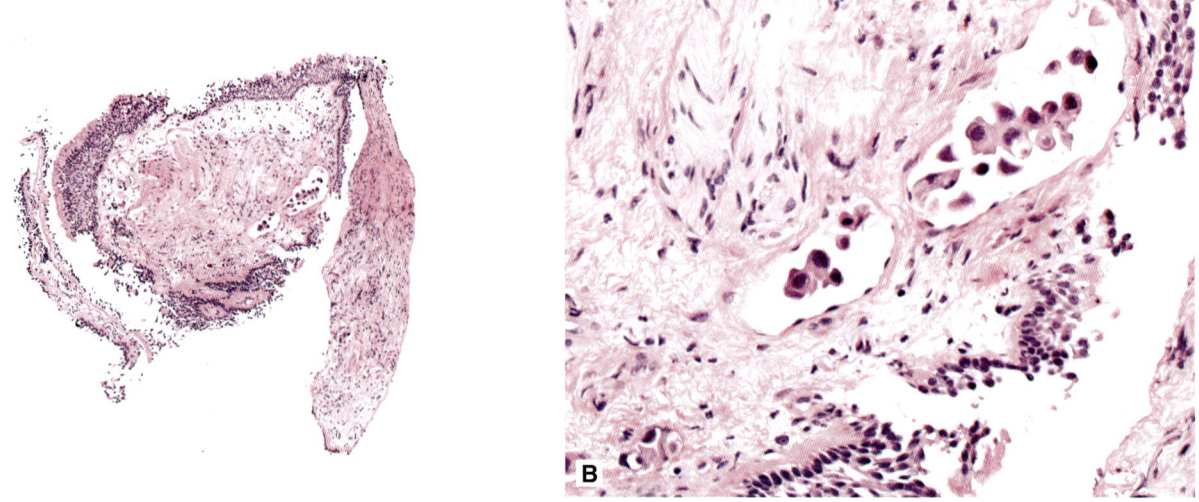

Figure 3.6: (*continued*) (E) A combined Alcian blue periodic acid-Schiff (PAS) stain (without nuclear counterstain) shows mixed acidic and neutral mucin in both an extracellular and intracellular locations. (F) Most lung adenocarcinomas, especially such as this case with a papillary architecture, show strong thyroid transcription factor-1 (TTF-1) positive nuclear staining. Normal bronchial epithelium does not stain. (G) Strong carcinoembryonic antigen (CEA) expression is typical in pulmonary adenocarcinoma.

Figure 3.7: (A) A small bronchial biopsy fragment covered by normal respiratory epithelium, unremarkable subepithelial stroma, and in the deep part of the biopsy dilated lymphatic-containing cells. (B) Adenocarcinoma cells within the dilated lymphatic were the only evidence of malignancy in this bronchial biopsy. Such an appearance is often associated with lymph node metastases.

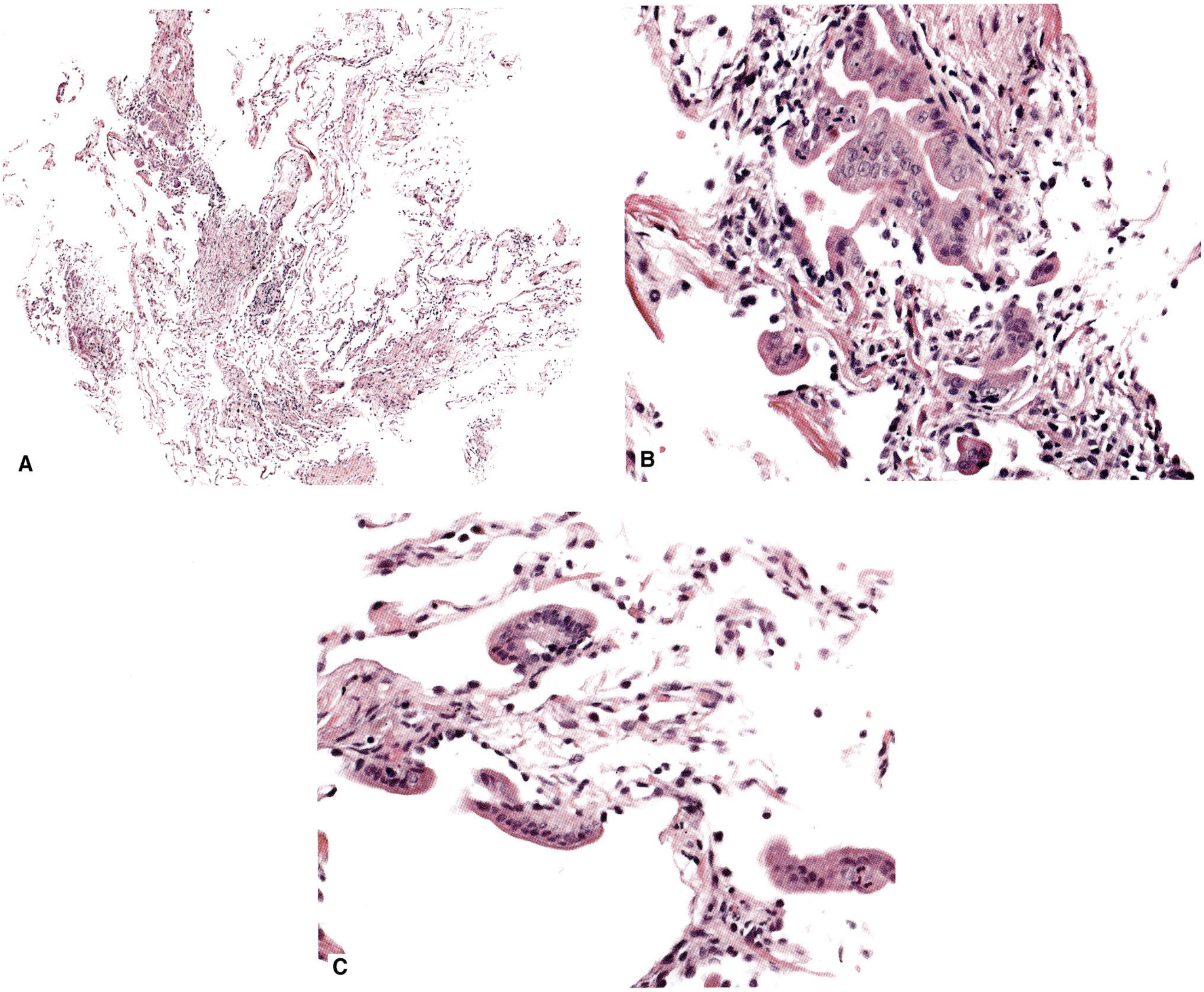

Chapter 3 • Non–Small Cell Carcinomas

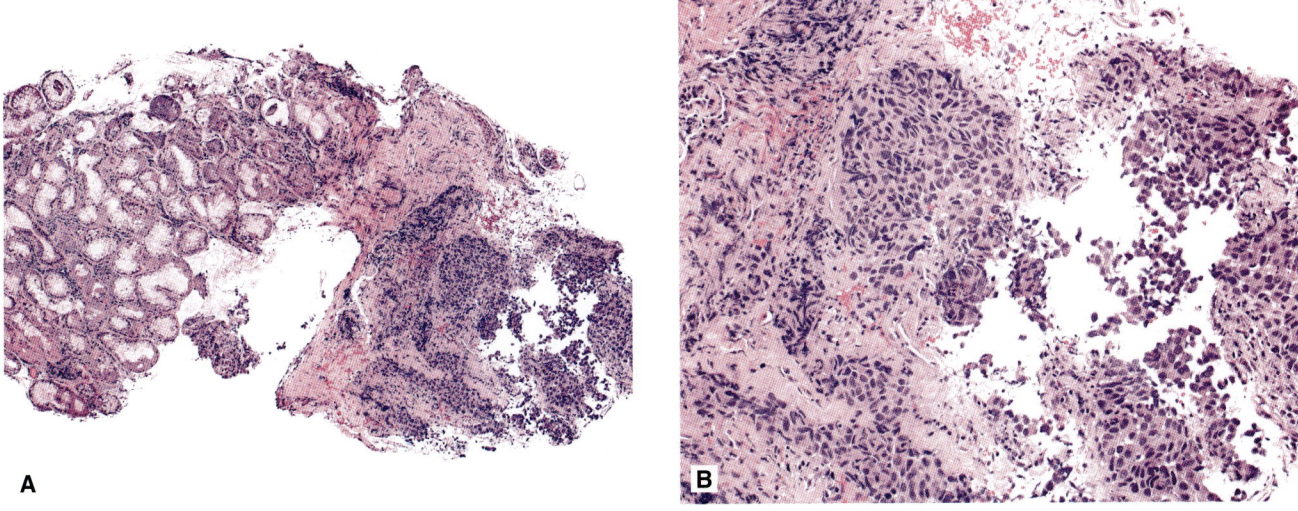

Figure 3.8: (A) A rather crushed transbronchial lung biopsy. Note the cluster of larger epithelial cells in the top left corner. (B) At higher power these columnar epithelial cells line alveolar walls in well-defined groups. There is some nuclear pleomorphism, and together the adjacent cell apices form a well-defined line. This is a small focus of mucinous bronchioloalveolar pattern of adenocarcinoma. (C) Tiny well-defined groups of columnar tumor cells stuck to alveolar walls, protruding in a mushroom-like fashion into the alveolar spaces, are characteristic of the mucinous bronchioloalveolar pattern of adenocarcinoma. In this particular example the mucin production is slight and confined to an intracellular location. In some cases tumor goblet cells are present; mucin is plentiful and may fill affected alveoli.

Figure 3.9: (A) Bronchial mucosal biopsy showing submucosal glands (left) and invasive carcinoma (right). (B) The invasive tumor has been traumatized during the biopsy process. There is no obvious evidence of architectural differentiation. (*Continued*)

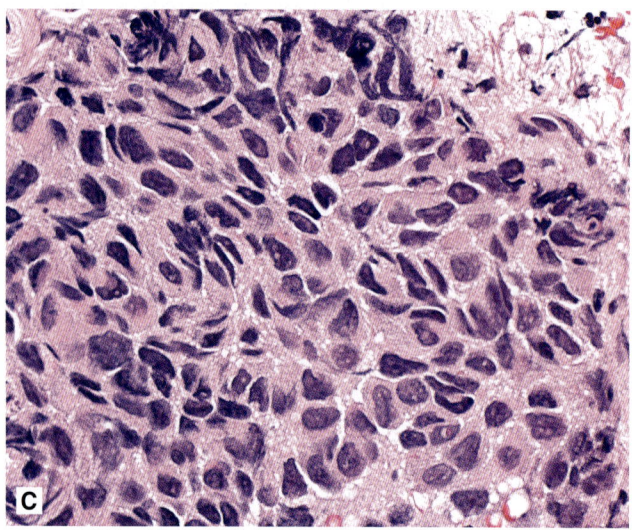

Figure 3.9: (*continued*) (C) At high power the tumor cells appear relatively large, nuclei pleomorphic with irregular clumped chromatin and no nucleoli. There is a moderate amount of cytoplasm. Keratinization and intercellular bridges are absent, as is any evidence of glandular differentiation. This is a case of non–small cell carcinoma, not further specified.

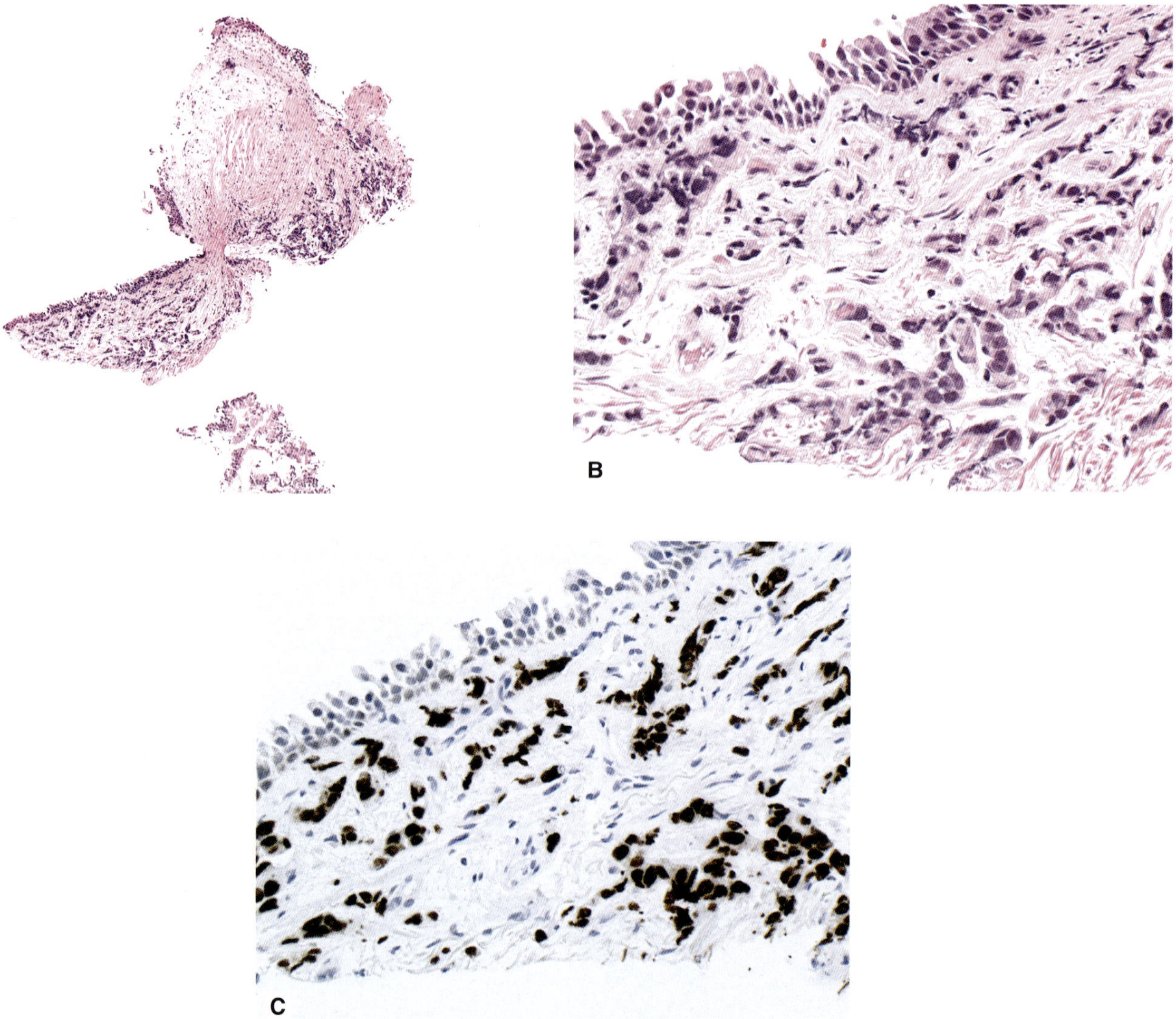

Figure 3.10: (A) Bronchial biopsy showing small amounts of invasive carcinoma in the subepithelial stroma. (B) Scattered groups and cords of malignant cells infiltrating below the normal bronchial epithelium. Note the prominent nucleoli in the tumor cells. This tumor appears undifferentiated but is clearly not small cell carcinoma. (C) There is insufficient tumor in this biopsy to allow identification of any pattern typical of adenocarcinoma, but there is strong thyroid transcription factor-1 (TTF-1) expression. This is highly likely to be pulmonary adenocarcinoma infiltrating the bronchial wall, although the correct diagnosis is, in this case, "non–small cell carcinoma, probably adenocarcinoma."

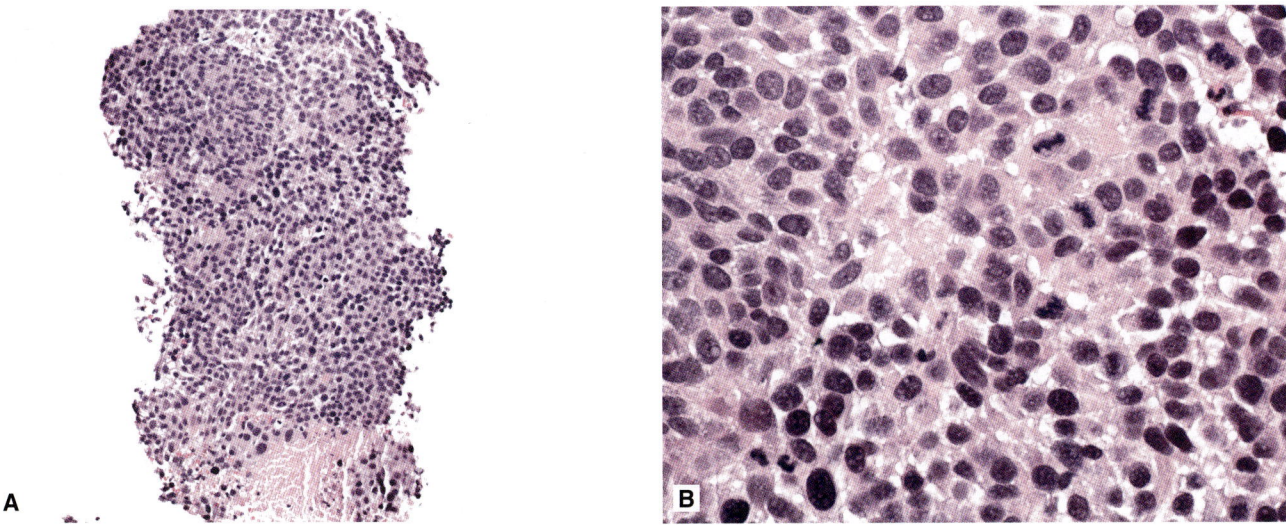

Figure 3.11: (A) This is a fragment of undifferentiated carcinoma in a bronchial biopsy. There is necrosis evident at the bottom of the fragment. (B) At higher power the tumor shows relatively small cells (smaller than in Fig. 3.9C) and several mitoses, but there is plentiful cytoplasm and no nuclear molding. Although this could be basaloid carcinoma, this diagnosis cannot be made with certainty on small biopsies, and the correct diagnosis on this material is non–small cell carcinoma, not further specified.

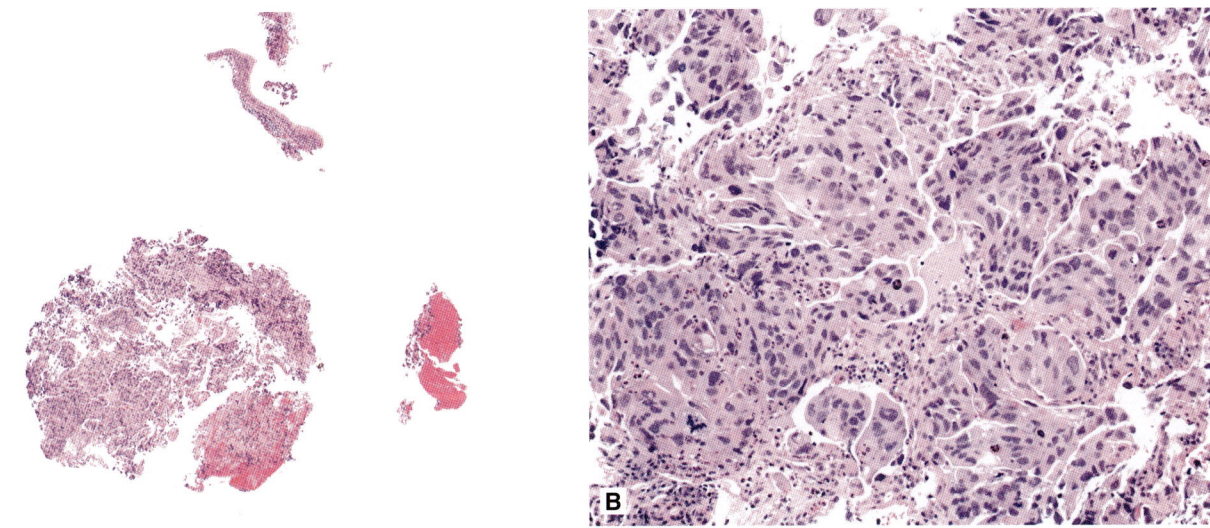

Figure 3.12: (A) Small bronchial mucosal biopsy with dissociated surface respiratory epithelium. (B) Invading the mucosa in this biopsy are sheets of pleomorphic carcinoma admixed with inflammatory cells. (*Continued*)

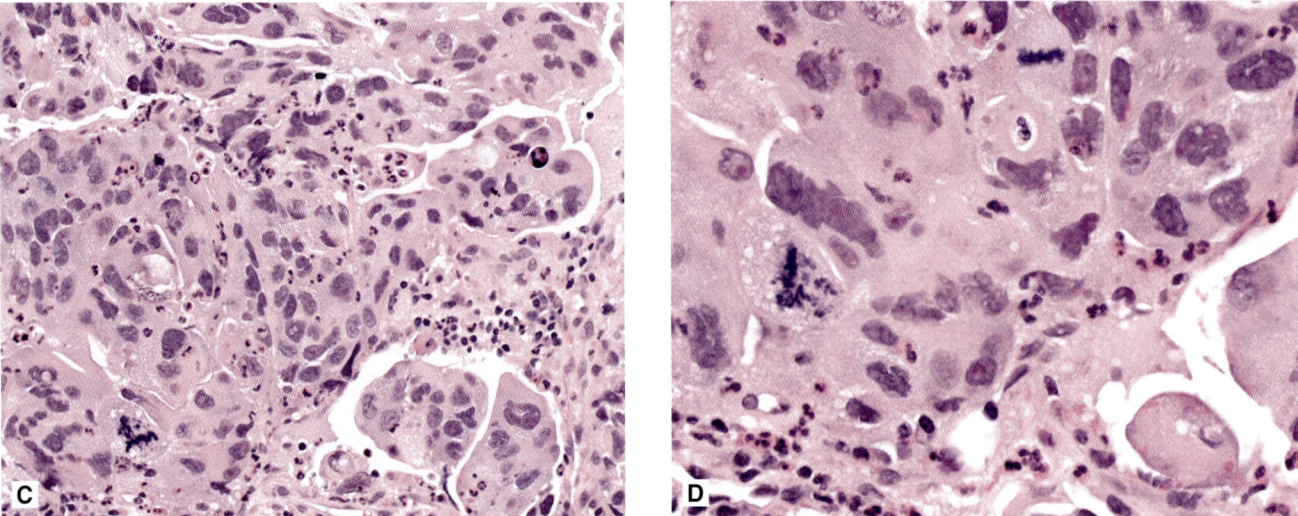

Figure 3.12: (*continued*) (C) At higher magnification the extremely large size and pleomorphism of the tumor cells is evident. The inflammatory infiltrate comprises both lymphocytes and neutrophils. Neutrophil emperipolesis (phagocytosis by tumor cells) is very characteristic in foci of pleomorphic tumor giant cells. (D) Huge tumor cells and bizarre mitotic figures are also features of sarcomatoid carcinoma, but this specific diagnosis cannot be made on small biopsies. The appropriate diagnosis in this case is non–small cell carcinoma with sarcomatoid features.

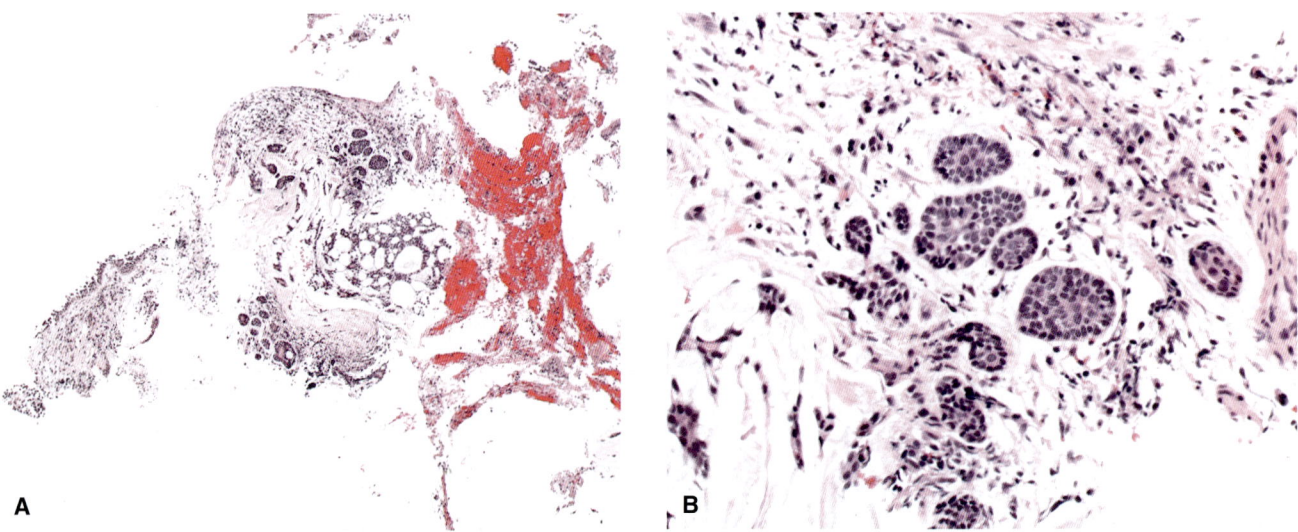

Figure 3.13: (A) Biopsy of main bronchus showing adenoid cystic carcinoma. (B) In places this adenoid cystic carcinoma shows small solid foci of small tumor cells. (*Continued*)

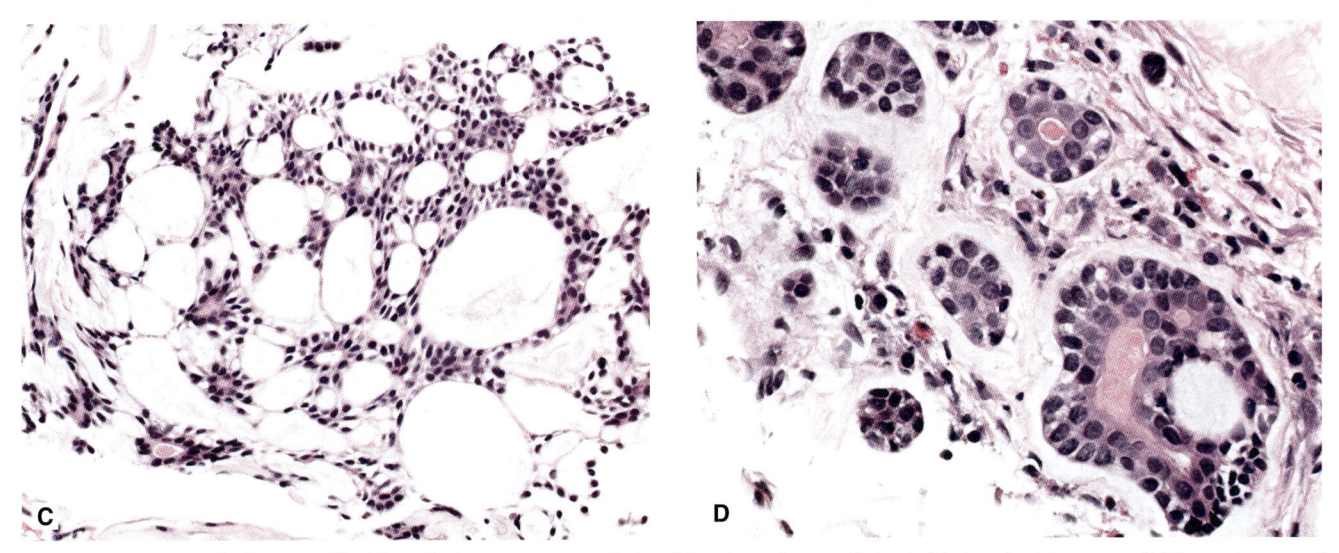

Figure 3.13: (*continued*) (C) Typical lacelike cribriform appearance of adenoid cystic carcinoma admixed with tiny glandular spaces. (D) In another area of this adenoid cystic carcinoma there are glandular spaces surrounded by a thick cuff of basement membrane material.

Suggested Readings

Detterbeck FC, Rivera MP, Socinski MA, et al., eds. *Diagnosis and Treatment of Lung Cancer: An Evidence-Based Guide for the Practicing Clinician.* Philadelphia, Pa: WB Saunders; 2001.

Edwards SL, Roberts C, McKean ME, et al. The preoperative histological diagnosis of lung cancer: accuracy of classification and use of the non–small cell category. *J Clin Pathol* 2000;53:537–540.

Kerr KM, Lyall MS, Chapman AD. The diagnosis of lung cancer on bronchoscopic biopsy. *CPD Bull Cell Pathol* 2006;6:20–30.

Schreiber G, McCrory DC. Performance characteristics of different modalities for diagnosis of suspected lung cancer. *Chest* 2003;123:S115–128.

Travis WD, Brambilla E, Muller-Hermelink HK, et al., eds. *World Health Organisation Classification of Tumours. Pathology and Genetics of Tumours of the Lung, Pleura, Thymus and Heart.* Lyon, France: IARC Press; 2004.

Travis WD, Garg K, Franklin WA, et al. Bronchioloalveolar carcinoma and lung adenocarcinoma: the clinical importance and research relevance of the 2004 World Health Organization pathologic criteria. *J Thorac Oncol* 2006;1:S13–19.

Neuroendocrine Tumors

▶ Keith M. Kerr, FRCPath
▶ Kun Y. Kwon, MD
▶ Jae Y. Ro, MD

The two separate categories of neuroendocrine tumors in the World Health Organization (WHO) classification of lung tumors are small cell carcinoma and carcinoid tumor. A further important tumor type is a variant of large cell carcinoma: large cell neuroendocrine carcinoma. Non–small cell lung carcinomas of various types, as described in Chapter 3, may exhibit neuroendocrine differentiation at a molecular level as detected by immunohistochemistry or electron microscopy. This finding is of no proven clinical or pathologic importance, and these so-called non–small cell carcinomas with neuroendocrine differentiation are not discussed any further in this chapter. Table 4-1 lists those neuroendocrine carcinomas included in the WHO classification.

Small cell lung carcinoma comprises around 15% to 25% of all lung cancers. It is typically a central bronchogenic tumor and as such is frequently encountered in endoscopic biopsy specimens. The cells in small cell lung carcinoma are generally small, no more than the diameter of three small resting lymphocytes side by side, and they form sheets and masses of tumor infiltrating the bronchi. Tumor may infiltrate between the bronchial glands without destroying them. Cords of cells may dissect between collagen in the bronchial submucosa. Crush artifact is extremely common in this tumor type, but a similar change may occur in lymphoid tissue when it presents an important differential diagnosis. In uncrushed areas of tumor, which may require careful searching to find when sparse, tumor cells characteristically show nuclear molding but otherwise, the sheets of tumor cells generally show little architecture and may appear as a rather haphazard mishmash of small spindle or fusiform cells with a high mitotic and apoptotic rate. Nuclei are round, oval, or spindle shaped, and nuclear features are very characteristic, showing a fine granular (salt and pepper) or even featureless chromatin. Nucleoli are absent or, if present, almost always inconspicuous. Cytoplasm is generally scanty. Some cases show more epithelioid, cuboidal cells, and some architecture with trabeculae; an organoid pattern or rosette formation may be in evidence. Coagulative necrosis may be identified, particularly if the tumor sample is relatively large. Some small cell lung carcinoma cases show scattered larger cells with open nuclei, clumped chromatin, and even nucleoli; and occasionally, tumor giant cells may be scattered among typical small cells. Lymphatic invasion is not uncommon in the bronchial mucosa, and tumor cells frequently infiltrate, in a pagetoid fashion, the overlying surface epithelium, which may be of normal pseudostratified respiratory type, show squamous metaplasia or even squamous dysplasia, or carcinoma in situ. The bronchial mucosal stroma adjacent to small cell lung carcinoma often shows quite marked vascular proliferation, a feature that may, however, also be seen with non–small cell carcinomas. Occasionally small cell lung carcinoma may be found in conjunction with some form of non–small cell carcinoma, so-called combined small cell lung carcinoma. If both components are represented in the samples, such a diagnosis could be made on endoscopic biopsy material because there is no stipulation in the WHO classification of a required minimum proportion of the small cell lung carcinoma in combined cases. Small cell lung

Table 4-1	WHO Histological Classification of Neuroendocrine Tumors	
Carcinoid tumor		
Typical carcinoid		8240/3
Atypical carcinoid		8249/3
Small cell carcinoma		8041/3
Combined small cell carcinoma		8045/3
Large cell neuroendocrine carcinoma		8013/3
Combined large cell neuroendocrine carcinoma		8013/3

carcinoma is a diagnosis that can be made very reliably and confidently on bronchial or occasionally transbronchial biopsy material stained by standard haematoxylin and eosin. Immunohistochemistry is not required to achieve a diagnostic accuracy of 90% and interobserver agreement among pathologists of 95%. These figures are better than those for non–small cell carcinomas, as described in Chapter 3. Where tumor is extremely crushed or there are some histologic features that raise the possibility of an alternative diagnosis, such as severe inflammation, lymphoma, or non–small cell carcinoma, immunohistochemistry may be useful. Confusion with benign lymphoid tissue may be compounded in cases that lack obvious mitotic activity or necrosis. Cytokeratin immunohistochemistry often shows paranuclear dot positivity, and this, together with negativity with CD45, may be sufficient to secure a diagnosis in a crushed sample, distinguishing small cell lung carcinoma from crushed benign or malignant lymphoid tissue. Small cell lung carcinoma expresses neuroendocrine markers in most cases; usually at least two of CD56, synaptophysin and chromogranin, are positive, but evidence of neuroendocrine differentiation as demonstrated by immunohistochemistry or electron microscopy is not required for a diagnosis of small cell lung carcinoma. Thyroid transcription factor-1 (TTF-1) is expressed in around 90% of cases. Neuroendocrine markers are obviously useful in differentiating small cell lung carcinoma from those nonneuroendocrine carcinomas, such as basaloid carcinoma and both basaloid and small cell variants of squamous cell carcinoma, which may mimic small cell lung carcinoma in small biopsy samples, especially when there is crush artifact. Useful adjuncts to diagnosis in this situation are the anti-HMW cytokeratin 34betaE12 and p63, which are not expressed in a range of neuroendocrine lung tumors but are frequently found in nonneuroendocrine carcinomas.

Large cell neuroendocrine carcinoma is a relatively rare tumor that biologically is similar to small cell lung carcinoma in some ways; it is smoking related and occurs in central airways but also in the lung periphery. As a variant of large cell carcinoma, the tumor cells have, on average, a diameter greater than three lymphocytes, large nuclei with an open chromatin pattern, and prominent nucleoli. Nuclear molding is generally not seen, and cytoplasm is usually abundant and may be eosinophilic. An organoid pattern with trabeculation and rosette formation with peripheral palisading of the cells is common. There are, by definition, more than ten mitoses present in 2 mm^2 of tumor (ten high-power fields); in practice most cases average 60 to 70 mitoses in such an area of tumor. It is most unlikely, however, that there would be sufficient tumor in an endoscopic biopsy to allow such an assessment. These features may be found in other large cell carcinomas, particularly in basaloid carcinoma, and in this case, by definition, neuroendocrine differentiation must be demonstrated by either electron microscopy or, more usually, by immunohistochemistry to secure a diagnosis of large cell neuroendocrine carcinoma. In the presence of hematoxylin and eosin (H&E) features as described earlier, clear immunopositivity with CD56, synaptophysin, or chromogranin is sufficient for diagnosis. Around 50% of large cell neuroendocrine carcinomas express TTF-1. Even with positive neuroendocrine immunohistochemistry, the other features may not be well represented in small tissue samples, and thus a definitive diagnosis of large cell neuroendocrine carcinoma is frequently not possible in endoscopic biopsies. Distinction from small cell lung carcinoma can be difficult, and nuclear features are the key to the diagnosis.

Carcinoid tumor is another infrequent malignant neuroendocrine tumor of the lung. Most occur in the large central bronchi, presenting as slow-growing endobronchial polypoid masses. They may also appear as peripheral coin lesions without any obvious association with a bronchus. Most cases show a variety of patterns of neuroendocrine tumor with an insular or trabecular architecture. Some cases show solid sheets of cells, little stroma but marked vascularity. Rosettes or acini may be seen. Occasionally the tumor stroma is abundant and may show bone or cartilage formation or even amyloid deposition. The cells are relatively small in most cases, uniform and polygonal with finely granular chromatin. Nucleoli are small or absent and cytoplasm may be even or granular, eosinophilic or basophilic, and abundant in oncocytic forms. Most cases show very few mitoses, and it is most unusual to see any in the small samples of tumor present in endoscopic biopsies. Approximately 10% of carcinoid tumors show spindle cells, but spindle cell carcinoids tend to occur in the lung periphery and consequently are less frequently found in endoscopic biopsies. By definition, the very much rarer atypical carcinoid tumor (<10% of lung carcinoid tumors) shows a mitotic count of between 2 and 10 per 2 mm^2 (ten high-power fields) of tumor and/or shows focal coagulative necrosis. Typical carcinoid tumors do not show necrosis, and the mitotic index is less than in atypical carcinoid (<2 per 2 mm^2 of tumor). Cellular and nuclear pleomorphism is not infrequent, even in typical carcinoid, and this does not indicate a diagnosis of atypical carcinoid. In bronchial or transbronchial biopsy, a diagnosis of carcinoid tumor may be made with confidence, supported by neuroendocrine marker immunohistochemistry as necessary, but there would rarely be sufficient features present to allow discrimination between typical and atypical forms. It is not unusual for the endobronchial component of a bronchial carcinoid tumor to be covered by a thin metaplastic squamous epithelium. Crush artifact in small biopsies can distort the histologic appearances, and occasionally it is difficult to distinguish carcinoid tumor from small cell lung carcinoma: If the tumor does not have any mitoses or areas of necrosis, the possibility of this tumor being a carcinoid tumor is higher. Tumors with prominent rosettes or pseudoacini may mimic adenocarcinoma. With the former distinction, neuroendocrine marker immunohistochemistry is unlikely to help, but in the latter instance it may; it is also worth remembering that although around 75% of lung adenocarcinomas (and up to 90% of small cell lung carcinomas) express TTF-1, this marker is rarely expressed strongly in insular and trabecular forms of carcinoid, although is more often found in spindle cell carcinoid tumors.

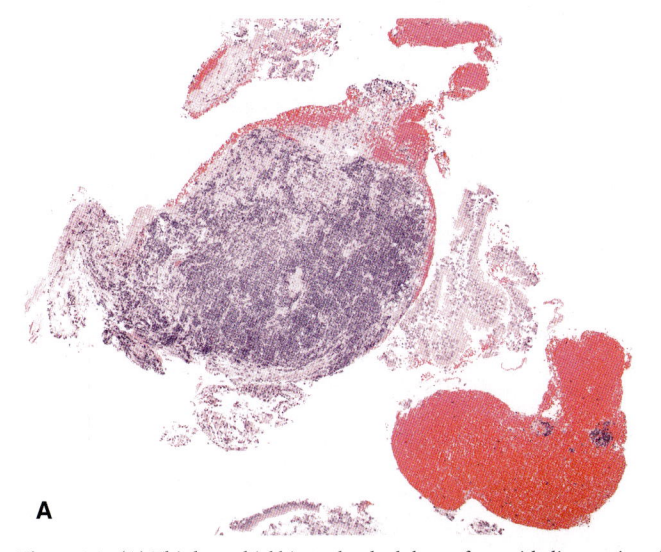

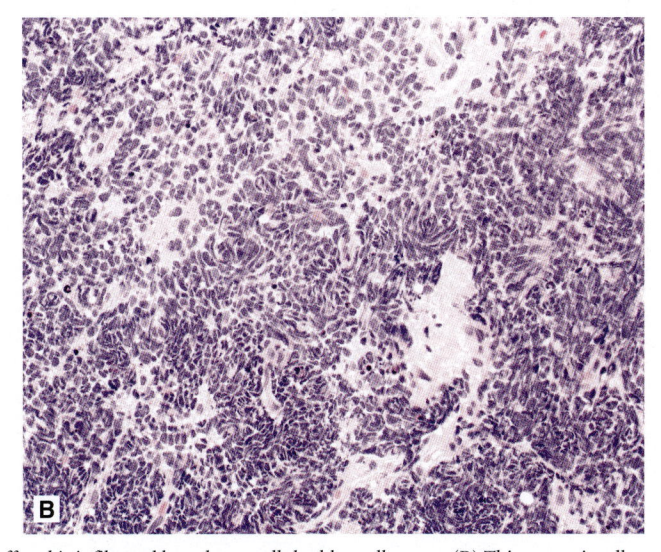

Figure 4.1: (A) This bronchial biopsy has had the surface epithelium stripped off and is infiltrated by a dense, cellular blue cell tumor. (B) This tumor is cellular and focally crushed. The pale areas usually represent capillary vessels, and apoptosis is easily identified. (*Continued*)

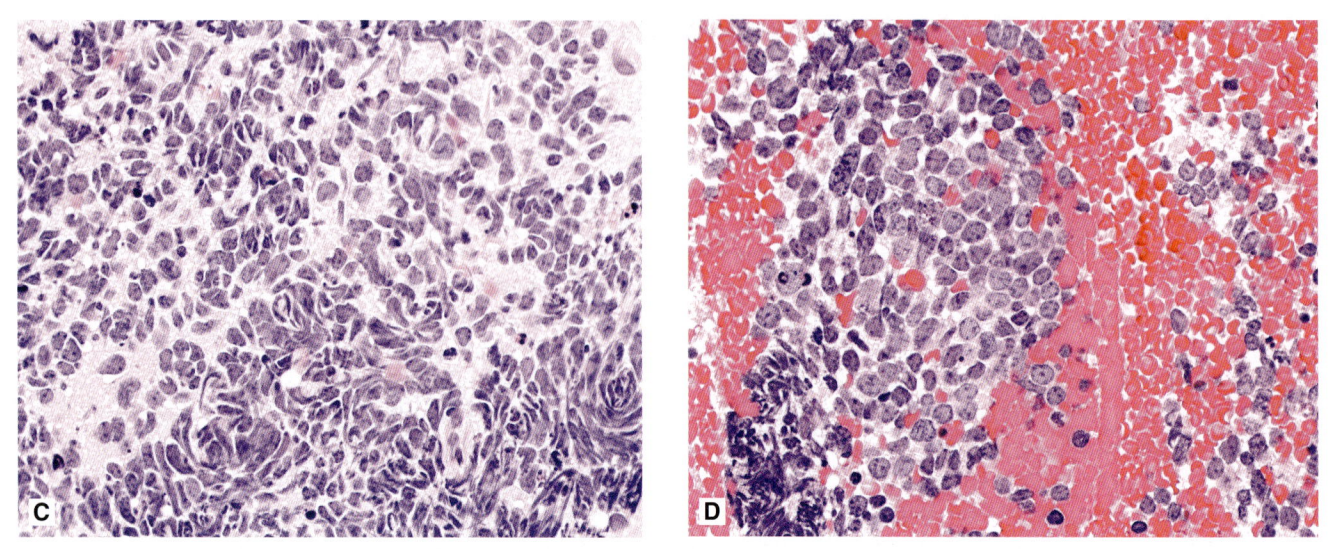

Figure 4.1: (*continued*) (C) Nuclear molding is clearly seen, even in areas that show some crush artifact. (D) In this area the cells are spared any crushing and the nuclear features typical of small cell carcinoma are readily seen; fine stippled chromatin and indistinct nucleoli in nuclei not much bigger than the few admixed small lymphocytes.

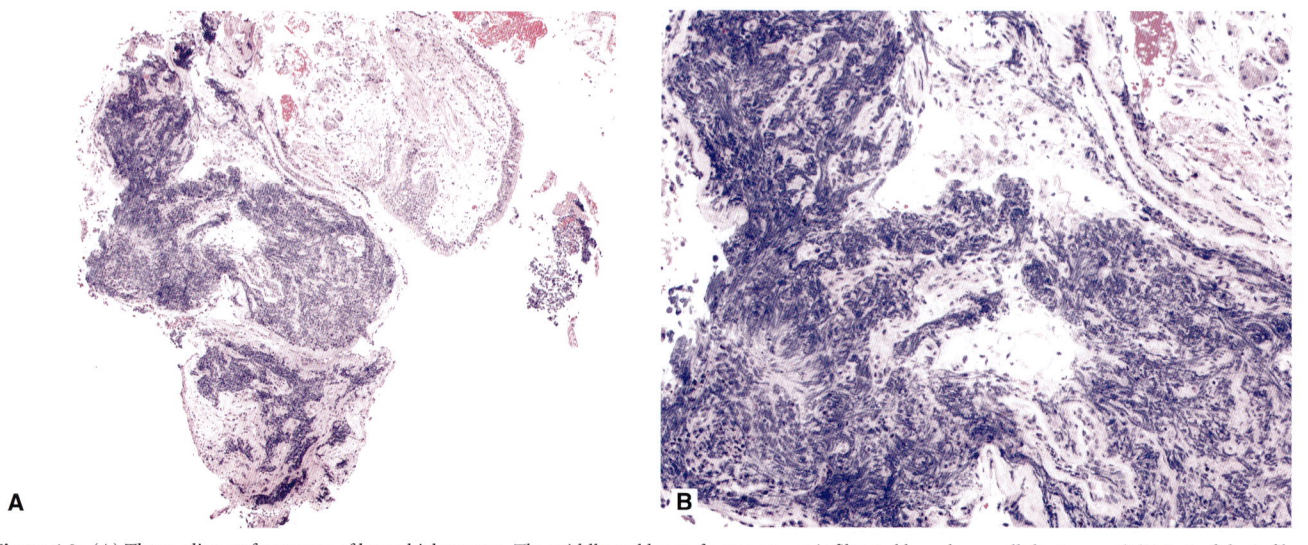

Figure 4.2: (A) Three adjacent fragments of bronchial mucosa. The middle and lower fragments are infiltrated by a dense cellular tumor. (B) Most of the infiltrating tumor shows crush artifact. Strips of bronchial epithelial basal cells resting on a thickened basement membrane and a focally dense capillary network stand out in the sea of crushed tumor nuclei. This is a very typical appearance in biopsied small cell carcinoma. (*Continued*)

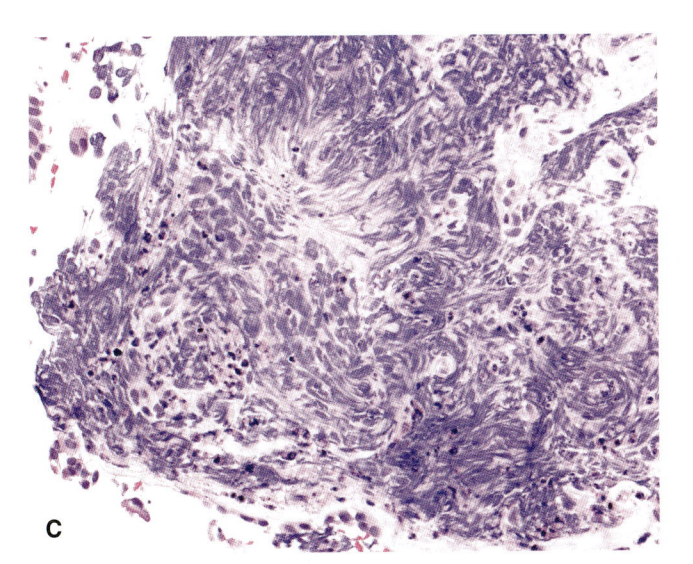

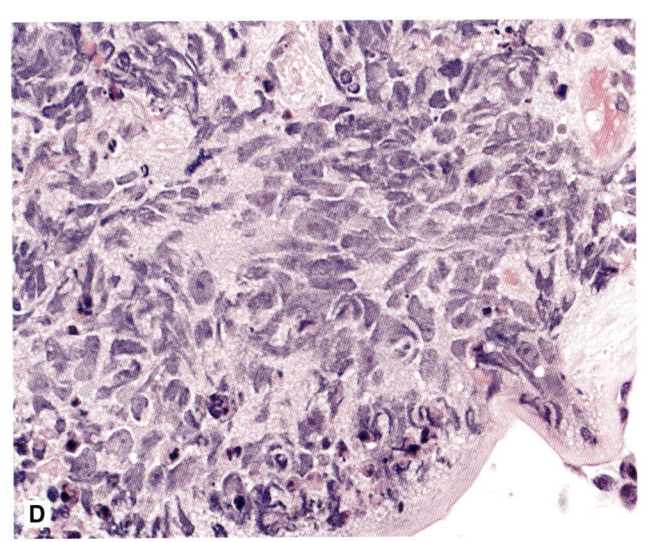

Figure 4.2: (*continued*) (C) Despite the lack of cellular or nuclear detail, apoptotic bodies are easily seen. (D) Careful examination usually reveals a few groups of uncrushed cells where almost featureless nuclei are molded together with indistinct cytoplasm. These features are sufficient for a diagnosis of small cell carcinoma. Immunohistochemistry is not required in the diagnosis of small cell lung carcinoma.

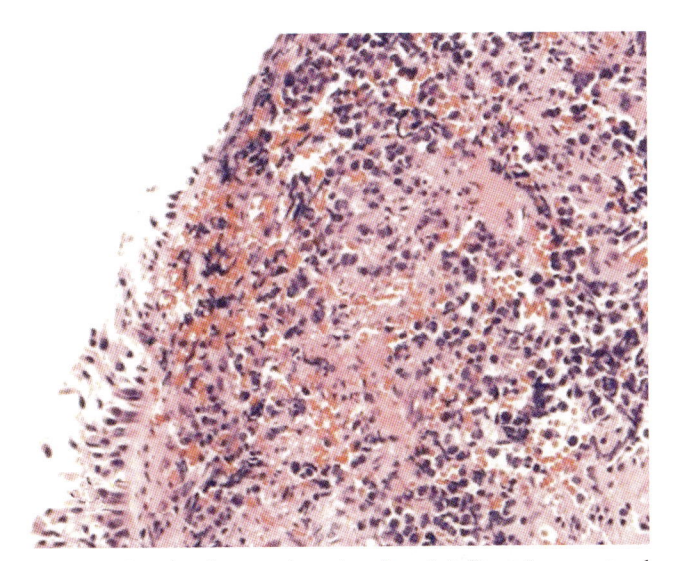

Figure 4.3: Occasionally a very heavy lymphocytic infiltrate is encountered in a bronchial biopsy, which may be confused with small cell lung carcinoma infiltrating the mucosa, although in the least traumatized areas the lymphoid nature of the cells may be apparent. Even crushed tumor stains by immunohistochemistry, and both cytokeratins and CD45 are useful in distinguishing small cell lung carcinoma from crushed lymphoid tissue.

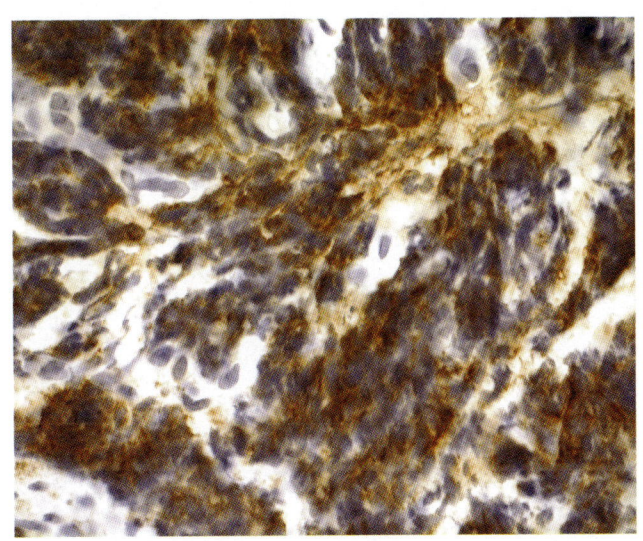

Figure 4.4: Neuroendocrine markers are also useful to confirm the neuroendocrine nature of the infiltrate. Recommended markers are chromogranin (most specific), synaptophysin, and CD56 (illustrated; least specific but most sensitive of the three). NSE and PGP9.5 are not recommended.

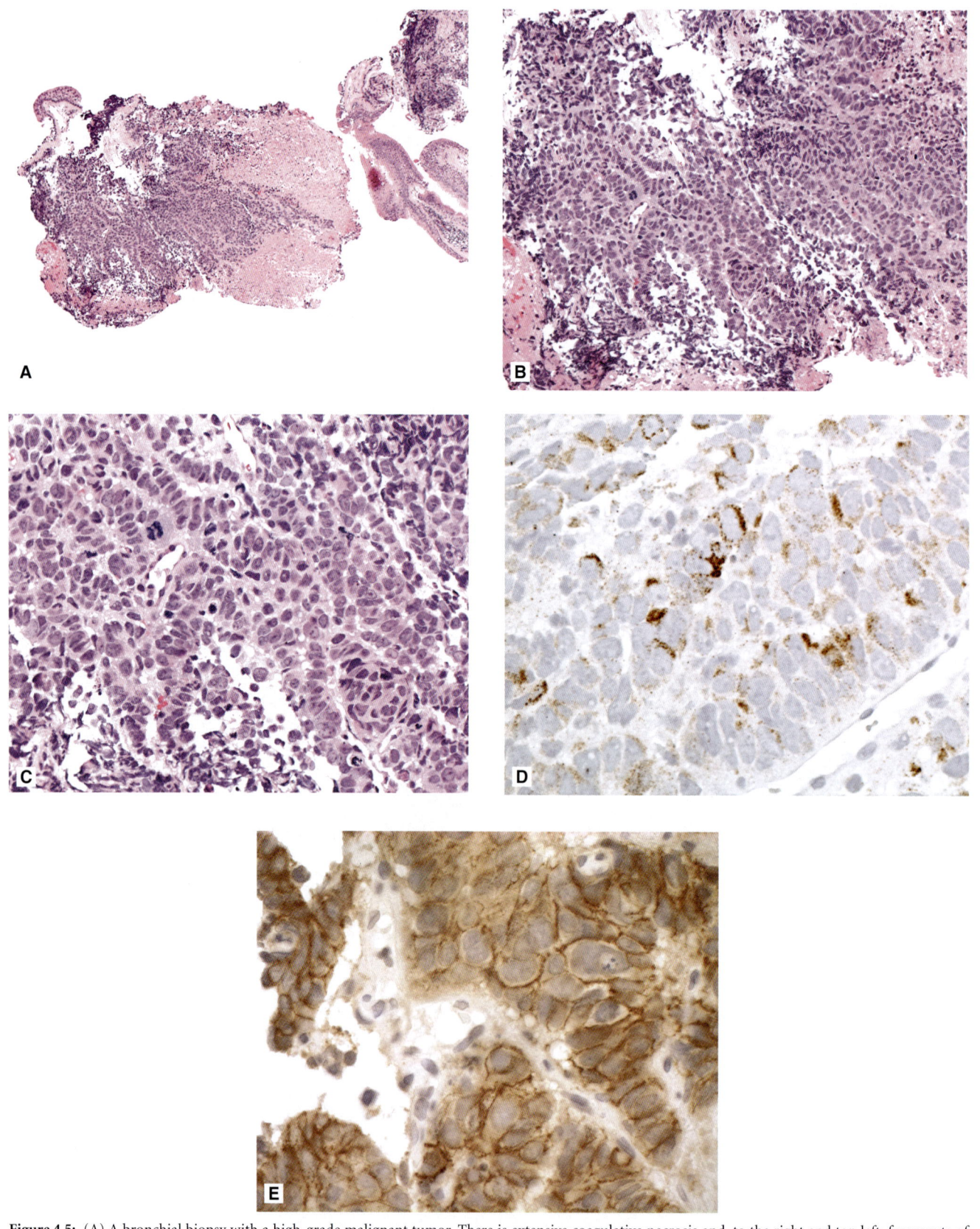

Figure 4.5: (A) A bronchial biopsy with a high-grade malignant tumor. There is extensive coagulative necrosis and, to the right and top left, fragments of normal respiratory epithelium. (B) This carcinoma has a clear trabecular architecture. (C) The tumor cells are relatively large, nuclei have an open chromatin pattern with obvious nucleoli, and there is obvious cytoplasm. Several mitoses are evident in this high-power field and there is apoptosis. These appearances all suggest a neuroendocrine tumor and are compatible with large cell neuroendocrine carcinoma. (D) High power of tumor cells showing granular cytoplasmic chromogranin expression. (E) Synaptophysin is also characteristically immunopositive in large cell neuroendocrine carcinoma. Such evidence of neuroendocrine differentiation is required for a diagnosis of large cell neuroendocrine carcinoma, and in this case a diagnosis of "probable large cell neuroendocrine carcinoma" would be justified.

Chapter 4 • Neuroendocrine Tumors

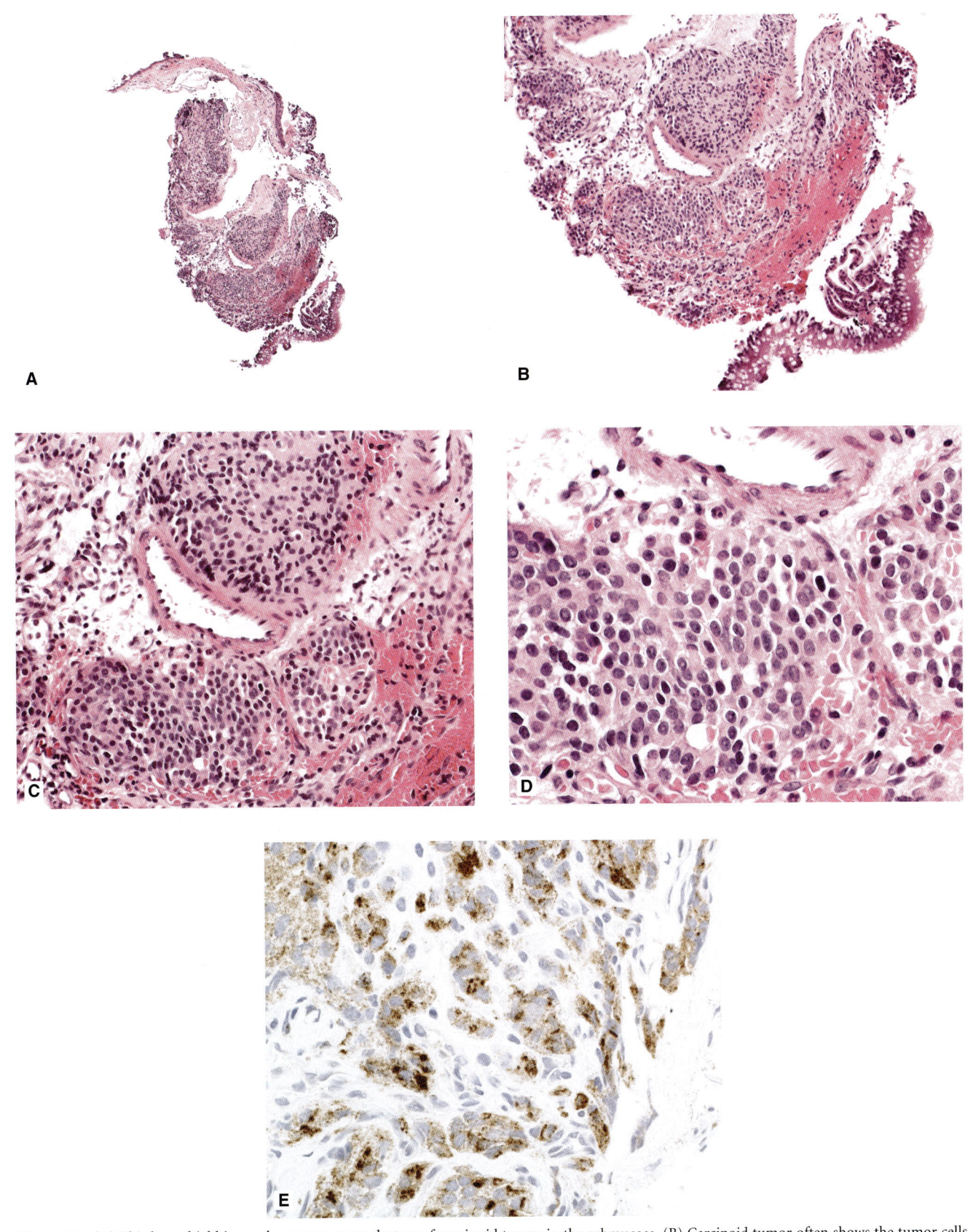

Figure 4.6: (A) This bronchial biopsy shows numerous clusters of carcinoid tumor in the submucosa. (B) Carcinoid tumor often shows the tumor cells distributed in well-circumscribed nests. (C) Bronchial carcinoid tumor cells are relatively small and regular. Little architecture is evident in the tumor cell nests in this case. (D) Carcinoid tumor nuclei are oval with little variation, chromatin is regular, and nucleoli are inconspicuous. There is relatively little cytoplasm, and the cells are evenly spaced. (E) Bronchial carcinoid tumors usually show strong granular expression of chromogranin in the tumor cell cytoplasm.

Suggested Readings

Burnett RA, Swanson Beck J, Howatson SR, et al. Observer variability in histopathological reporting of malignant bronchial biopsy specimens. *J Clin Pathol* 1994;47:711–713.

Detterbeck FC, Rivera MP, Socinski MA, et al., eds. *Diagnosis and Treatment of Lung Cancer: An Evidence-Based Guide for the Practicing Clinician.* Philadelphia, Pa: WB Saunders; 2001.

Kerr KM, Lyall MS, Chapman AD. The diagnosis of lung cancer on bronchoscopic biopsy. *CPD Bulletin Cell Pathol* 2006;6:20–30.

Schreiber G, McCrory DC. Performance characteristics of different modalities for diagnosis of suspected lung cancer. *Chest* 2003;123:S115–128.

Travis WD, Brambilla E, Muller-Hermelink HK, et al., eds. *World Health Organisation Classification of Tumours. Pathology and Genetics of Tumours of the Lung, Pleura, Thymus and Heart.* Lyon, France: IARC Press; 2004.

Metastatic Cancers

▶ Keith M. Kerr, FRCPath

The lungs are the most common site, after the liver, for metastatic cancer, and, as a clinical problem, pulmonary metastases are more frequently encountered than primary carcinoma of the lung. In around 15% to 25% of cases, the lung is the sole site of metastatic disease. In most instances, metastases are multiple. When they are solitary they may present an important differential diagnosis with primary carcinoma. Approximately 28% of lung metastases originate from the gastrointestinal and genitourinary tracts, respectively, 17% from the female breast, and 11% are metastatic sarcomas.

Most lung metastases are peripheral subpleural lesions that are not accessible to bronchial biopsy but may be sampled by transbronchial biopsy, especially if the bronchoscopist knows which bronchopulmonary segment to target. Atypical patterns of metastases occur in 9% of patients and include solitary lesions, cavitation, central/hilar location, endobronchial tumor, hilar/mediastinal lymphadenopathy, and superior sulcus lesions with neurologic syndromes; all features suggestive of primary carcinoma.

Around 30% to 40% of solitary pulmonary metastases are colorectal in origin with breast, kidney, bladder, and testis accounting, in descending order of frequency, for many of the remainder. Endobronchial metastases are most frequently from breast, colorectal, and renal cell carcinomas, melanoma, or sarcoma, again in descending order of frequency. This is very much reflected in the experience of metastatic disease encountered in bronchial biopsy samples. Metastases from pancreas, colon, and stomach may grow in a bronchioloalveolar pattern and thus may be found in transbronchial biopsy samples. Metastatic disease may be encountered in bronchial or transbronchial biopsies in the context of a number of differing clinical scenarios, such as multiple pulmonary lesions, solitary lung lesions mimicking primary tumor, known history of previous extrapulmonary malignancy, previous history of metastases at other sites, no known history of extrapulmonary malignancy either current or in the past, and useful or indicative history not communicated to the reporting pathologist.

Relatively few metastatic carcinomas are so distinctive that, even in the absence of a full history, the correct diagnosis will be made from the histologic examination of hematoxylin and eosin (H&E)-stained sections. Almost all the commonly encountered metastatic tumors have close equivalent primary lung tumors. Thus in the absence of any clinical history, many metastatic tumors may not be recognized because their features are perfectly acceptable as primary disease. Equally, even if the pathologist knows about the possibility of metastatic disease, it may be a challenge to distinguish it from primary carcinoma. Diagnostic difficulty is compounded by the small amount of tumor usually available for examination.

Most lung metastases are adenocarcinomas. Primary lung adenocarcinoma is an extremely heterogeneous tumor and may show an acinar, cribriform, or even signet-ring cell pattern as seen in breast or many upper gastrointestinal carcinomas; the enteric pattern of adenocarcinoma with so-called dirty necrosis, typical of colorectal cancer, may occur as a primary lung tumor, and clear cell variants of adenocarcinoma and large cell carcinoma may easily mimic metastatic renal cell carcinoma. Not all metastatic melanomas show melanin, and they can simulate large cell lung carcinoma with abundant eosinophilic cytoplasm and prominent nucleoli. Sarcomatoid carcinomas are named precisely for the reason that they are similar in appearance to a variety of true sarcomas, whereas neuroendocrine and squamous cell carcinomas look the same regardless of their origin.

Without an appropriate history, and accepting that primary lung cancer can show a very wide range of appearances, the pathologist should be aware of the possibility of metastatic disease and have a high index of suspicion if the tumor in a bronchial or transbronchial biopsy is in any way unusual. Apart from seeking further clinical or radiologic detail, immunohistochemistry is of vital importance in this area of differential diagnosis. Immunohistochemical profiles of different primary tumors are published in detail elsewhere, including descriptions of the relative discriminating power of various markers or groups of markers. There is no immunohistochemical solution to the problem of (possible) metastatic neuroendocrine or squamous cell carcinoma. Lung adenocarcinomas express CK7 but only rarely CK20, carcinoembryonic antigen (CEA) in 95% of cases and thyroid transcription factor-1 (TTF-1) in 75% of cases. TTF-1 is particularly useful in identifying primary lung cancer when thyroid or neuroendocrine carcinoma is ruled out by other means. The CK20+/CK7–/CDX2+/MUC2+ profile of most colorectal carcinomas is very useful, but enteric-pattern primary lung adenocarcinoma may also show this combination, although CDX2 is less often positive. TTF-1 may be present in the lung version of this tumor, and both CK20 and MUC2 are found only occasionally. Mucinous bronchioloalveolar carcinomas are frequently CK20 positive but do not express CDX2. Renal cell carcinomas do not produce mixed neutral and acidic mucins and may express CD10. Prostate and breast carcinomas may be identified by the presence of PSA (or prostatic acid phosphatase) and ERalpha, respectively. S-100, MelanA, and HMB45 are most useful in the identification of melanoma.

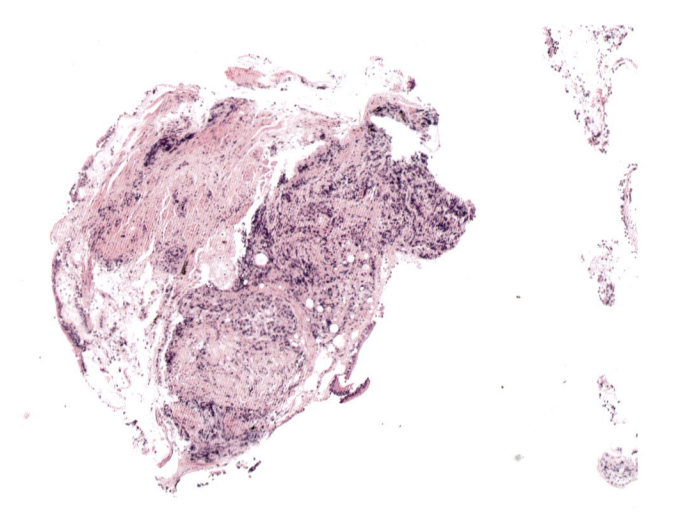

Figure 5.1: Metastatic breast cancer. Bronchial biopsy covered by respiratory epithelium and infiltrated by tumor. This biopsy was accompanied by a history of previous ductal carcinoma of the breast.

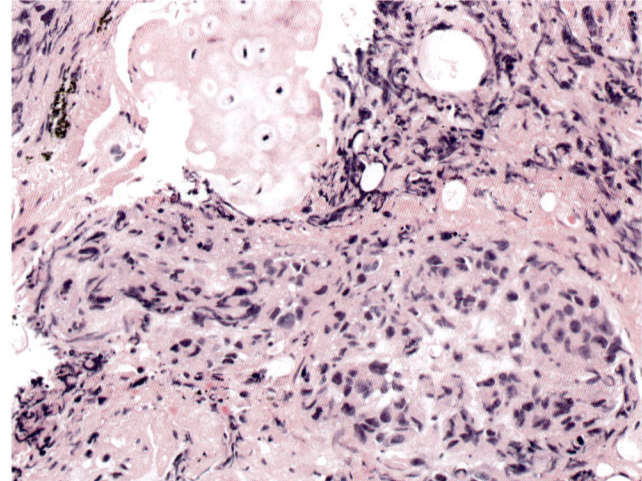

Figure 5.2: Metastatic breast cancer. Rather undifferentiated tumor infiltrates the bronchial mucosa in the lower part of this field. The bronchial cartilage appears eroded.

Chapter 5 • Metastatic Cancers

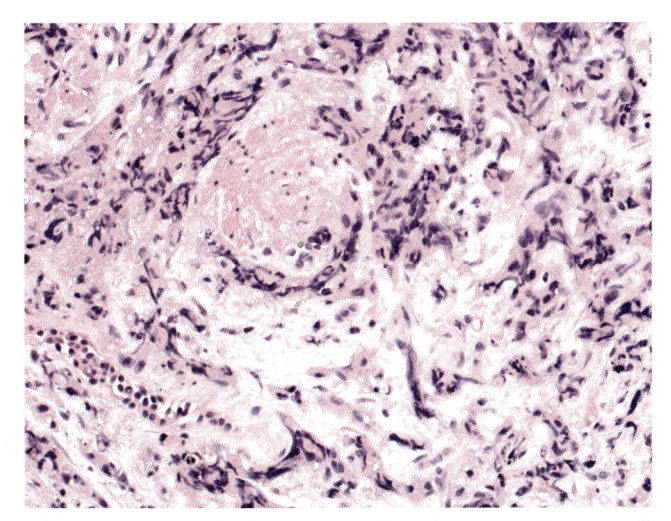

Figure 5.3: Metastatic breast cancer. Crush artifact is not unique to small cell lung carcinoma, as can been seen here where the tumor also shows perineural infiltration.

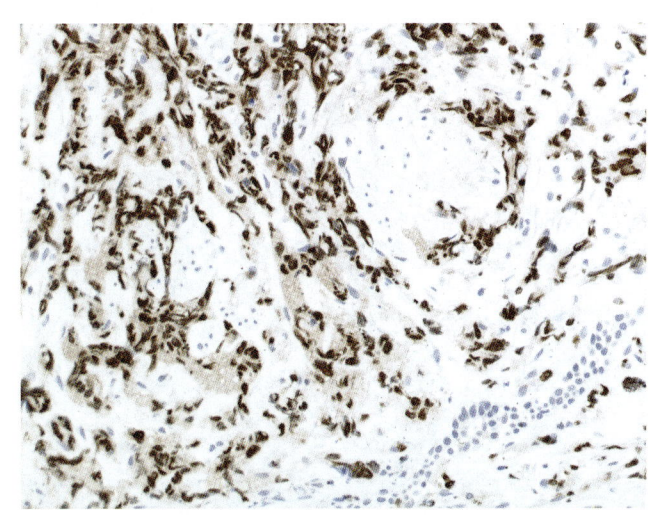

Figure 5.4: Metastatic breast cancer. The tumor strongly expresses nuclear ER alpha on immunohistochemistry, entirely in keeping with this tumor being metastatic carcinoma of the breast.

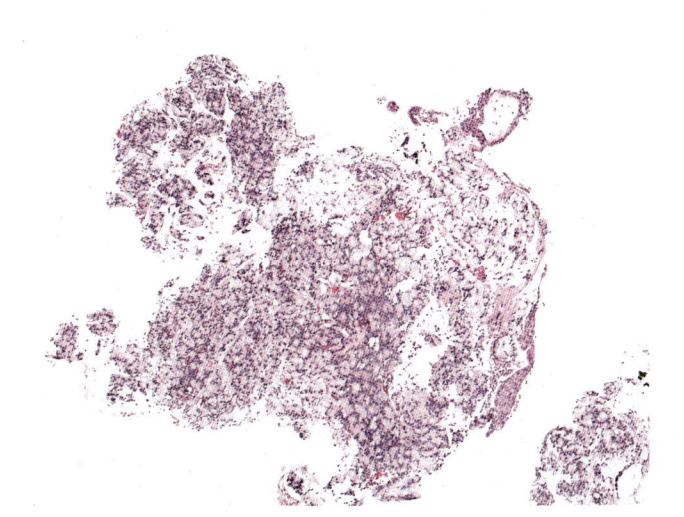

Figure 5.5: Metastatic colorectal cancer. This bronchial biopsy is infiltrated by a gland-forming tumor. Clinical history suggested primary lung carcinoma.

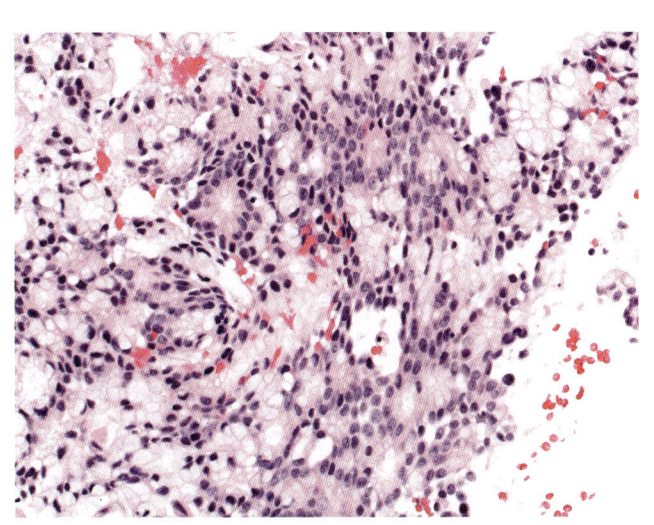

Figure 5.6: Metastatic colorectal cancer. This biopsy shows invasive adenocarcinoma with a glandular and cribriform pattern with goblet cells and some signet-ring cells. This unusual pattern of tumor for primary lung adenocarcinoma raised suspicion of metastatic disease.

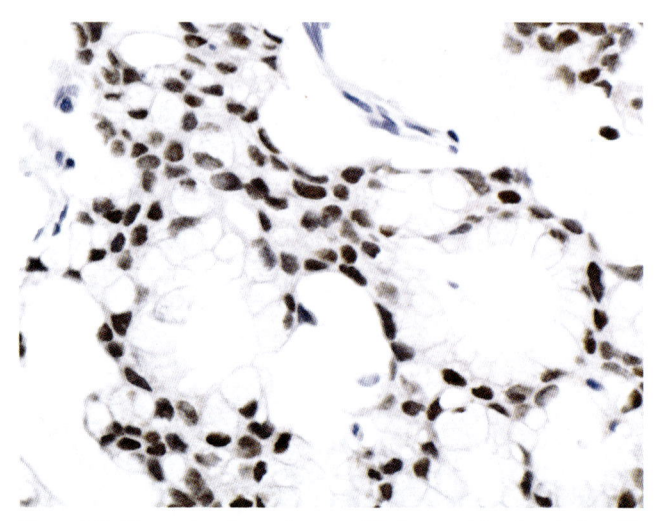

Figure 5.7: Metastatic colorectal cancer. The immunohistochemical profile of this tumor was CK7–/CK20+/CEA+/TTF-1– and, as illustrated in the photograph, CDX2 positive in tumor cell nuclei. This suggested a gastrointestinal carcinoma metastasis rather than primary pulmonary adenocarcinoma, and further investigation of the patient revealed a primary tumor in the ascending colon.

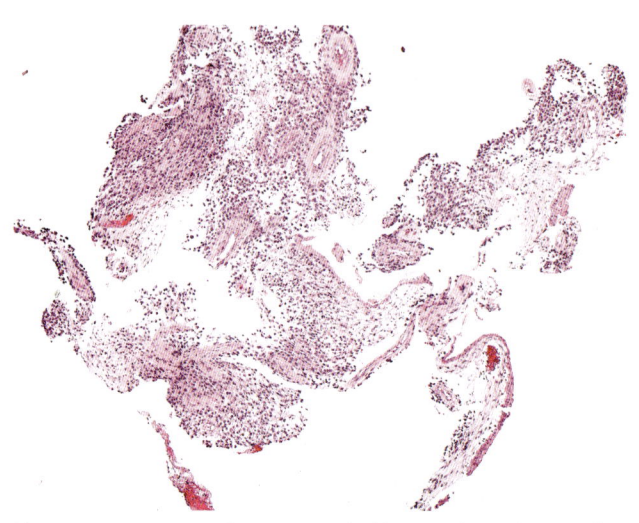

Figure 5.8: Metastatic melanoma. Bronchial biopsy infiltrated by undifferentiated tumor. Note the thin squamous metaplasia of the surface epithelium (far right). This is a common finding overlying a variety of endobronchial tumors.

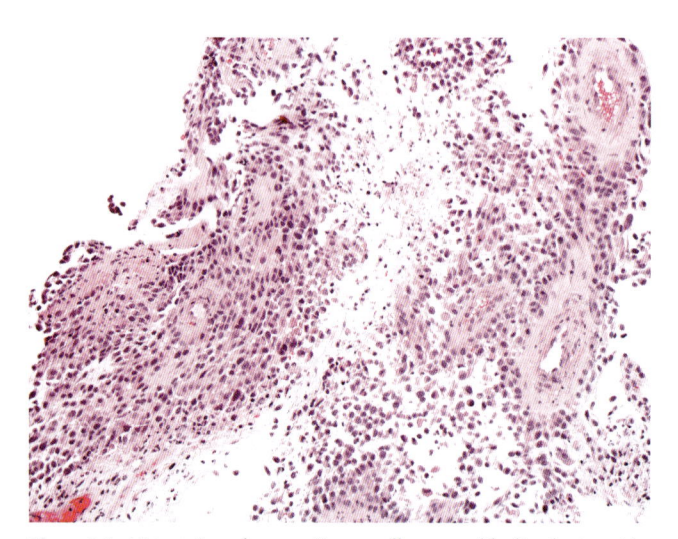

Figure 5.9: Metastatic melanoma. Tumor cells are notably discohesive without any discernable architecture and have plentiful eosinophilic cytoplasm.

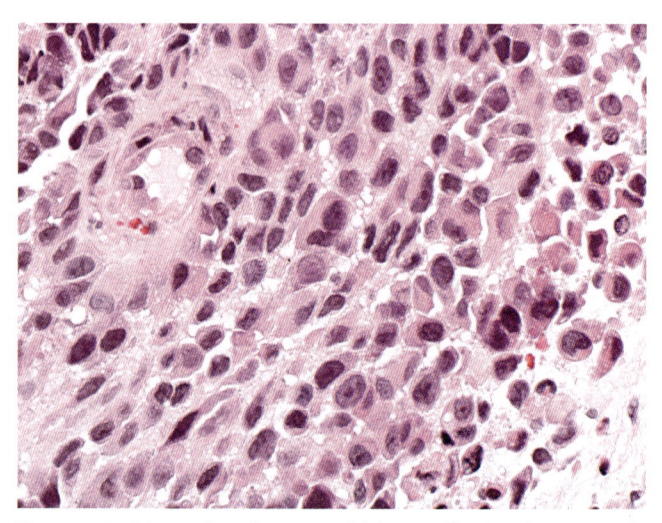

Figure 5.10: Metastatic melanoma. At high magnification the tumor cells are not very large and have rather dense chromatin, but in some areas there are prominent nucleoli. Cytoplasm is abundant and eosinophilic with no evidence of mucin vacuoles.

Chapter 5 • Metastatic Cancers

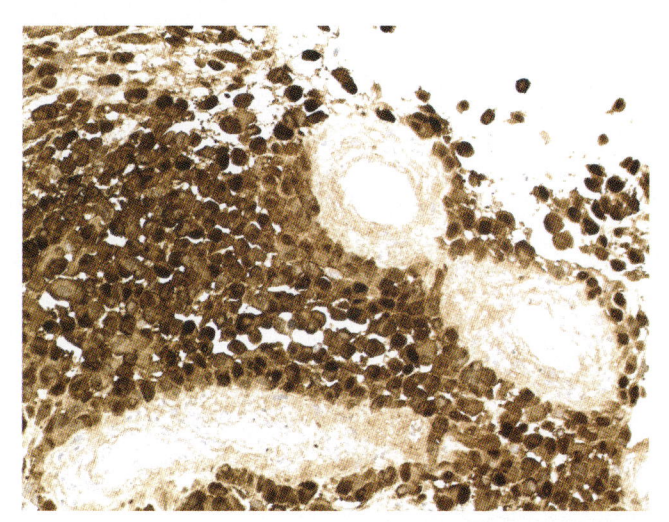

Figure 5.11: Metastatic melanoma. The features on the H&E-stained sections raised a question about metastatic malignant melanoma despite the working clinical diagnosis of primary lung cancer. S-100 protein was strongly expressed in this tumor, which did not express cytokeratins or MelanA but showed focal expression of HMB45. After the diagnosis of malignant melanoma in the bronchus was rendered, the patient's history revealed a discription of melanoma excised from the scalp 8 years previously.

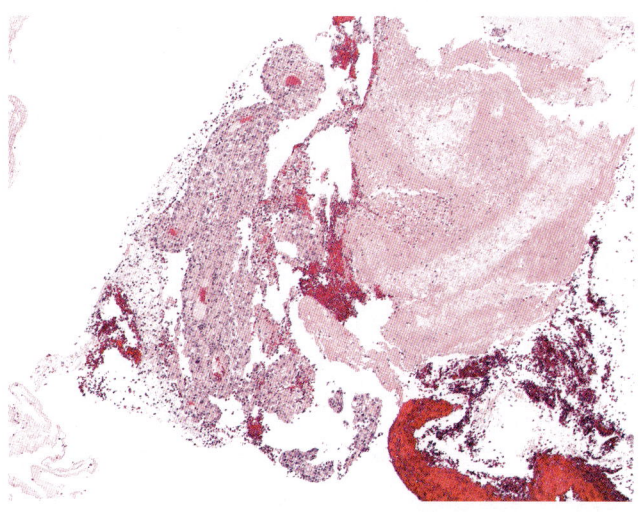

Figure 5.12: Metastatic renal cell cancer. Bronchial biopsy taken from a patient who presented with hemoptysis and radiographically had a central tumor mass that was visible at bronchoscopy. A computed tomography body scan also showed a large renal mass consistent with primary carcinoma of the kidney.

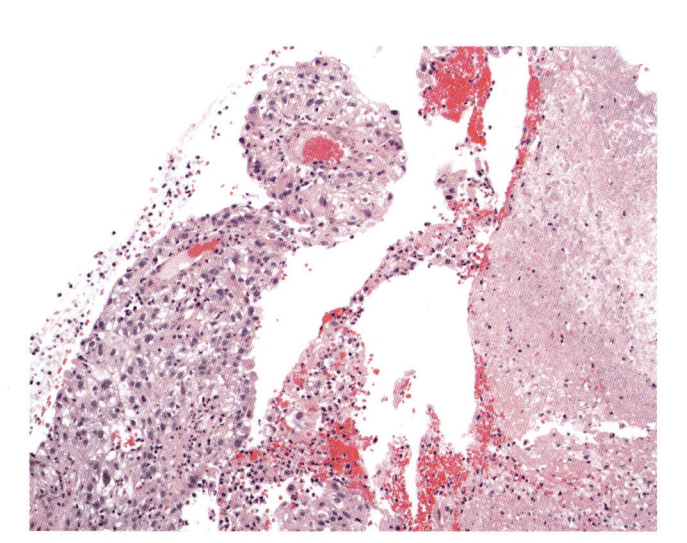

Figure 5.13: Metastatic renal cell cancer. This tumor shows extensive necrosis (right) and a prominent vascular pattern. The tumor has a solid architecture, lacking differentiation.

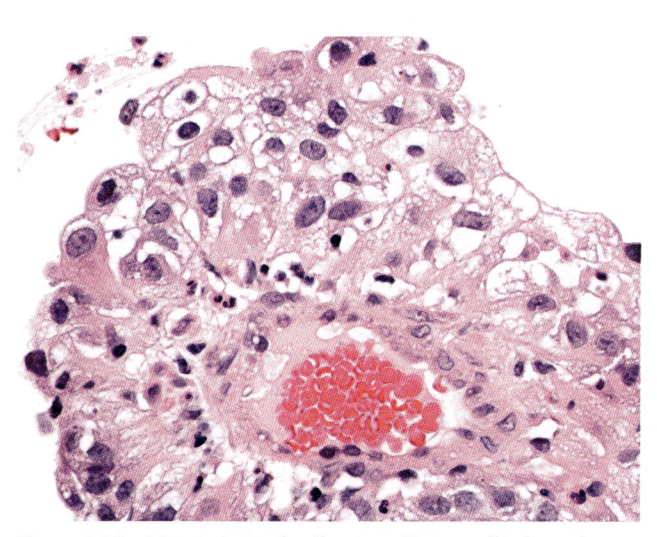

Figure 5.14: Metastatic renal cell cancer. Tumor cells show clear or eosinophilic cytoplasm and moderate nuclear pleomorphism. There was no evidence of tumor mucin production on Alcian blue/PAS staining. Although primary carcinoma of the lung may look like this tumor, given the radiologic finding of a renal mass, metastatic renal cell carcinoma to the bronchus was suspected. The bronchial tumor expressed CD10 but not TTF-1 or CEA. Needle biopsy of the renal mass confirmed renal cell carcinoma.

Suggested Readings

Dail D, Cagle PT, Marchevskey A, et al. Metastases to the lung. In: Travis WD, Brambilla E, Muller-Hermelink HK, et al., eds. *World Health Organisation Classification of Tumours. Pathology and Genetics of Tumours of the Lung, Pleura, Thymus and Heart.* Lyon, France: IARC Press; 2004.

Dail DH. Metastases to and from the lung. In: Dail DH, Hammar SP, eds. *Pulmonary Pathology.* 2nd ed. New York: Springer-Verlag; 1993.

De Lott LB, Morrison C, Suster S, et al. CDX2 is a useful marker of intestinal-type differentiation: a tissue microarray-based study of 629 tumours from various sites. *Arch Pathol Lab Med* 2005;129:1100–1105.

Dennis JL, Hvidsten TR, Wit EC, et al. Markers of adenocarcinoma characteristic of the site of origin: development of a diagnostic algorithm. *Clin Cancer Res* 2005;11:3766–3772.

Filderman AE, Coppage L, Shaw C, et al. Pulmonary and pleural manifestations of extrathoracic malignancies. *Clin Chest Med* 1989;10:747–807.

Lau SK, Weiss LM, Chu PG. Differential expression of MUC1, MUC2 and MUC5AC in carcinomas of various sites: an immunohistochemical study. *Am J Clin Pathol* 2004;122:61–69.

Nash JW, Morrison C, Frankel WL. The utility of estrogen receptor and progesterone receptor immunohistochemistry in the distinction of breast carcinoma from other tumours of the liver. *Arch Pathol Lab Med* 2003;127:1591–1595.

Rossi G, Murer B, Cavazza A, et al. Primary mucinous (so-called colloid) carcinomas of the lung: a clinicopathological and immunohistochemical study with special reference to CDX2 homeobox gene and MUC2 expression. *Am J Surg Pathol* 2004;28:442–452.

Skinnider BF, Amin MB. An immunohistochemical approach to the differential diagnosis of renal tumours. *Semin Diagn Pathol* 2005;22:51–68.

Tsuta K, Ishii G, Nitadonri J, et al. Comparison of the immunophenotypes of signet-ring cell carcinoma, solid adenocarcinoma with mucin production, and mucinous bronchioloalveolar carcinoma of the lung characterised by the presence of cytoplasmic mucin. *J Pathol* 2006;209:78–87.

Yousem SA. Pulmonary intestinal-type adenocarcinoma does not show enteric differentiation by immunohistochemical study. *Mod Pathol* 2005;18:816–821.

Preinvasive Lesions

▶ Keith M. Kerr, FRCPath

Three recognized preinvasive lesions are precursors of invasive tumors in the bronchial tree and lung: squamous dysplasia and carcinoma in situ (SD/CIS) of the tracheobronchial mucosa, atypical adenomatous hyperplasia (AAH), and diffuse idiopathic pulmonary neuroendocrine cell hyperplasia (DIPNECH). Both AAH and DIPNECH occur in the lung periphery.

SD/CIS lesions are generally invisible to the bronchoscopist during standard bronchoscopy but may be identified as nonspecific areas of abnormality at autofluorescence bronchoscopy (AFB). Bronchial biopsies taken from abnormal AFB mucosa generate more SD/CIS lesions but also inflamed or even normal mucosa. Squamous dysplasia is graded as mild, moderate, or severe by the degree of cytological atypia (mild dysplasia showing slight nuclear atypia; severe disease shows marked atypia) and architectural alteration of the bronchial epithelium. By definition, SD/CIS occurs in a full-thickness squamous (metaplastic) epithelium in which the distribution of atypical, often basaloid cells with vertically oriented nuclei occurs in the lower third, lower two thirds, or extends into the upper third in mild, moderate, and severe disease, respectively. Mitoses are found off the basal layer of the epithelium but confined to its lower third in moderate dysplasia and at higher levels in severe dysplasia. Carcinoma in situ is characterized by a completely chaotic epithelium of highly atypical cells and little or no evidence of organization or maturation. The basement membrane remains intact but varies in thickness and tends to be relatively straight, which is helpful in differentiation from invasive disease when subepithelial tissue is scant. Occasionally SD/CIS adopts a papillary architecture with vascular pegs of connective tissue protruding into the epithelium, so-called angiogenic squamous dysplasia.

Both AAH and DIPNECH are lesions of the peripheral lung, and neither is visible to the endoscopist or diagnosable on bronchial biopsy. It is conceivable that some alveoli showing AAH could, by chance, be sampled at transbronchial biopsy, but, depending on the degree of atypia, distinction between reactive changes or even bronchioloalveolar carcinoma may be impossible, so a certain diagnosis of AAH cannot be made at transbronchial biopsy. Similarly with DIPNECH, a carcinoid tumorlet or focus of bronchiolar neuroendocrine cell hyperplasia may be sampled by transbronchial biopsy, but the significance of such a finding cannot be ascertained.

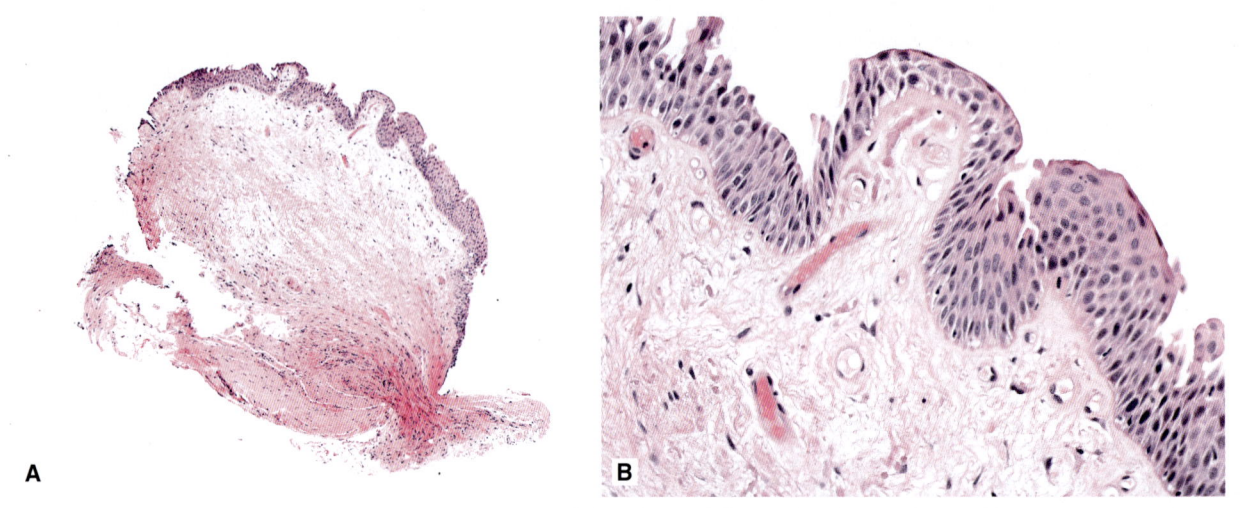

Figure 6.1: (A) Bronchial biopsy showing a papillary organization of the surface epithelium. (B) High power shows mild atypia in a squamous type epithelium that also exhibits so-called angiogenic squamous dysplasia.

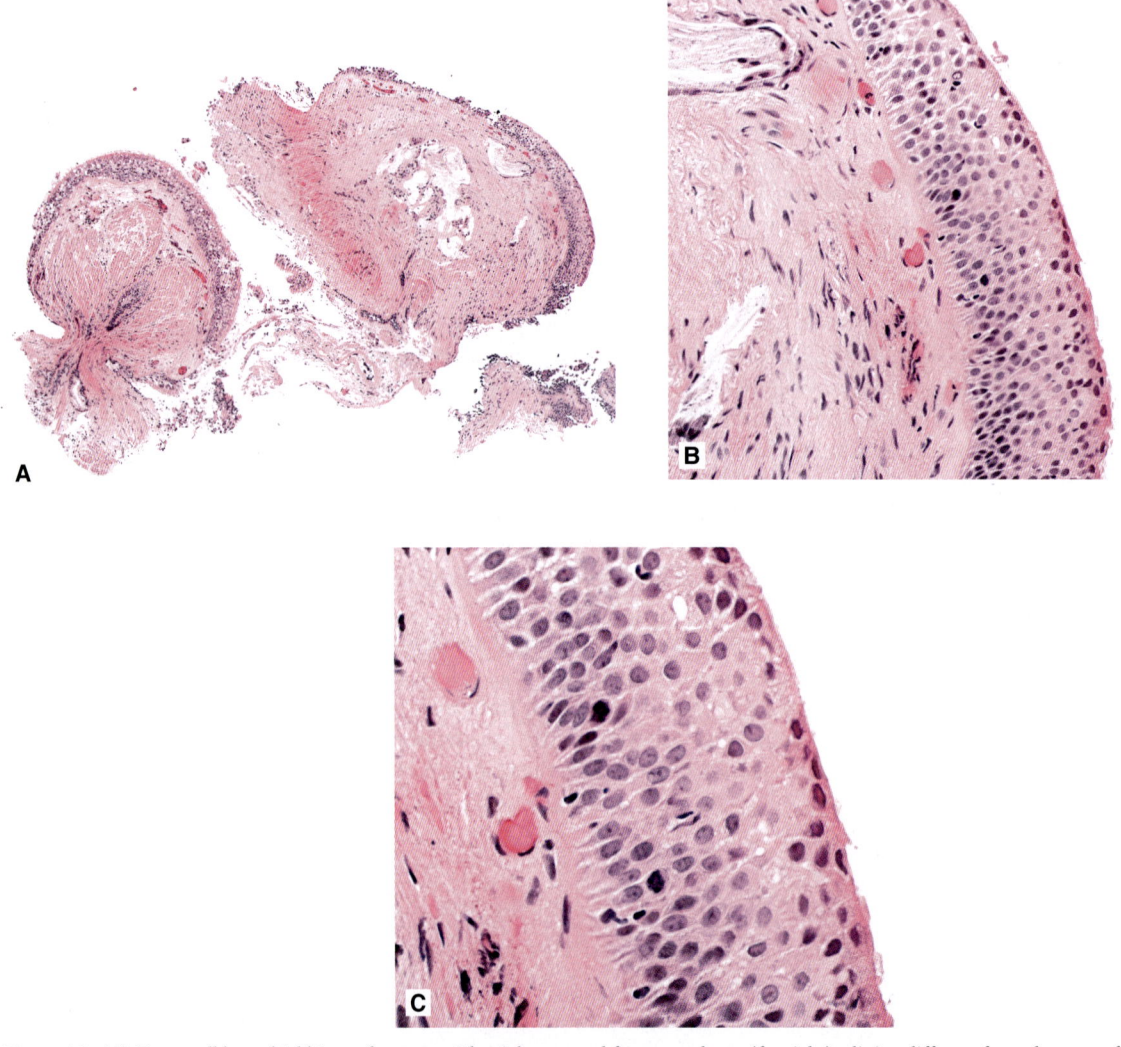

Figure 6.2: (A) Two small bronchial biopsy fragments. The right mucosal fragment shows (far right) a lining different from the normal bronchial respiratory epithelium. (B) At medium power this epithelium shows squamous differentiation (although columnar epithelial cells persist on the surface, a not uncommon occurrence) with vertical nuclei in the lower third. (C) At high power there is some nuclear irregularity extending into the middle third and mitoses are present off the base in the lower third of the epithelium. In this area, moderate dysplasia is present.

Chapter 6 • Preinvasive Lesions

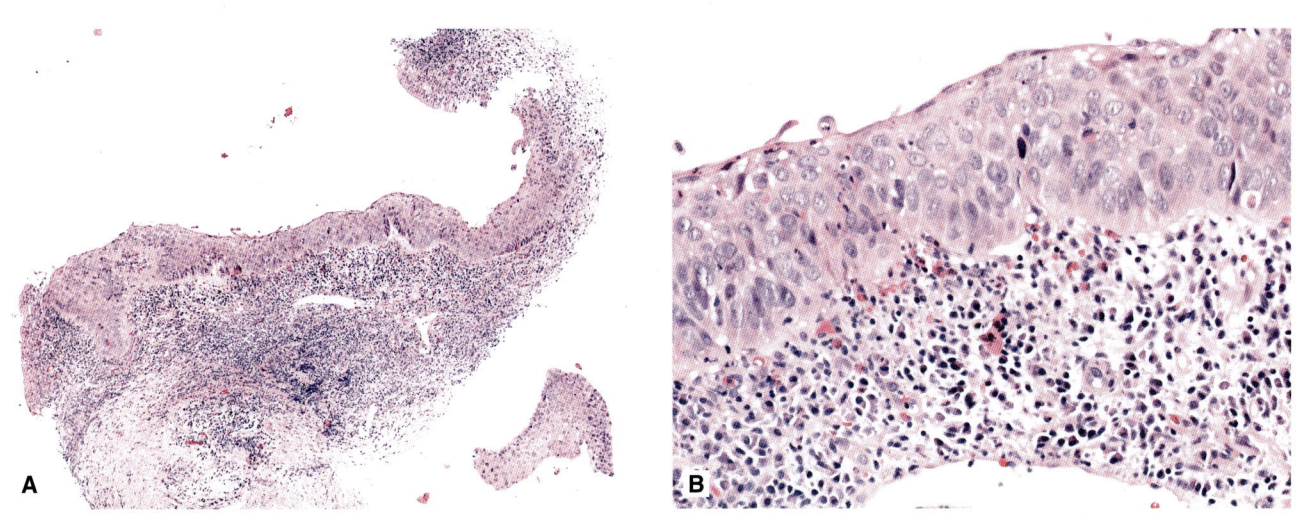

Figure 6.3: (A) This very inflamed bronchial biopsy shows a cellular squamous lining that is atypical. Note also the dissociated atypical squamous fragment. With such an appearance, it may be difficult to distinguish in-situ from invasive carcinoma. (B) High power of severe dysplasia shows marked atypia with a hint of maturation.

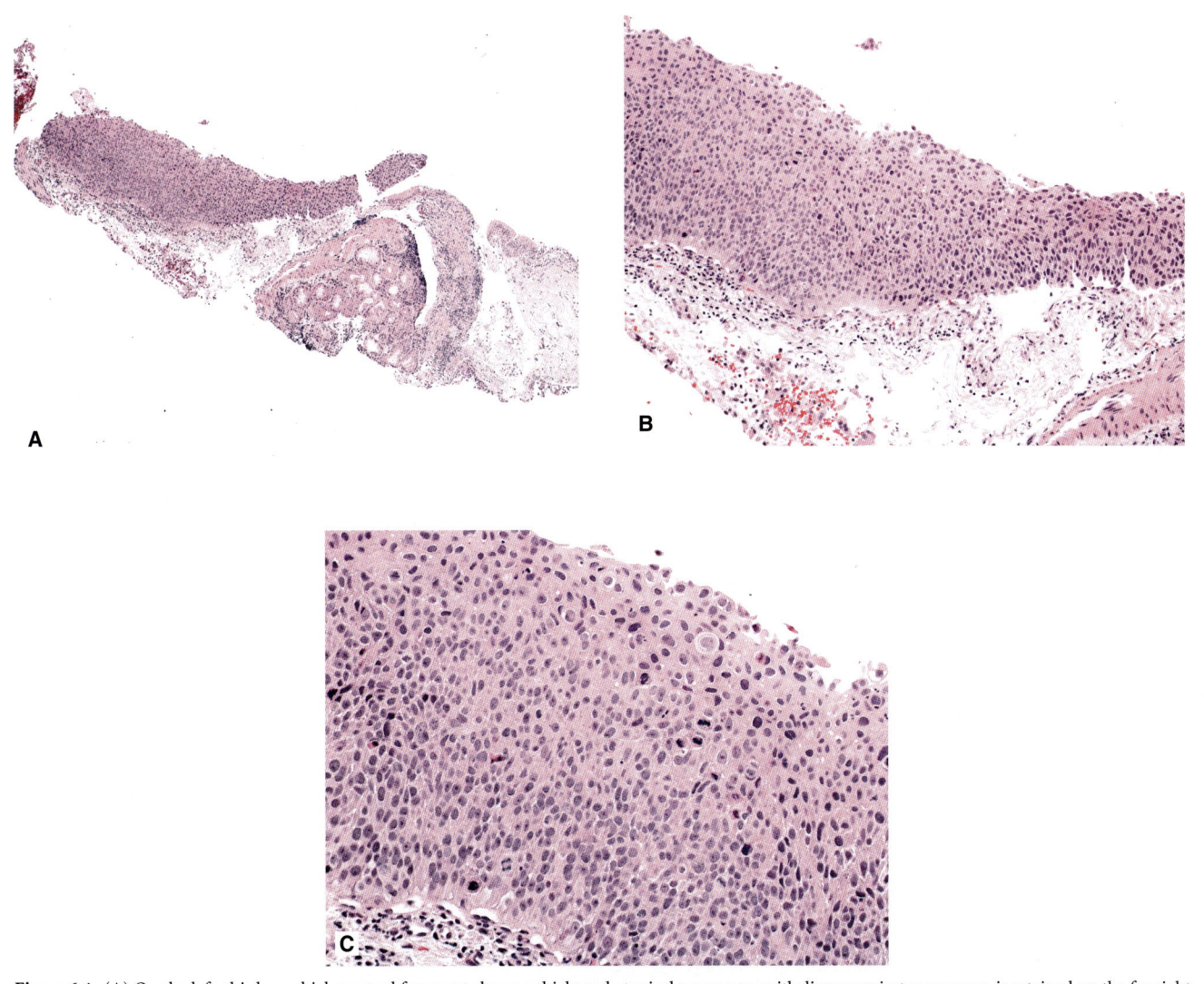

Figure 6.4: (A) On the left, this bronchial mucosal fragment shows a thickened atypical squamous epithelium; respiratory mucosa is retained on the far right. (B) The atypical squamous epithelium shows no maturation and appears chaotic and jumbled. (C) Mitoses are present at all levels in this case of carcinoma in situ.

Suggested Readings

Franklin WA, Wistuba II, Geisinger K, et al. Squamous dysplasia and carcinoma in situ. In: Travis WD, Brambilla E, Muller-Hermelink HK, et al., eds. *World Health Organisation Classification of Tumours. Pathology and Genetics of Tumours of the Lung, Pleura, Thymus and Heart.* Lyon, France: IARC Press; 2004:68–72.

Kerr KM. Pulmonary preinvasive neoplasia. *J Clin Pathol* 2001;54:257–271.

Kerr KM, Popper HH. The differential diagnosis of pulmonary pre-invasive lesions. In: Timens W, Popper HH, eds. *European Respiratory Monographs: Pathology of the Lung.* Vol 12, Monograph 39; 2007:37–62.

Lam S, MacAulay C, LeRiche JC, et al. Detection and localization of early lung cancer by fluorescence bronchoscopy. *Cancer* 2000;89:2468–2473.

Nagamoto N, Saito Y, Sato M, et al. Clinicopathological analysis of 19 cases of isolated carcinoma in situ of the bronchus. *Am J Surg Pathol* 1993;17:1234–1243.

Hematolymphoid Malignancies

7

▸ Timothy C. Allen, MD, JD
▸ Keith M. Kerr, FRCPath
▸ Jaishree Jagirdar, MD

Bronchial-associated lymphoid tissue is an ordinary finding in bronchial biopsies, and benign lymphocytic infiltrates are very common in bronchial biopsies as a nonspecific reaction or as part of an infection or specific inflammatory disease. Therefore, benign reactive lymphoid infiltrates are relatively common on endobronchial and transbronchial biopsies, whereas lymphomas are uncommon.

The lung is rarely the site of primary hematologic malignancies. Primary pulmonary non-Hodgkin lymphomas are rare, making up <1% of primary pulmonary neoplasms, with extranodal marginal zone B-cell lymphoma of mucosa-associated lymphoid tissue (MALT lymphoma) arising as the most common primary pulmonary hematologic malignancy. Lymphomatoid granulomatosis and large B-cell lymphomas may also occur infrequently. Hodgkin lymphoma and other non-Hodgkin lymphomas are rarely found as pulmonary primary malignancies. MALT lymphomas occur most commonly in older patients, many of whom are asymptomatic. The lesion may be composed of varying proportions of small lymphocytes and intermediate-size lymphocytes, plasmacytoid lymphocytes, and plasma cells. Although lymphocytic infiltration of bronchial mucosa, with the formation of lymphoepithelial lesions, is characteristic of MALT lymphoma, the feature is not specific and may be found in various reactive lesions. Primary large B-cell lymphoma of the lung occurs less frequently as a primary pulmonary neoplasm than MALT lymphoma, but nonetheless it may occasionally be encountered. It occurs over a wide range of ages, and diagnosis is often accompanied by symptoms such as dyspnea and chest pain. It typically consists of sheets of discohesive large cells that efface pulmonary architecture. Lymphomatoid granulomatosis is the term used for a T-cell-rich, large B-cell lymphoma with malignant B-cell immunopositivity with Epstein-Barr virus. It is associated with immunodeficiency. The differential diagnosis for lymphomatoid granulomatosis includes infections, Wegener granulomatosis, necrotizing sarcoidosis, and bronchocentric granulomatosis. Primary pulmonary Hodgkin lymphoma patients often present symptomatically, usually with multiple pulmonary lesions. Because of extensive associated granulomatous inflammation, differential diagnosis includes infection, large-cell non-Hodgkin lymphoma, and poorly differentiated carcinoma.

A MALT lymphoma may histologically show various morphologic features throughout the lesion. Lymphomatoid granulomatosis may have only focal diagnostic areas containing large cells. Features necessary to diagnose Hodgkin lymphoma, including the appropriate inflammatory background, may be widely or focally distributed throughout the lesion. Other hematologic neoplasms such as T-cell lymphomas frequently exhibit a polymorphous inflammatory background. As such, definitive diagnosis of these diseases on endobronchial or transbronchial biopsy may be extremely difficult or impossible. Findings on endobronchial or transbronchial biopsy may be suggestive of a hematolymphoid process and lead to an open biopsy such as wedge biopsy to obtain enough tissue for adequate histologic, immunohistochemical, and flow cytometric workup of the lesion.

In contrast to the infrequency of primary pulmonary hematologic neoplasms, the lung is a common site of involvement by systemic lymphomas, plasma cell dyscrasias, and leukemias. These neoplasms frequently exhibit histologic features similar to those found in primary nodal lesions. Careful attention to clinical history, radiographic findings, and previous tissue diagnoses may occasionally suggest the appropriate diagnosis. An appropriate panel of immunostains may be very helpful to render a diagnosis of lung involvement by systemic lymphoma, leukemia, or plasma cell dyscrasia on endobronchial or transbronchial biopsy.

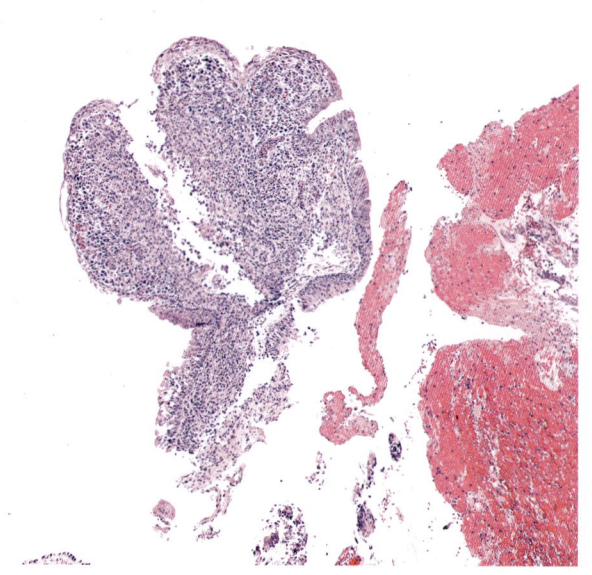

Figure 7.1: Small fragment of bronchial mucosa appears cellular at low power.

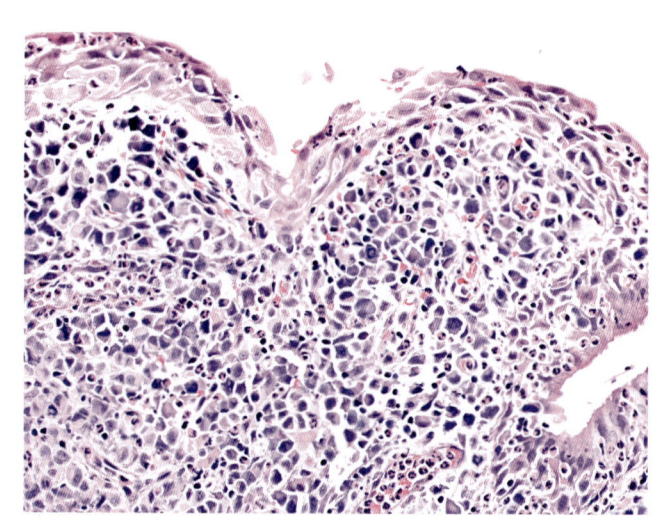

Figure 7.2: Bronchial submucosa is infiltrated by a discohesive population of large pleomorphic malignant cells with indistinct nuclear features. The tumor infiltrates the overlying epithelium, some of which shows squamous metaplasia. Neutrophils are also present.

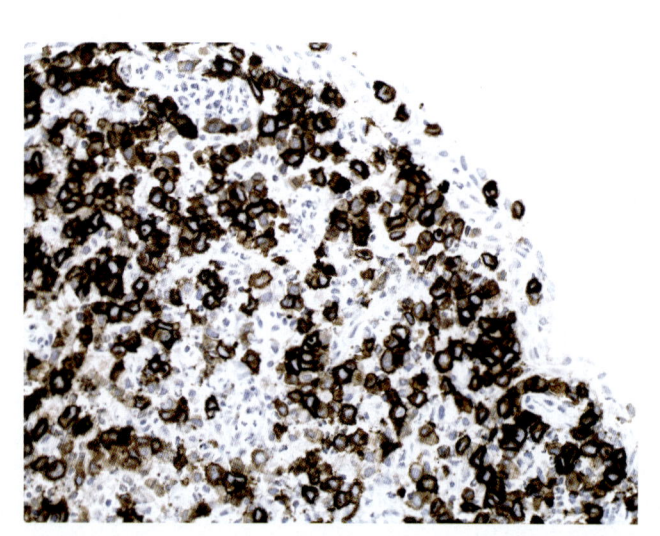

Figure 7.3: The tumor cells are CD30 positive, consistent with a diagnosis of anaplastic large cell lymphoma (B- and T-cell markers were negative).

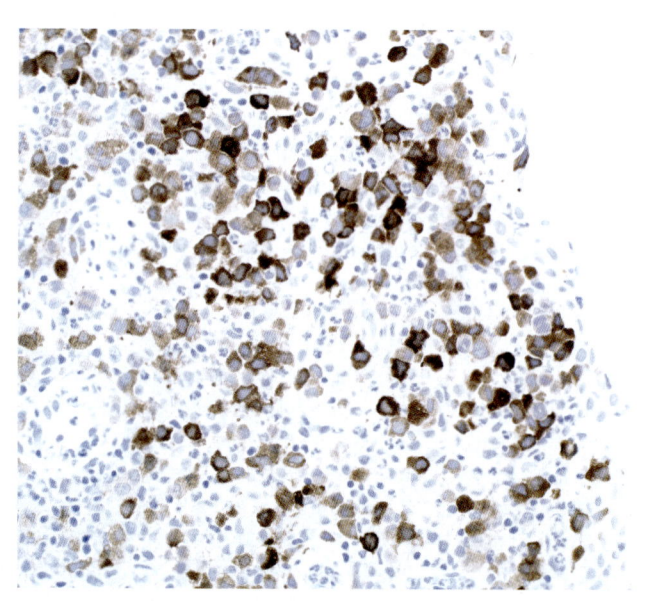

Figure 7.4: The tumor cells are also ALK-1 positive, confirming the diagnosis of anaplastic large cell lymphoma.

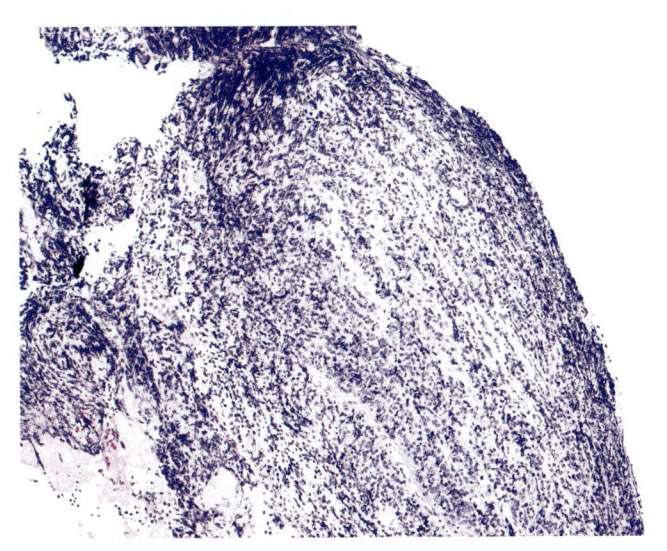

Figure 7.5: Low power of endobronchial biopsy shows intense submucosal lymphoid infiltrate.

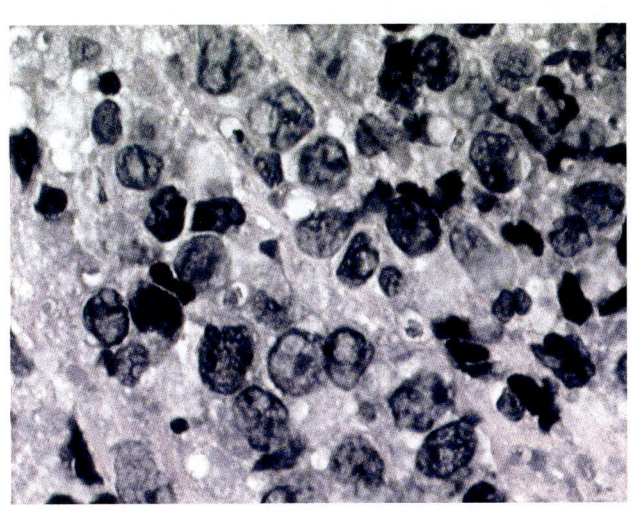

Figure 7.6: High power shows that the lymphoid cells are cytologically atypical with large nuclei and prominent nucleoli.

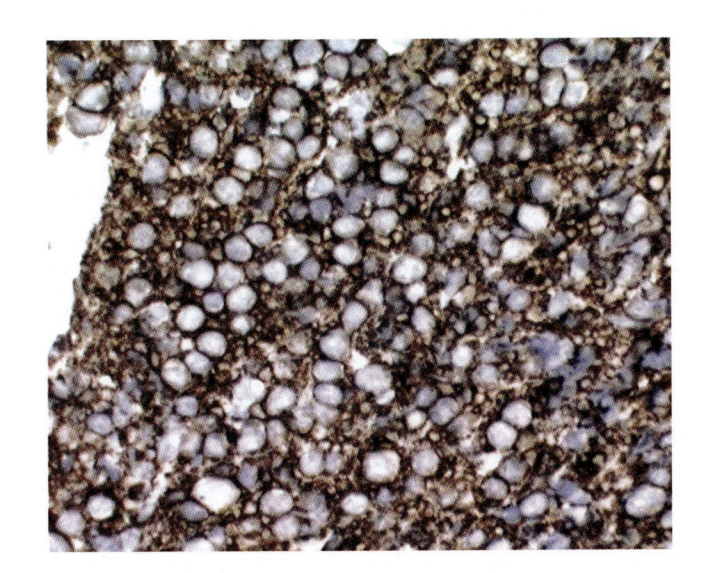

Figure 7.7: An overwhelming majority of the atypical lymphoid cells are immunopositive for the B-cell marker CD20, supporting a diagnosis of large B-cell lymphoma.

Suggested Readings

Cattelani L, Sooli P, Rusca M, et al. Primary pulmonary lymphoma: report of a case diagnosed by transbronchial biopsy. *J Cardiovasc Surg (Torino)* 1996;37:539–541.

Hematologic malignancies. In: Cagle PT, ed. *Color Atlas and Text of Pulmonary Pathology.* Philadelphia, Pa: Lippincott Williams & Wilkins; 2004.

Phadke SM, Chini BA, Patton D, et al. Relapsed non-Hodgkin's lymphoma diagnosed by flexible bronchoscopy. *Pediatr Pulmonol* 2002;34:488–490.

Benign Neoplasms

▶ Keith M. Kerr, FRCPath

Benign neoplasms of the lung are numerous, heterogeneous, and rare. Most occur in the lung periphery, neither visible to the bronchoscopist nor likely to be sampled by bronchial biopsy. Transbronchial biopsy could access a tiny portion of tumor tissue, but in all but the most exceptional case, it is highly unlikely that material will be obtained exhibiting sufficient features to allow a specific diagnosis. Some benign lung tumors do involve more central bronchi and may be encountered at bronchoscopy. These include squamous cell papilloma, glandular papilloma or mixed lesions, mucous gland adenoma, pleomorphic adenoma, chondroid hamartoma, and lipoma.

Squamous cell papillomas are mostly exophytic lesions but may be inverted, and they are usually solitary in adult men. The bronchi may be involved by multiple papillomas in juvenile laryngotracheal papillomatosis. Biopsy shows well-differentiated stratified squamous epithelium covering a loose fibrovascular stroma. Some keratinize, others show transitional epithelium, and 20% show koilocytosis. Dyskeratosis, focal atypia, and mitoses occur, and caution must be taken to distinguish them from well-differentiated squamous cell carcinoma. Glandular and mixed lesions are exceptionally rare. The glandular epithelium may be ciliated, mucigenic or mixed, pseudostratified, or simple columnar.

Mucous gland adenoma is extremely rare and comprises glands, tubules, and cystic mucin-filled spaces lined by cytologically bland cuboidal, columnar, or flattened cells, and occasionally papillae. As with other bronchial tumors, the overlying mucosa may show squamous metaplasia. Definitive diagnosis usually requires an excision specimen.

Biopsy of pleomorphic adenoma may reflect the biphasic nature of this lesion with fibromyxoid stroma and sheets or cords of epithelial and/or myoepithelial cells. Glands and chondroid stroma are less common.

Chondroid hamartoma, also referred to as mesenchymoma, is endobronchial in 10% of cases. Lesions comprise a variable mixture of mature cartilage, fat (common in endobronchial lesions), connective tissue, smooth muscle, and even bone, together with bland epithelial cell-lined cleft-like spaces. In biopsy samples the challenge is to recognize the abnormal disposition and quantity of elements that are otherwise normal bronchial constituents. The cartilage is more cellular than normal but not atypical. Lipoma, possibly related to hamartoma, comprises only mature adipocytes and, rarely, occasional lipoblast-like cells.

Chapter 8 • Benign Neoplasms

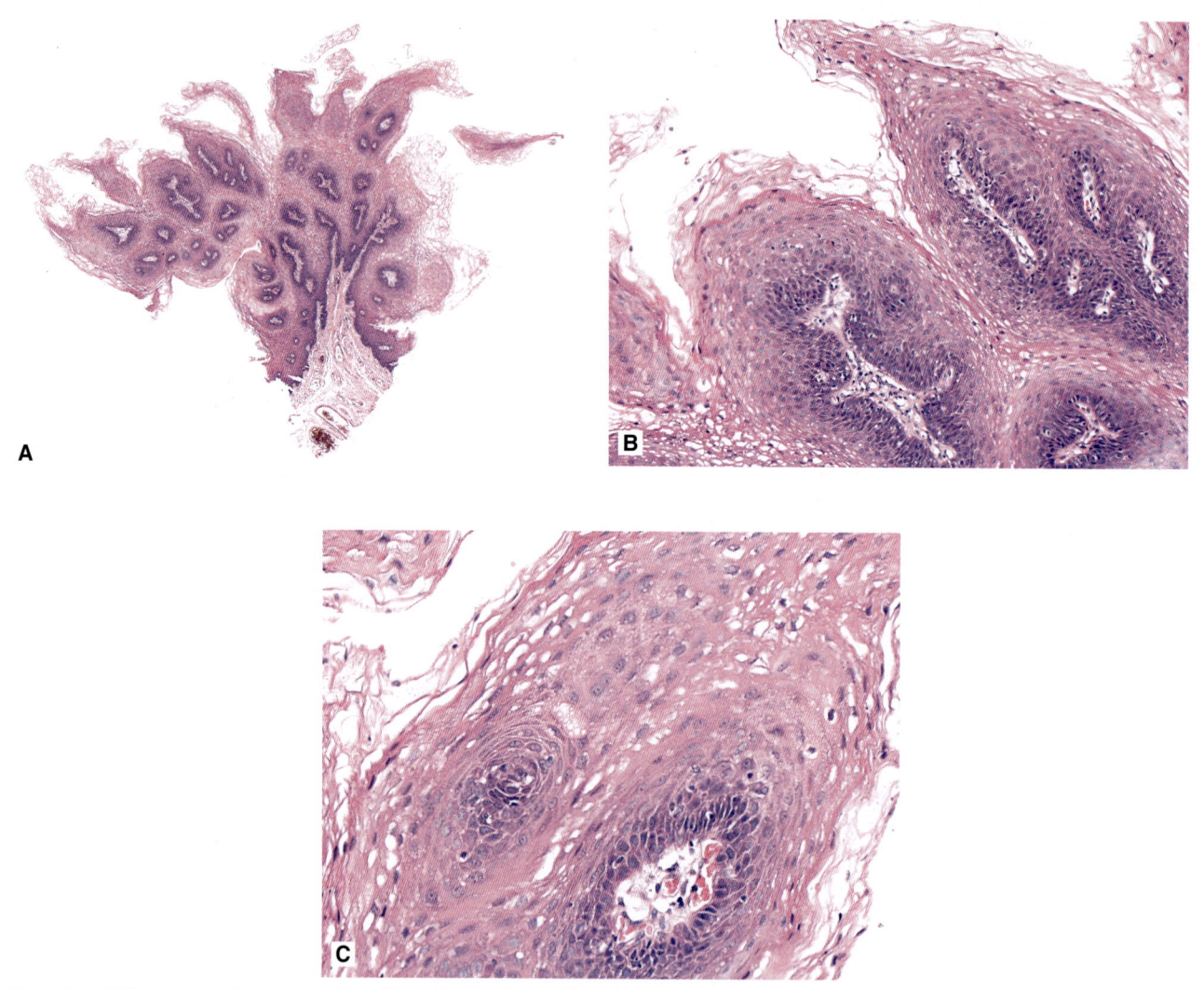

Figure 8.1: (A) Low power of squamous cell papilloma biopsy. The papillary pattern can be appreciated. (B) Thin fronds of squamous cell papilloma lined by a bland squamous epithelium. (C) High power shows well-differentiated stratified squamous epithelium covering a loose fibrovascular stroma.

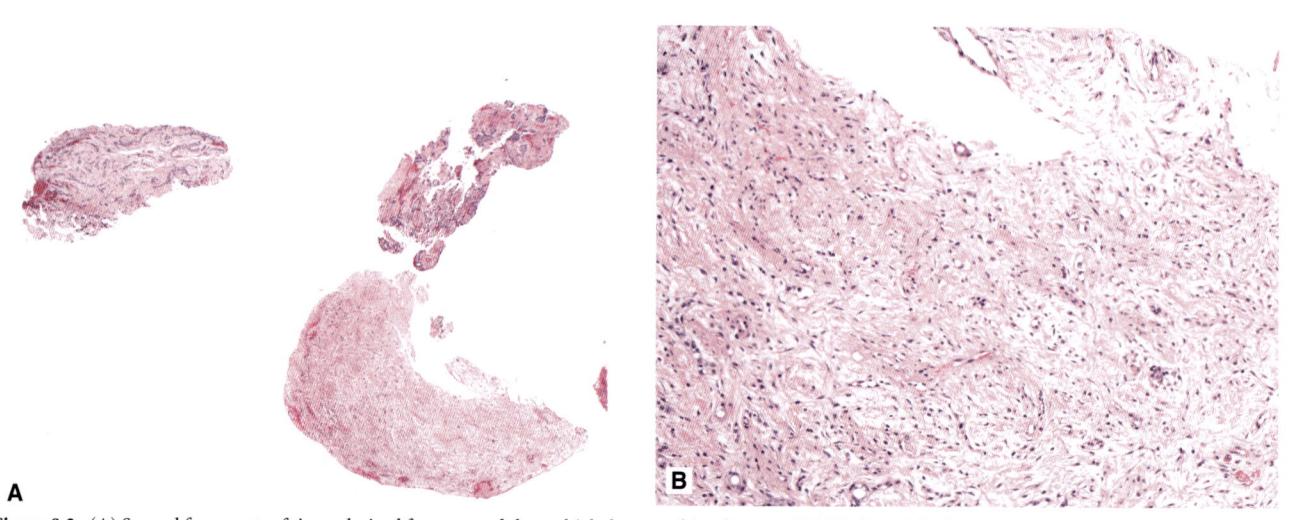

Figure 8.2: (A) Several fragments of tissue derived from an endobronchial pleomorphic adenoma. (B) The low right fragment shown in Figure 8.2A shows only the fine fibroblastic stromal component of the tumor. (*Continued*)

Chapter 8 • Benign Neoplasms

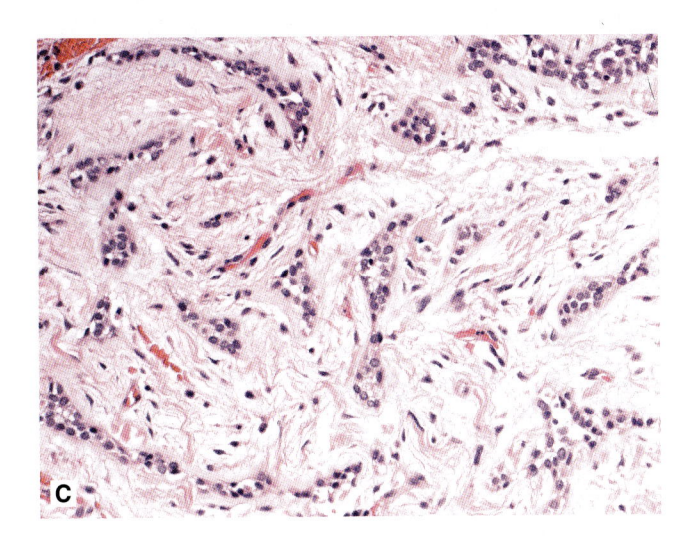

Figure 8.2: (*continued*) (C) The small fragment to the left in Figure 8.2A shows stroma and delicate cords of bland epithelial cells.

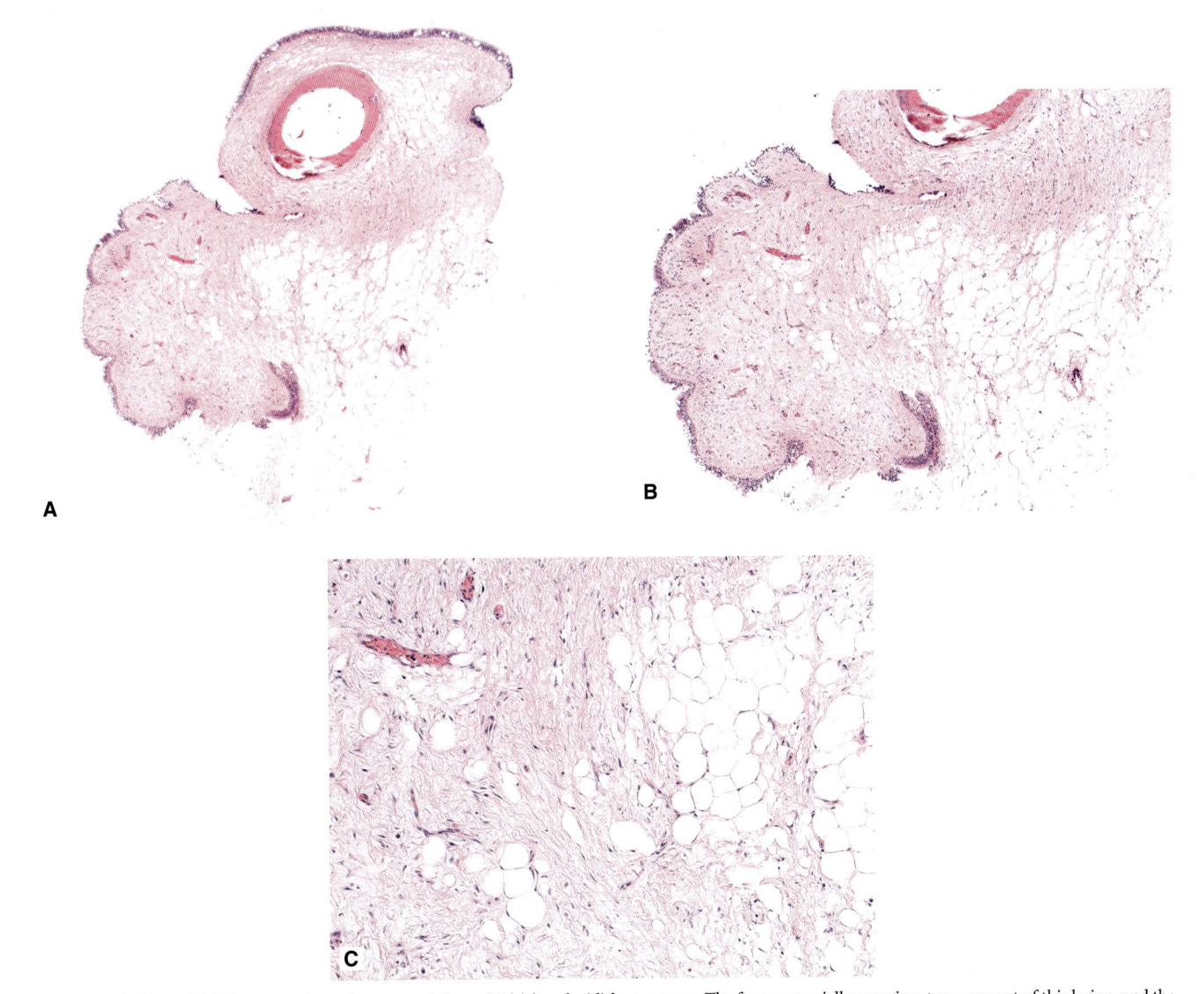

Figure 8.3: (A) Bronchial biopsy specimen from an endobronchial (chondroid) hamartoma. The fat, an especially prominent component of this lesion, and the fibroconnective tissue are well represented in this biopsy. Although cartilage was a significant component of the resected tumor, large cartilage fragments are difficult to sample at endobronchial biopsy, and the tissue in this biopsy is probably normal bronchial cartilage. (B) Fat admixed with a fibroblastic stroma unlike that usually found in the bronchus extends up to the bronchial epithelium. (C) Mature adipose tissue is abundant in endobronchial hamartoma and makes distinction from lipoma (see Fig. 8.4) difficult.

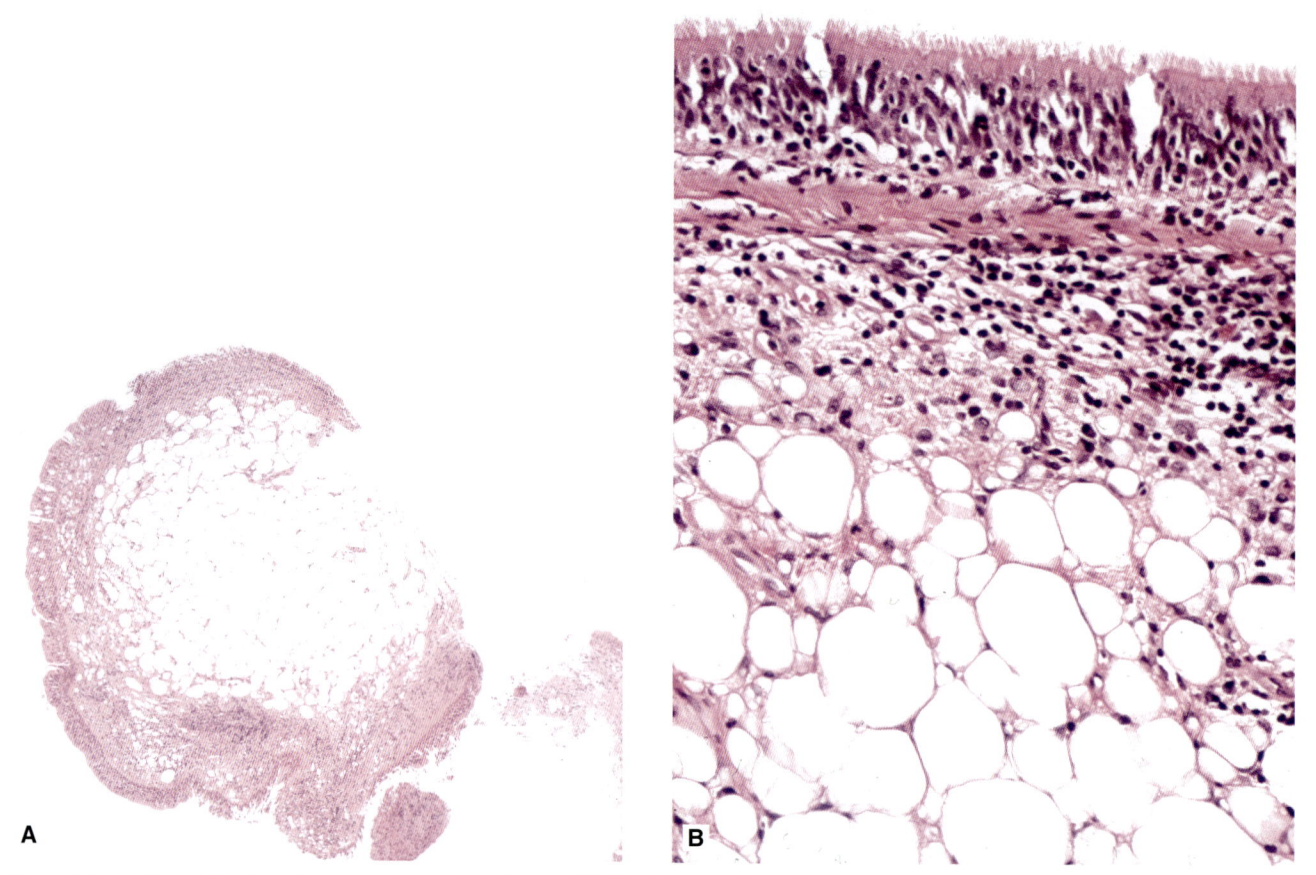

Figure 8.4: (A) Bronchial biopsy from an endobronchial lipoma. (B) The lesion consists only of mature adipocytes lying deep to a normal respiratory epithelium.

Suggested Readings

Flieder DB, Koss MN, Nicholson AG, et al. Solitary pulmonary papillomas in adults: a clinicopathologic and in situ hybridisation study of 14 cases combined with 27 cases in the literature. *Am J Surg Pathol* 1998;22:1328–1342.

Moran CA, Suster S, Askin FB, et al. Benign and malignant salivary gland-type mixed tumours of the lung. Clinicopathologic and immunohistochemical study of eight cases. *Cancer* 1994;73:2481–2490.

Moran CA, Suster S, Koss MN. Endobronchial lipomas: a clinicopathologic study of four cases. *Mod Pathol* 1994;7:212–214.

Tomashefski JF Jr. Benign endobronchial mesenchymal tumours: their relationship to parenchymal pulmonary hamartomas. *Am J Surg Pathol* 1982;6:531–540.

Travis WD, Brambilla E, Muller-Hermelink HK, et al., eds. *World Health Organisation Classification of Tumours. Pathology and Genetics of Tumours of the Lung, Pleura, Thymus and Heart.* Lyon, France: IARC Press; 2004.

van den Bosch JM, Wagenaar SS, Corrin B, et al. Mesenchymoma of the lung (so called hamartoma): a review of 154 parenchymal and endobronchial cases. *Thorax* 1987;42:790–793.

Viruses

▶ Abida Haque, MD
▶ Philip T. Cagle, MD

Viral infections of lung are common, and often latent and self-limited except in immunocompromised patients, who can develop extensive pulmonary infections with severe respiratory compromise. Diagnosis of viral infection in nonimmunocompromised individuals is made by serology and viral cultures. In immunocompromised patients, time is of the essence, and transbronchial biopsy may yield a quick diagnosis based on the detection of typical viral inclusions. The diagnosis can be confirmed by immunohistochemical stains for viruses. In situ hybridization and polymerase chain reaction (PCR) tests are available for common viruses for further confirmation.

Almost all viruses induce cytopathic effects in the infected cells, some so morphologically distinct as to provide a diagnosis with confidence.

The viral pulmonary infections commonly seen in general surgical pathology practice include adenovirus, cytomegalovirus, herpes simplex virus, measles virus, respiratory syncytial virus, and, less commonly, varicella-zoster, influenza, and parainfluenza virus.

Some viral inclusions are associated with intranuclear or cytoplasmic inclusions and others with both. In the early stages of infection, the viral inclusions of different members of the herpesvirus family, that is, cytomegalovirus, herpes simplex, and varicella zoster, are difficult to distinguish from each other, and initially a specific diagnosis may not be made on transbronchial biopsy (Table 9-1).

Table 9-1. Morphologic Features of Viral Inclusions

Virus	Nuclear	Cytoplasm	Cytologic Features
Adenovirus	+	−	Early inclusions HSV-like, Cowdry A, late inclusions deep basophilic with smudged nuclei
Cytomegalovirus	+	+	Large cells, single Cowdry A nuclear inclusion, cytoplasmic inclusions small, basophilic, multiple
Herpes simplex	+	−	Multinucleated large cells, eosinophilic Cowdry A inclusions, ground-glass nuclei, molding
Measles	+	+	Multinucleated giant cells, nuclear inclusions HSV-like, cytoplasmic inclusions deep, eosinophilic, hyalinized, tallow-like
Respiratory syncytial virus	−	+	Multinucleated giant cells, deep eosinophilic, multiple, smooth contoured inclusions
Varicella-zoster virus	+	−	HSV-like inclusions
Influenza	−	−	No inclusions
Parainfluenza	−	+	Multinucleated giant cells, indistinct eosinophilic, pleomorphic inclusions

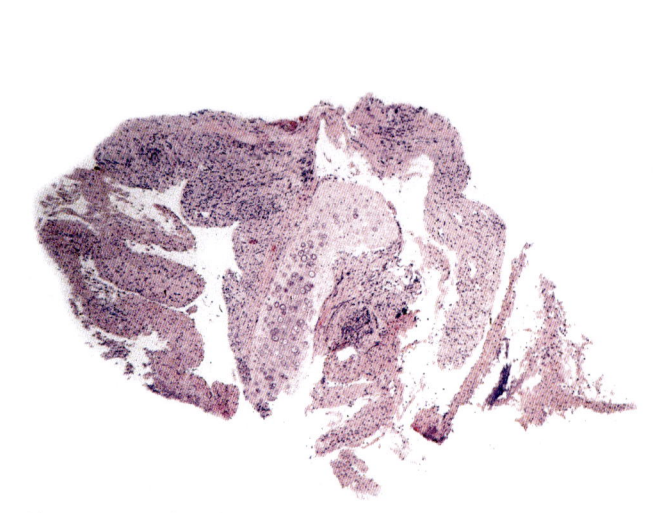

Figure 9.1: Transbronchial biopsy from a lung transplant patient with adenovirus infection shows airway mucosa and cartilage with increased mucosal cellular infiltrate.

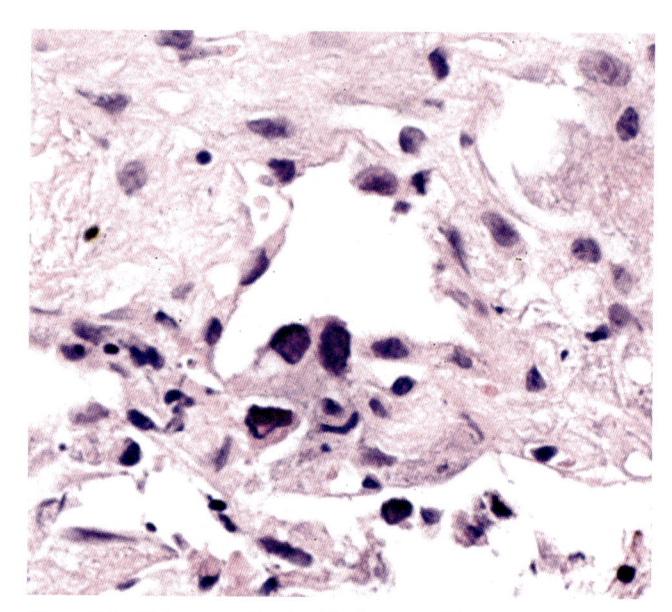

Figure 9.2: Higher magnification illustrates a mild increase in pneumocyte size and deeply basophilic enlarged "smudged" nuclei, characteristic of adenovirus infection.

Chapter 9 • Viruses

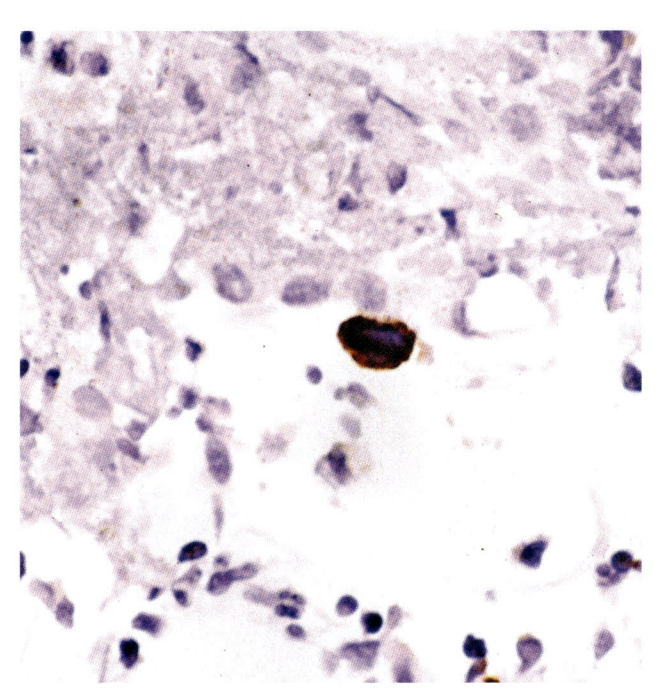

Figure 9.3: Immunostain for adenovirus is positive in a "smudge" cell within the transbronchial biopsy.

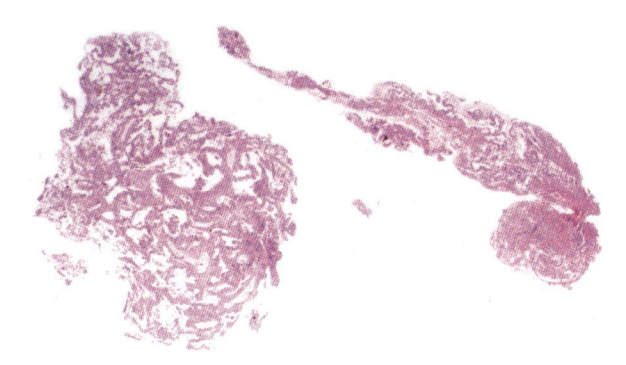

Figure 9.4: Transbronchial biopsy from a patient with acquired immunodeficiency syndrome and cytomegalovirus pneumonia shows open alveoli and suggestion of an increased alveolar interstitial cellularity.

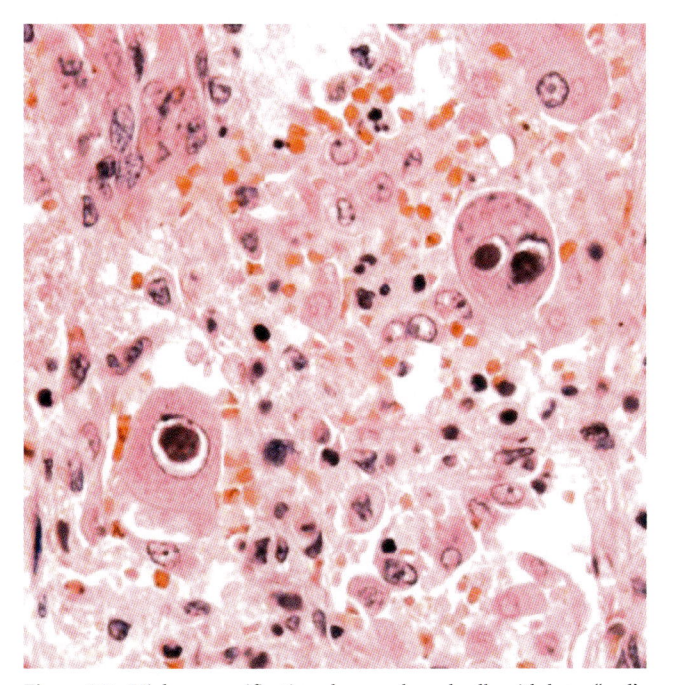

Figure 9.5: Higher magnification shows enlarged cells with large "owl's eyes" nuclear inclusions, consistent with cytomegalovirus infection.

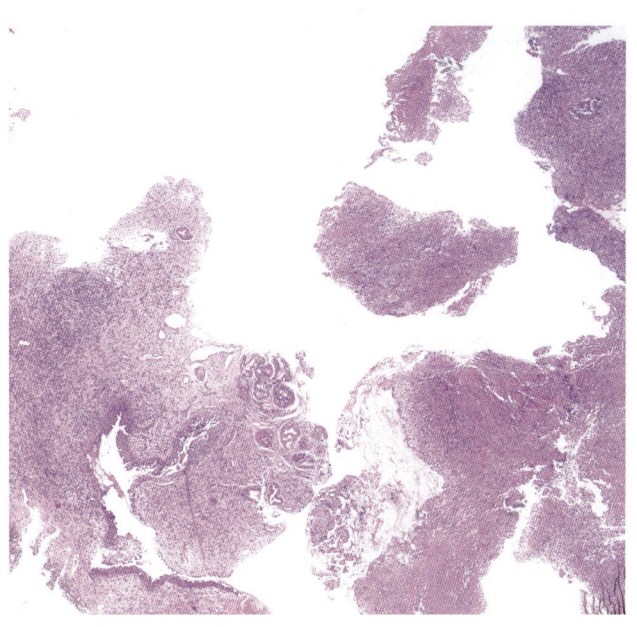

Figure 9.6: Low power of transbronchial biopsy shows extensive necrosis and inflammation of bronchial wall and lung parenchyma in a patient with herpes pneumonia.

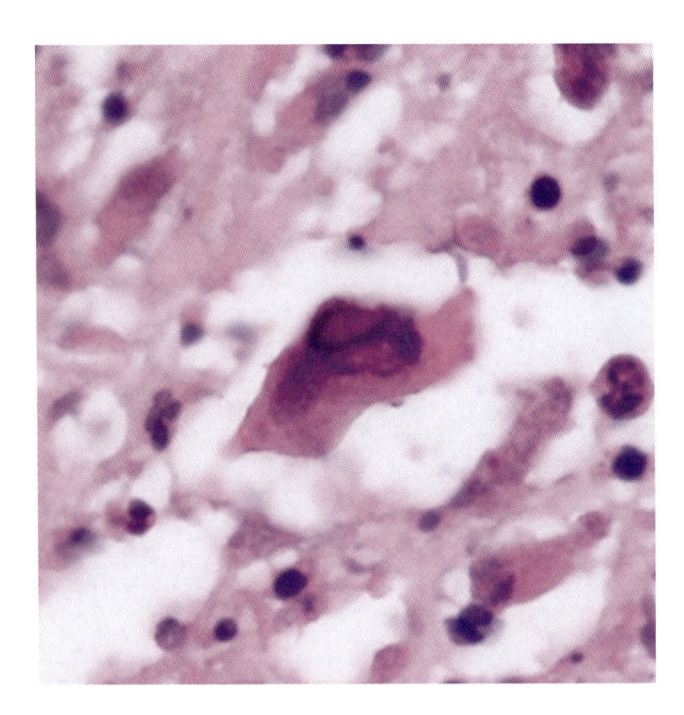

Figure 9.7: High power of necrotizing pneumonia shows cell with multiple ground-glass eosinophilic nuclei characteristic of herpes infection.

Suggested Readings

Chakinala MM, Walter MJ. Community acquired respiratory viral infections after lung transplantation: clinical features and long term consequences. *Semin Thorac Cardiovasc Surg* 2004;16:342–349.

Snelgrove R, Williams A, Thorpe C, et al. Manipulation of immunity to and pathology of respiratory infections. *Expert Rev Anti Infect Ther* 2004;2:413–426.

Viruses. In: Cagle PT, ed. *Color Atlas and Text of Pulmonary Pathology*. Philadelphia, Pa: Lippincott Williams & Wilkins; 2004.

Bacterial Pneumonia

▶ Armando E. Fraire, MD
▶ Abida Haque, MD
▶ Clifford G. Risk, MD

Several decades after the introduction of modern antimicrobials, bacterial pneumonia remains a major cause of morbidity and mortality. Two major types of pneumonia are recognized: lobar pneumonia, presenting with a diffuse uniform inflammation of an entire lobe of the lung, and the more frequent bronchopneumonia, in which the inflammation primarily involves the terminal airways and the secondary lobules. Causative organisms include Gram-positive cocci as well as Gram-negative rods. Among the Gram positive, *Staphylococcus aureus* and *Streptococcus pneumoniae* predominate. Among the Gram negatives, *Klebsiella pneumoniae, Haemophilus influenzae, Pseudomonas* organisms, and *Escherichia coli* are commonly encountered. The histopathological hallmark of pneumonia is an acute inflammatory and/or fibrinous exudate with secondary necrosis of the alveolar epithelium. A biopsy is seldom required for diagnosis, but bronchoscopists may elect to perform a biopsy when attempting to obtain sterile material for culture and sensitivity. In these instances, and depending on whether pneumonia or bronchopneumonia is present, an acute inflammatory process will be evident in biopsy material.

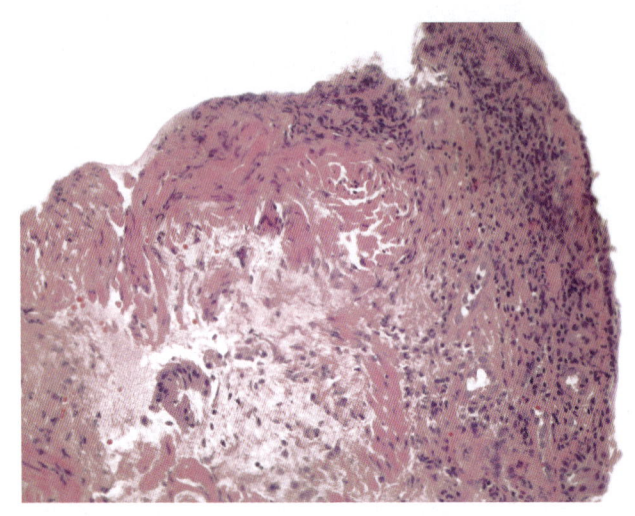

Figure 10.1: Medium power of transbronchial biopsy shows acute and chronic inflammatory infiltrates in the submucosal tissue in a case of *Pseudomonas* bronchopneumonia confirmed by microbiologic culture.

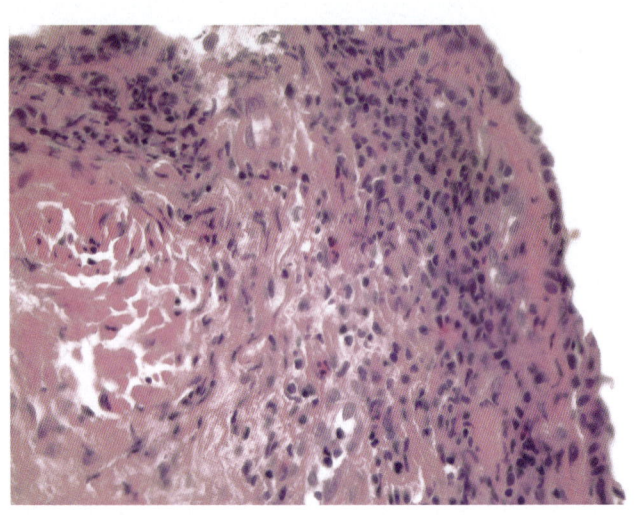

Figure 10.2: Higher power shows the acute and chronic inflammatory infiltrates in the submucosal tissue in biopsy from patient with *Pseudomonas* pneumonia.

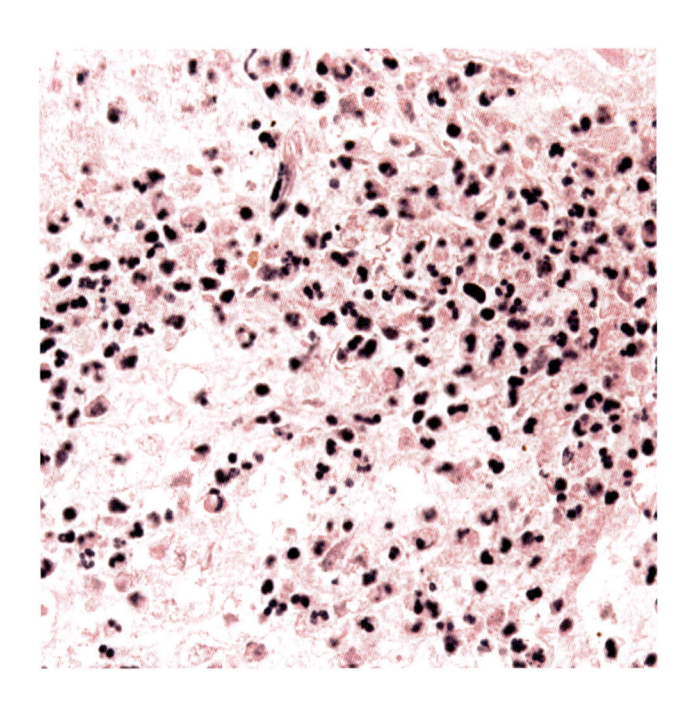

Figure 10.3: High power shows neutrophils, neutrophil "bands," lymphocytes, and macrophages in the alveolar spaces in a case of culture-proven *Pseudomonas* bronchopneumonia. The findings in the transbronchial biopsy shown in these three figures are consistent with an acute bacterial pneumonia.

Suggested Readings

Easmon CSF, Goodfellow M. Staphylococcus and micrococcus. *Systematic Bacteriology.* Parker MT, Collier LH, eds. *Topley and Wilson's Principles of Bacteriology, Virology and Immunity*; vol. 2. 8th ed. London: Edward Arnold; 1990:162.

Leslie KO, Wick MR, eds. *Practical Pulmonary Pathology: A Diagnostic Approach.* Philadelphia, Pa: Churchill Livingstone; 2005:108–113.

Pääkko P, Särkioja T, Hirvonen J, et al. Postmortem radiographic, histological and bacteriological studies in terminal respiratory infections and other pulmonary lesions in hospital and non-hospital necropsies. *J Clin Pathol* 1984;37:1281–1288.

Polsky B, Gold JWM, Whimbey E. Bacterial pneumonia in patients with the acquired immunodeficiency syndrome. *Ann Intern Med* 1986;104:38–41.

Public Health Laboratory Service. Necropsy survey of staphylococcal infection in patients dying in hospitals. *Br Med J* 1966;1:313–319.

Mycoplasma Pneumonia

▶ Armando E. Fraire, MD

Pneumonia due to *Mycoplasma pneumoniae* ranks among the most common variants of community-acquired pneumonia, affecting primarily children, adolescents, and young adults, notably more frequently in the fall and early winter. The lung damage seen in lung infections due to *Mycoplasma* is believed to be secondary to a direct cytotoxic effect, a host immune reaction, or a combination of the two. The disease is rarely fatal, and bronchoscopic biopsies are seldom performed for diagnosis. Therefore, knowledge of the disease remains limited to that derived from cases in which a biopsy is performed with subsequent diagnostic serologic or enzyme immunoassay testing revealing *Mycoplasma* infection. A major histopathologic manifestation of the disease is an acute bronchiolitis with permeation of the bronchiolar walls by mixed inflammatory infiltrates consisting of lymphocytes, neutrophils, and histiocytes. From the bronchioles, a lymphoplasmacytic infiltrate extends into the surrounding interstitium, with a resultant widening of the interalveolar walls. In contrast to bacterial pneumonias, a neutrophilic exudate does not occur.

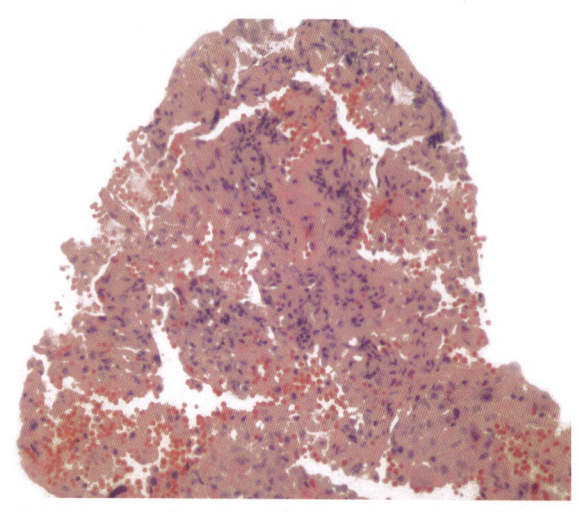

Figure 11.1: Low power of transbronchial biopsy from patient with proven mycoplasma pneumonia shows lymphoplasmacytic and macrophage infiltrates.

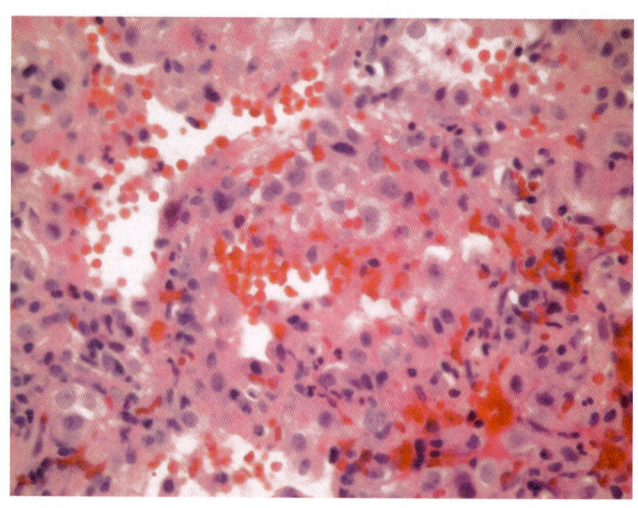

Figure 11.2: High power of transbronchial biopsy shows lymphoplasmacytic infiltrates in the interstitium and macrophages in the alveolar spaces in mycoplasma pneumonia. Neutrophils are present but are relatively sparse compared with bacterial pneumonias.

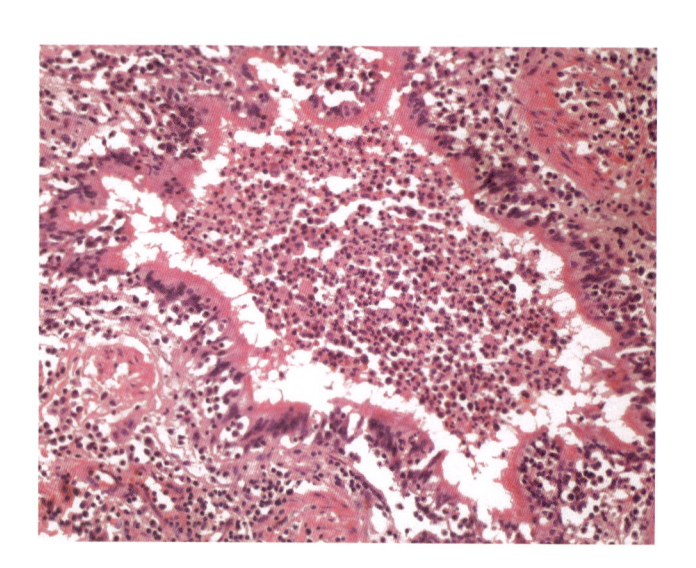

Figure 11.3: High power shows neutrophils and macrophages in the lumen of a bronchiole and infiltration of the bronchiolar wall by neutrophils, lymphocytes, and macrophages, typical of the acute bronchiolitis seen in mycoplasma pneumonia.

Suggested Readings

Hasleton P. Atypical pneumonias. In: Hasleton P, ed. *Spencer's Pathology of the Lung.* New York: McGraw-Hill; 1996:179.

Kaufman JM, Cuvelier CA, Van der Straeten M. Mycoplasma pneumonia with fulminant evolution into diffuse interstitial fibrosis. *Thorax* 1980;35:140.

Koletsky RJ, Weinstein AJ. Fulminant *Mycoplasma pneumoniae* infection: report of a fatal case and a review of the literature. *Am Rev Respir Dis* 1980;122:491.

Maisel JC, Babbitt LH, John TJ. Fatal *Mycoplasma pneumoniae* infection with isolation of organisms from lung. *JAMA* 1967;202:287.

Petitjean J, Vabret A, Gourin VS. Evaluation of four commercial immunoglobulin G (IgG) and IgM-specific enzyme immunoassays for the diagnosis of *Mycoplasma pneumoniae* infections. *J Clin Microbiol* 2002;40:165–171.

Rollins S, Colby T, Clayton F. Open lung biopsy in *Mycoplasma pneumoniae* pneumonia. *Arch Pathol Lab Med* 1986;110:34.

Pneumocystis jiroveci

▶ Abida Haque, MD
▶ Anna Sienko, MD
▶ Philip T. Cagle, MD

Pneumocystis pneumonia is one of the most common pulmonary infections in patients with acquired immunodeficiency syndrome (AIDS) and in immunosuppressed organ transplant recipients. *Pneumocystis jiroveci* infection is acquired by inhalation of trophozoites or cysts and their subsequent development in the lungs. The cysts are thick walled, 5 to 8 μm, with round to oval and navicular boat-shaped partially collapsed cysts forms, and stain with Gomori methenamine silver (GMS), cresyl violet, and toluidine blue stains. In the vegetative forms of *P. jiroveci*, the trophozoites are 2 to 8 μm. They are attached to the alveolar epithelial cells and do not stain with GMS, but rather with Romanowsky stains (Giemsa, Wright, Diff-Quick). Trophozoites and cysts may be seen within the foamy alveolar exudates by using special stains.

Transbronchial biopsy is often useful in the diagnosis of pulmonary *Pneumocystis* infection. The presence of eosinophilic foamy or bubbly alveolar exudates in the biopsy is highly suggestive of *Pneumocystis* infection and should be confirmed with GMS stain. Interstitial and alveolar fibrosis with type 2 alveolar epithelial cell hyperplasia and granulomas may be seen in chronic infections. Occasionally in patients who have received treatment, cysts do not stain with GMS and are demonstrated only with immunostain.

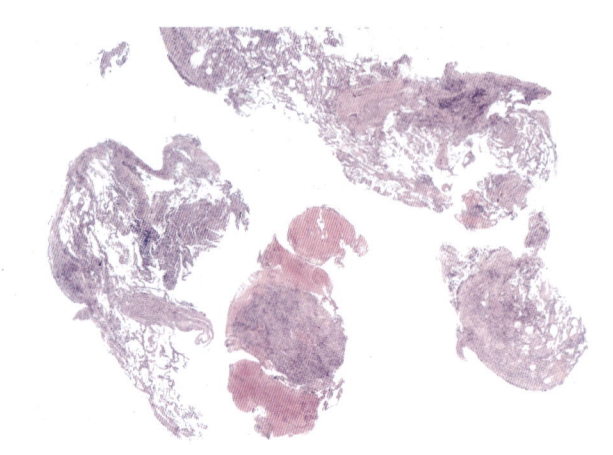

Figure 12.1: Transbronchial biopsy from patient with *Pneumocystis* infection has multiple cellular areas within the lung parenchyma at low magnification.

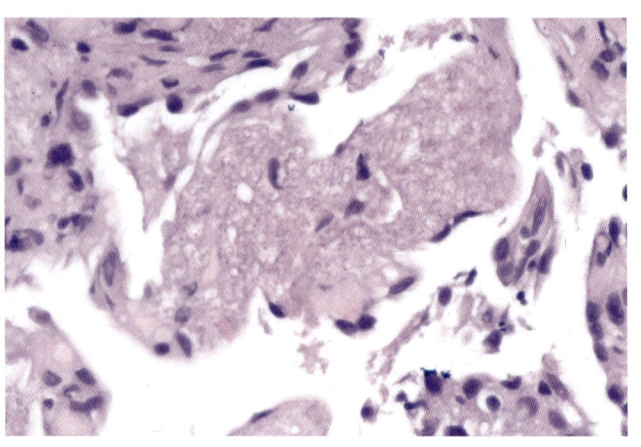

Figure 12.2: High magnification shows the characteristic foamy/bubbly alveolar exudates of *Pneumocystis* infection. Rare dots may be seen in the exudates representing localized thickening of the inner cyst wall, better seen with Gomori methenamine silver stain.

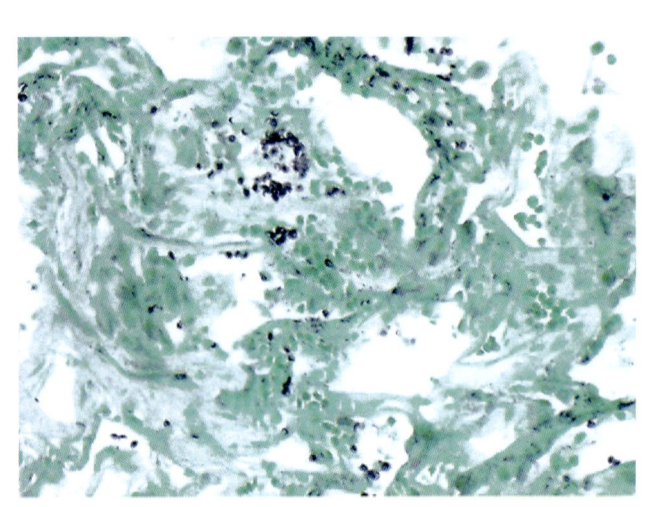

Figure 12.3: Gomori methenamine silver stain shows typical cysts of *Pneumocystis*.

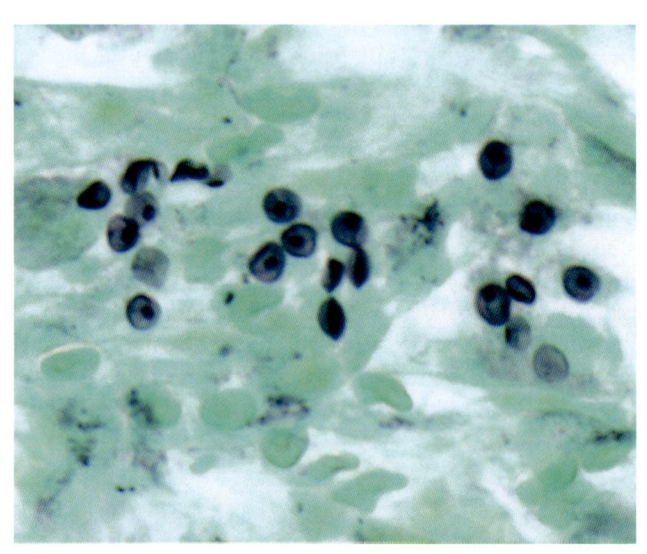

Figure 12.4: Higher power of Gomori methenamine silver stain shows cup-shaped cysts of *Pneumocystis* with thickening of wall and central "dot."

Suggested Readings

Feldman C. Pneumonia associated with HIV infection. *Curr Opin Infect Dis* 2005;18:165–170.

Fungus. In: Cagle PT, ed. *Color Atlas and Text of Pulmonary Pathology*. Philadelphia, Pa: Lippincott Williams & Wilkins; 2004.

Gal AA, Koss MN, Strigle S, et al. *Pneumocystis carinii* infection in the acquired immune deficiency syndrome. *Semin Diagn Pathol* 1989;6:287–299.

Saldana MJ, Mones JM. Pulmonary pathology in AIDS: atypical *Pneumocystis carinii* infection and lymphoid interstitial pneumonia. *Thorax* 1994;49:S46–55.

Thomas CF Jr, Limper AH. Current insights into the biology and pathogenesis of *Pneumocystis* pneumonia. *Nat Rev Microbiol* 2007;5:298–308.

Mycobacteria

▶ Abida Haque, MD
▶ Anna Sienko, MD
▶ Philip T. Cagle, MD

Mycobacterium tuberculosis is an acid-fast bacillus (AFB), 0.5 × 4 to 5 μm, and the etiologic agent of tuberculosis in debilitated individuals. *M. tuberculosis* infection produces necrotizing granulomas, with a few bacilli found in the necrotic center and within the epithelioid cells and Langerhans multinucleated giant cells. The bacilli are slender, often beaded, and stain bright red with carbol fuchsin. The bacteria also stain with Gomori methenamine silver, Gram, and periodic acid-Schiff (PAS) stains. Transbronchial biopsy may demonstrate the necrotizing granulomas; however, identification of the acid-fast bacilli often requires a diligent search under oil immersion.

Atypical mycobacteria are nontuberculous acid-fast bacilli, <1.0 μm × 4 to 6 μm, and etiologic agents of multisystem human infection in immunocompromised patients. Multiple strains include *Mycobacterium avium-intracellulare* complex (MAC), *M. kansasii*, *M. scrofulaceum*, and *M. xenopi*. Infection in immunocompetent individuals is uncommon and may show caseating or noncaseating granulomas in the transbronchial biopsy. In immunocompromised patients, the atypical mycobacteria often present as stacks of AFB-positive bacilli within the cytoplasm of histiocytes.

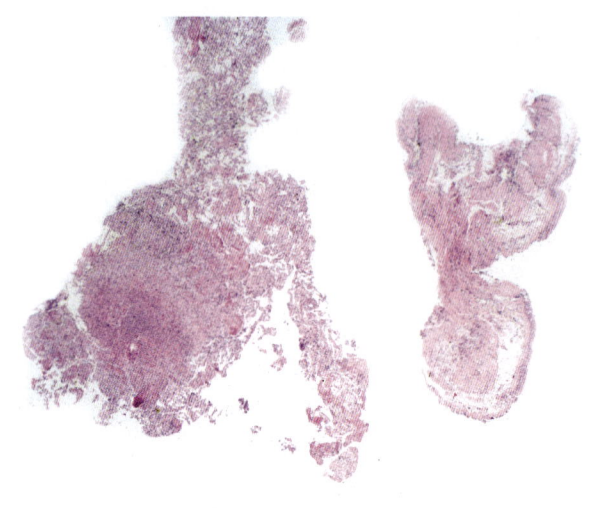

Figure 13.1: Transbronchial biopsy from a patient with mycobacterial infection has dense cellular areas with obliteration of normal alveolar pattern.

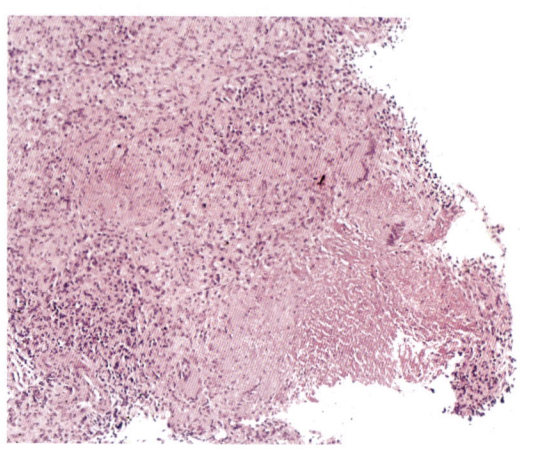

Figure 13.2: Higher magnification shows multiple caseating and noncaseating granulomas with Langerhans giant cells typical of mycobacterial infection.

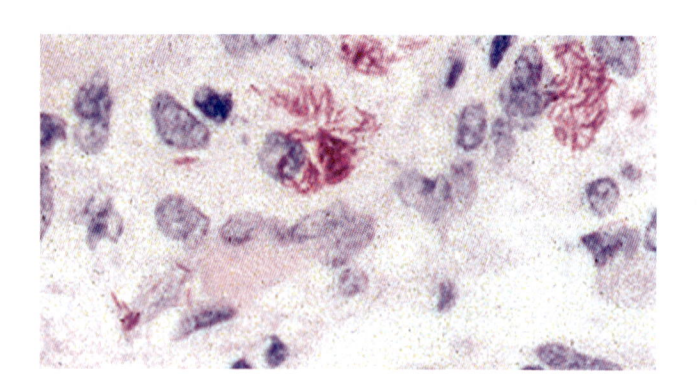

Figure 13.3: High magnification of acid-fast stain from a patient with acquired immunodeficiency syndrome has histiocytes packed with *Mycobacterium avium-intracellulare* complex, confirmed by culture.

Suggested Readings

El Zammar OA, Katzenstein AL. Pathological diagnosis of granulomatous lung disease: a review. *Histopathology* 2007;50:289–310.

Mycobacteria. In: Cagle PT, ed. *Color Atlas and Text of Pulmonary Pathology.* Philadelphia, Pa: Lippincott Williams & Wilkins; 2004.

Popper HH. Granulomas and granulomatous inflammation. In: Cagle PT, ed. *Diagnostic Pulmonary Pathology.* New York: Marcel Dekker; 2000.

Fungus

▶ Abida Haque, MD
▶ Anna Sienko, MD
▶ Philip T. Cagle, MD

Fungi are eukaryotic, unicellular organisms that are abundant in nature but rarely cause disease. Fungi are larger and genomically more complex than bacteria. Tubular aggregates of fungal cells are called *hyphae*, and if the hyphae show constrictions, they are called *pseudohyphae*. Discrete fungal cells are called *yeast* or *spores*, and spore-forming fruiting bodies are known as *conidia* or *sporangia* (Table 14-1). The diagnosis of pulmonary fungal infections depends on the demonstration of fungi in tissue and the confirmation of species by culture. Fungi can infect healthy individuals, although most infections by far are seen in an immunocompromised host. Infection occurs with inhalation of the airborne fungal hyphae, resulting in an exudative or a granulomatous response. Chronic infection can cause fibrosis with bronchiectasis and distortion of lung architecture. Transbronchial biopsy can be useful in the diagnosis of many fungal infections, including histoplasmosis, cryptococcosis, coccidioidomycosis, candidiasis, and aspergillosis. Some fungi are visible on hematoxylin and eosin stains; however, special stains such as Gomori methenamine silver (GMS), Grocott silver stain, and periodic acid-Schiff (PAS) stains are often needed for screening and confirmation. Fungi may be seen in the lung as yeast forms, spherules, hyphae, or pseudohyphae. A diagnosis of a particular fungus can be made based on the morphology and size.

Table 14-1	Diagnostic Features of Fungi			
Fungus	Morphology	Yeast	Hyphae	Pseudohyphae
Aspergillus	45-degree dichotomous branching (3–6 μm)	−	+ septate	−
Blastomyces	Broad-based budding	+	−	−
Candida	Dimorphic yeast	+	−/+	+
Coccidiosis	Spherules with endospores (20–60 μm)	−	−	−
Cryptococcus	Budding yeast with capsule (2–20 μm)	+	−	−
Histoplasma	Budding yeast (2–5 μm)	+	−	−
Mucormyces	Broad, irregular wide-angle branching (10–20 μm)	−	+ pauciseptate	−
Paracoccidioides	Spherules with external budding (10–60 μm)	−	−	−
Phaeohyphomycosis	Brown, melanin + (2–6 μm)	+/−	+ septate	−
Sporotrichosis	Dimorphic yeast (26 μm)	+	+	−

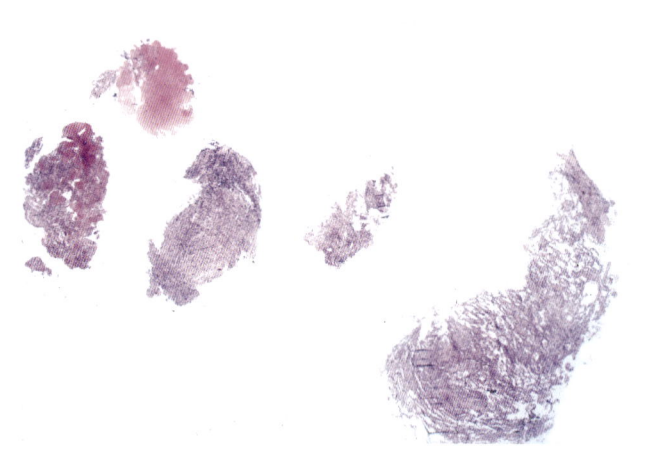

Figure 14.1: Transbronchial biopsy with *Histoplasma* shows multiple fragments, some appearing very cellular at this low magnification.

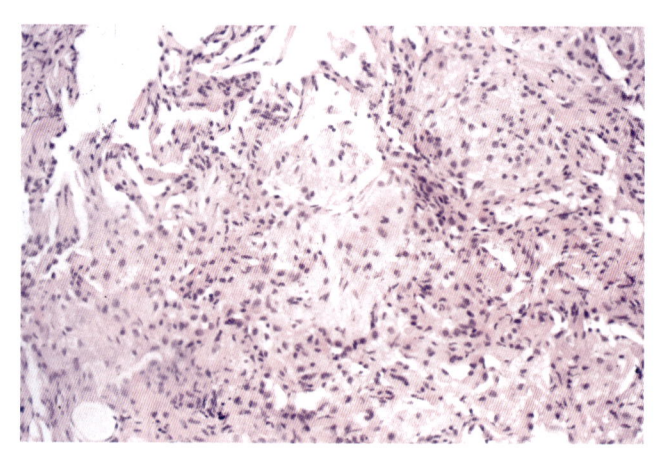

Figure 14.2: Higher magnification with many alveolar histiocytes in patient with *Histoplasma* infection.

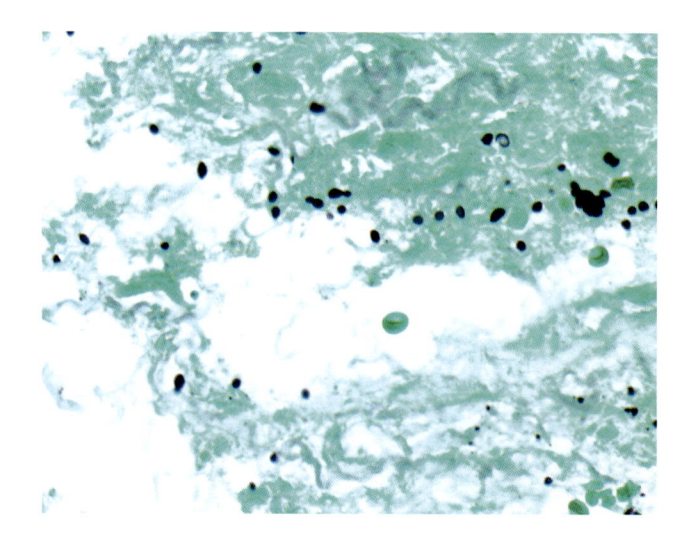

Figure 14.3: High power of GMS stain shows small fungal yeast forms, including budding yeast, consistent with *Histoplasma*.

Suggested Readings

El Zammar OA, Katzenstein AL. Pathological diagnosis of granulomatous lung disease: a review. *Histopathology* 2007;50:289–310.

Fungus. In: Cagle PT, ed. *Color Atlas and Text of Pulmonary Pathology.* Philadelphia, Pa: Lippincott Williams & Wilkins; 2004.

Litzky LA. The pathology of fungal disease in the lung. *Semin Roentgenol* 1996;31:4–13.

Popper HH. Granulomas and granulomatous inflammation. In: Cagle PT, ed. *Diagnostic Pulmonary Pathology.* New York: Marcel Dekker; 2000.

Other Infections

▶ Timothy C. Allen, MD, JD
▶ Philip T. Cagle, MD

Other infections occasionally occur in the lung and some may be identified on transbronchial biopsy. Rickettsiae, obligate intracellular bacteria, occur in the United States most commonly with tick-transmitted Rocky Mountain spotted fever, caused by *Rickettsia rickettsii*, and flea-transmitted endemic typhus, caused by *Rickettsia typhi*. Because these infections target the endothelial lining of the microvasculature systemically, cerebral and pulmonary edema due to increased microvasculature permeability is generally the cause of morbidity and mortality. Ehrlichiae are also obligate intracellular bacteria. *Ehrlichia chaffeensis* and *E. ewingii* target cells in the mononuclear phagocytic system and target polymorphonuclear neutrophils, respectively, and they are systemic diseases that may cause lung injury. Histologically, both rickettsiae and Ehrlichiae are small Gram-negative bacilli. These infections are most often diagnosed by open biopsy; however, transbronchial biopsy may show features of diffuse alveolar damage with edema, hyaline membranes, and interstitial pneumonitis. Immunostains or immunofluorescent techniques may occasionally show rickettsiae within the endothelial cells of the microcirculation, or ehrlichiae as intracytoplasmic bacterial aggregates within intravascular monocytes or pulmonary macrophages and neutrophils.

A variety of parasites is found in the lungs, and they are generally diagnosed by open biopsy. Some parasitic infections are amenable to diagnosis by transbronchial biopsy, however. Strongyloides infection is endemic in some countries, and infection may result from travel there. *Strongyloides stercoralis* lung infection occurs when migrating larvae molt within alveolar capillaries. Within immunocompromised patients, various stages of the life cycle may be identified, including filariform and rhabditiform larvae and eggs. Transbronchial biopsy of an involved area of lung parenchyma may show a mixture of hemorrhage, acute inflammation, and necrosis. Granulomas may be present and granulomatous inflammation may involve airways. Definitive diagnosis on transbronchial biopsy requires identification of filariform or rhabditiform larvae or eggs. Only very rarely is an adult female worm identified in the lung, even on open biopsy.

Malarial protozoa trophozoites may heavily parasitize red blood cells during the erythrocytic cycle. These red blood cells adhere to microvascular endothelium systemically, including in the lung. Transbronchial biopsy may occasionally be performed in an undiagnosed patient and can show marked pulmonary capillary congestion with a variable alveolar septal infiltrate of lymphocytes, plasma cells, and macrophages. Occasionally parasitized erythrocytes may be identified in the capillaries.

Toxoplasma gondii, an obligatory intracellular protozoon, may cause tissue cysts, including within the lung, containing infective bradyzoites. Histologically, lung parenchyma contains chronic interstitial pneumonia with alveolar pneumocytes and macrophages. Tachyzoites, identified more easily on Giemsa stain, may occasionally be found within cytoplasmic vacuoles of pneumocytes and macrophages or within the interstitium or foci of coagulative necrosis.

Acanthamoeba and Balamuthia are free-living amebae that may infect immunocompromised patients and cause chronic granulomatous inflammation, including in the lung. Trophozoite and cyst forms may occur within alveolar spaces, and septal widening with a mixed chronic inflammatory infiltrate may be found.

Pulmonary leishmaniasis may occur in immunocompromised patients, with *Leishmania donovani* amastigotes present within macrophages within pulmonary interstitium. Noncaseating granulomas may occur.

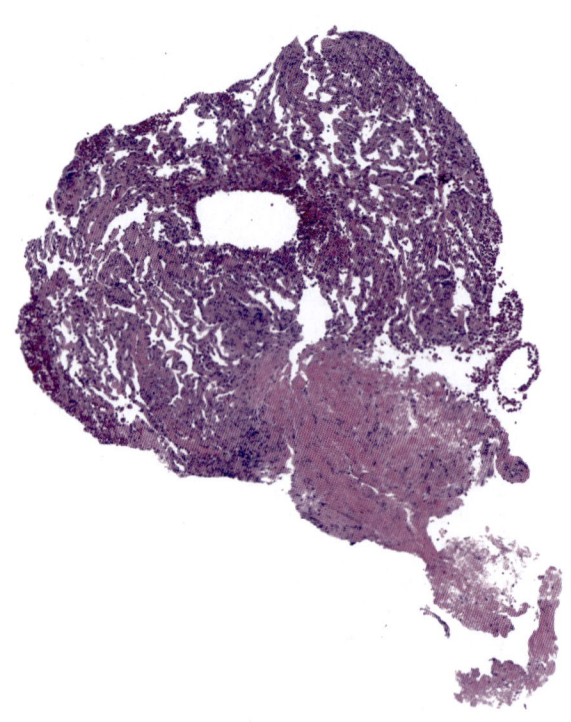

Figure 15.1: Low power of transbronchial biopsy from patient with toxoplasma infection shows interstitial lymphocytic infiltrates.

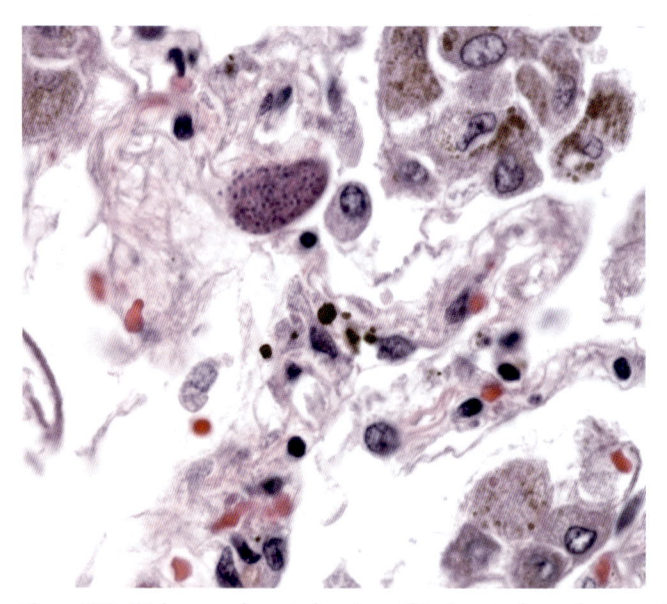

Figure 15.2: High power shows tachyzoites within the cytoplasm of a macrophage.

Suggested Readings

Anton RC, Cagle PT. Intra- and extracellular structures. In: Cagle PT, ed. *Diagnostic Pulmonary Pathology*. New York: Marcel Dekker; 2000.

Chitkara RK, Krishna G. Parasitic pulmonary eosinophilia. *Semin Respir Crit Care Med* 2006;27:171–184.

Kilani T, El Hammami S. Pulmonary hydatid and other lung parasitic infections. *Curr Opin Pulm Med* 2002;8:218–223.

Kuzucu A. Parasitic diseases of the respiratory tract. *Curr Opin Pulm Med* 2006;12:212–221.

Parasites. In: Cagle PT, ed. *Color Atlas and Text of Pulmonary Pathology*. Philadelphia, Pa: Lippincott Williams & Wilkins; 2004.

Rickettsia and related organisms. In: Cagle PT, ed. *Color Atlas and Text of Pulmonary Pathology*. Philadelphia, Pa: Lippincott Williams & Wilkins; 2004.

Taylor WR, White NJ. Malaria and the lung. *Clin Chest Med* 2002;23:457–468.

Diffuse Alveolar Damage

▶ Anna Sienko, MD
▶ Timothy C. Allen, MD, JD

Diffuse alveolar damage, clinically represented as acute respiratory distress syndrome, can be idiopathic. But it is more often due to other causes that cover an extensive list and can include infection both bacterial and viral, drugs, collagen vascular disease, inhalants/toxins, shock, and pulmonary vasculitis/pulmonary hemorrhage syndromes (Table 16-1). The lung injury, which is acute, shows similar histologic features regardless of the underlying cause or initiating event. Depending on the time interval of the underlying insult and transbronchial biopsy, the histologic features show variable morphology with an early acute phase, an organizing or proliferative phase, and a late fibrotic phase. The early acute phase is seen on biopsy as interstitial and intra-alveolar edema associated with variable hemorrhage and deposits of fibrin with the characteristic hyaline membranes forming several days after injury. Usually a week after injury the hyaline membranes are well formed and seen as eosinophilic fibrinous material of variable thickness, outlining the intra-alveolar spaces. The proliferative phase is seen at this time (usually 7 days after injury) associated with the hyaline membranes, type II pneumocyte hyperplasia, and demonstrates in the interstitium features of organization with formation of fibroblastic foci and associated acute inflammation. Diffuse alveolar damage can regress with treatment; however progression can also occur with fibrosis characterized by cellular infiltrates with proliferation of fibroblasts and deposition of collagen.

Table 16-1 Causes of Diffuse Alveolar Damage

Shock
- Cardiogenic
- Neurogenic
- Sepsis

Trauma
- Head
- Bone fractures
- Crush injuries
- Lung contusions
- Fat embolism

Infections
- Viral
- Bacterial
- Fungal

Aspiration
- Gastric contents
- Near-drowning
- Hydrocarbons

Drugs
- Chemotherapy
- Penicillamine
- Amiodarone
- Narcotics
- Nitrofurantoin

Pulmonary hemorrhage syndromes
- Wegener granulomatosis
- Polyarteritis nodosa
- Goodpasture syndrome
- Microscopic polyangiitis

Metabolic disorders
- Uremia
- Pancreatitis

Inhalation injury
- Oxygen
- Smoke
- Numerous toxic chemicals, fumes, and gases

Hematologic disorders
- Transfusion-associated lung injury
- Cardiopulmonary bypass
- Disseminated intravascular coagulation

Collagen vascular diseases
- Rheumatoid arthritis
- Scleroderma
- Systemic lupus erythematosus
- Polymyositis/dermatomyositis
- Mixed connective tissue disease

Idiopathic
- Acute interstitial pneumonia (Hamman-Rich syndrome)

Others
- Toxic shock syndrome
- Intravenous administration of contrast material
- Gestational trophoblastic disease
- Heat
- Radiation
- High altitude
- Burns

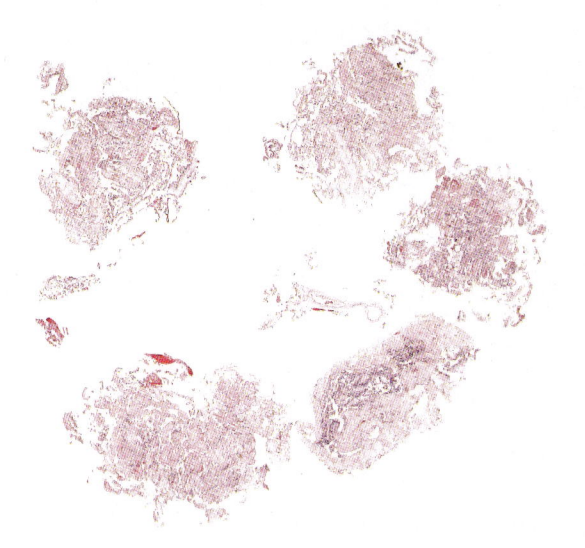

Figure 16.1: Low power of transbronchial biopsy from a patient with diffuse alveolar damage shows dense pink hyaline membranes outlining alveolar spaces.

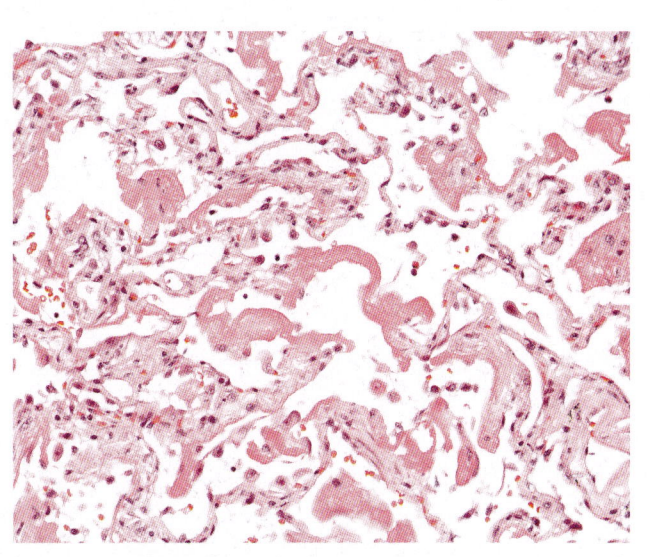

Figure 16.2: High power shows dense eosinophilic hyaline membranes and fibrinous material outlining alveolar spaces.

Suggested Readings

Barrios R. Diffuse alveolar damage. In: Cagle PT, ed. *Color Atlas and Text of Pulmonary Pathology.* Philadelphia, Pa: Lippincott Williams & Wilkins; 2004.

Penuelas O, Aramburu JA, Frutos-Vivar F, et al. Pathology of acute lung injury and acute respiratory distress syndrome: a clinical-pathologic correlation. *Clin Chest Med* 2006;27:571–578.

Pulmonary Edema

▶ Timothy C. Allen, MD, JD
▶ Roberto Barrios, MD

Pulmonary edema, the accumulation of extravascular fluid in the lungs, often accompanies passive heart failure such as left heart failure and valvular heart disease, where it is termed *cardiogenic pulmonary edema*. Pulmonary edema may relate to increased capillary or venule hydrostatic pressure or to a breakdown in alveolar septal-vascular integrity due to direct injury. Pulmonary edema may result from a wide variety of potential etiologies, including infections; acute respiratory distress syndrome; inhalation of smoke, chemical agents, and other fumes and toxins; cocaine and heroin abuse; high altitude; fluid overload; and renal failure; among others. It develops as an early interstitial phase, with fluid accumulation within the alveolar interstitium, followed by a second phase with fluid accumulating within alveolar spaces. Pulmonary edema is often seen on transbronchial biopsy as part of a spectrum of changes in cases of bronchopneumonia and cases of diffuse alveolar damage of varying causes. It may occasionally be the only histologic feature present on transbronchial biopsy in these conditions. Histologically, edema fluid involves alveolar spaces and may be associated with interstitial widening, vascular congestion, and lymphatic widening. The protein that accompanies the leaked fluid stains pink with hematoxylin and eosin (H&E) stain.

Differential diagnosis includes clear fluid within alveolar spaces as occurs with near-drowning or other clear fluid aspiration; however, clinical history will help differentiate these cases. Pulmonary alveolar proteinosis may superficially resemble edema; however, it contains course granules that are periodic acid-Schiff (PAS) positive, as well as scattered cholesterol clefts. *Pneumocystis* pneumonia may contain eosinophilic material within alveoli, but the material surrounding the cysts has a characteristic foamy appearance. Intra-alveolar mucin associated with a mucin-secreting tumor may occasionally mimic edema on a limited biopsy, but it can be distinguished with mucin stains.

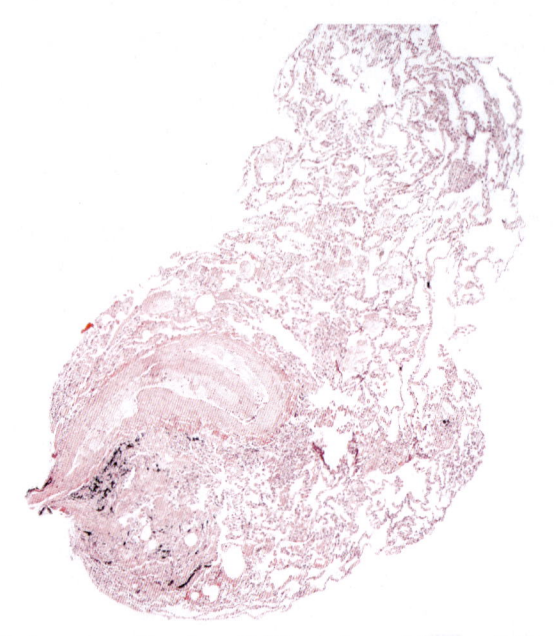

Figure 17.1: Low power of transbronchial biopsy shows pink edema fluid within some of the alveolar spaces.

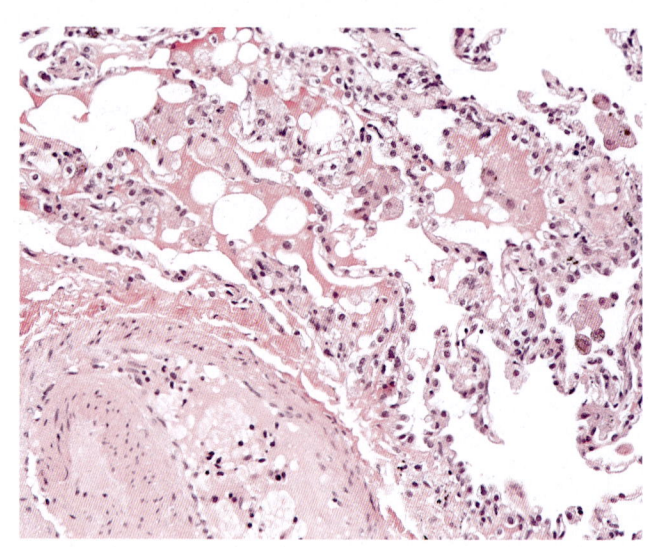

Figure 17.2: Medium power shows pink edema fluid focally within alveolar spaces. The rounded holes within the fluid are artifactual.

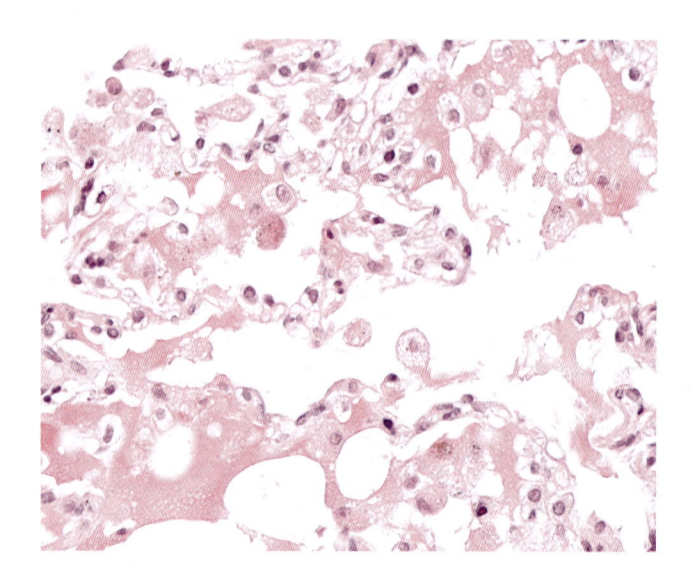

Figure 17.3: High power shows pink edema fluid and foamy macrophages within alveolar spaces.

Suggested Readings

Bailey ME, Fraire AE, Greenberg SD, et al. Pulmonary histopathology in cocaine abusers. *Hum Pathol* 1994;25:203–207.

Barrios R. Diffuse alveolar damage. In: Cagle PT, ed. *Color Atlas and Text of Pulmonary Pathology.* Philadelphia, Pa: Lippincott Williams & Wilkins; 2004.

Dail DH. Intraalveolar exudates/infiltrates. In: Cagle PT, ed. *Diagnostic Pulmonary Pathology.* New York: Marcel Dekker; 2000.

Lee-Chong T Jr, Matthay RA. Drug-induced pulmonary edema and acute respiratory distress syndrome. *Clin Chest Med* 2004;25:95–104.

Maggiorini M. High altitude-induced pulmonary edema. *Cardiovasc Res* 2006;72:41–50.

Organizing Pneumonia

▶ Philip T. Cagle, MD
▶ Timothy C. Allen, MD, JD

Organizing pneumonia was previously referred to as *bronchiolitis obliterans organizing pneumonia*, or BOOP. It may occur in organizing acute bacterial infections, viral infections, or other infections, as a reaction to fumes and toxins, in postobstructive lung, with aspiration, in drug reactions, as a result of chemotherapy or radiation therapy, and as a component of specific lung diseases including hypersensitivity pneumonitis, collagen vascular diseases, eosinophilic pneumonia, and Wegener granulomatosis (Table 18-1). It may also be seen as an idiopathic clinical syndrome called *cryptogenic organizing pneumonia* (COP), previously recognized as idiopathic BOOP. Transbronchial biopsies show lung parenchyma with scattered foci or "plugs" of granulation tissue in the lumens of alveoli. If sampled on the transbronchial biopsy, the granulation tissue may also be seen in alveolar ducts and/or bronchioles. The granulation tissue consists of edematous, myxoid stroma, often with a bluish or grayish tinge on hematoxylin and eosin (H&E), and variable numbers of fibroblasts and sometimes capillaries. The granulation tissue foci or "plugs" may be of variable size and relatively inconspicuous at low power in some biopsies. There may be additional findings of interstitial pneumonia, often lymphocytes, and occasionally specific findings that indicate the cause of the organizing pneumonia such as viral inclusions, fungal organisms, aspirated food or material, infectious granulomas, poorly formed granulomas of hypersensitivity pneumonitis, numerous eosinophils, and so on. Intra-alveolar foamy macrophages suggest small airway obstruction and may be seen in association with organizing pneumonia or may be the only indication of small airway obstruction in a clinically suspected case of COP or BOOP.

Table 18-1	Causes of Organizing Pneumonia

Organizing infections: viral, bacterial, mycoplasma, mycobacterial
Drugs: bleomycin, gold, amiodarone, others
Radiation therapy
Toxic fumes and inhalants
Aspiration
Idiopathic (cryptogenic organizing pneumonia)
Distal to proximal bronchial obstruction: tumors, foreign bodies
Periphery of mass lesions: tumors, granulomas, infarcts, other
Component of other specific diseases
    Collagen vascular diseases
    Chronic eosinophilic pneumonia
    Hypersensitivity pneumonitis
    Pulmonary Langerhans cell histiocytosis
    Wegener granulomatosis

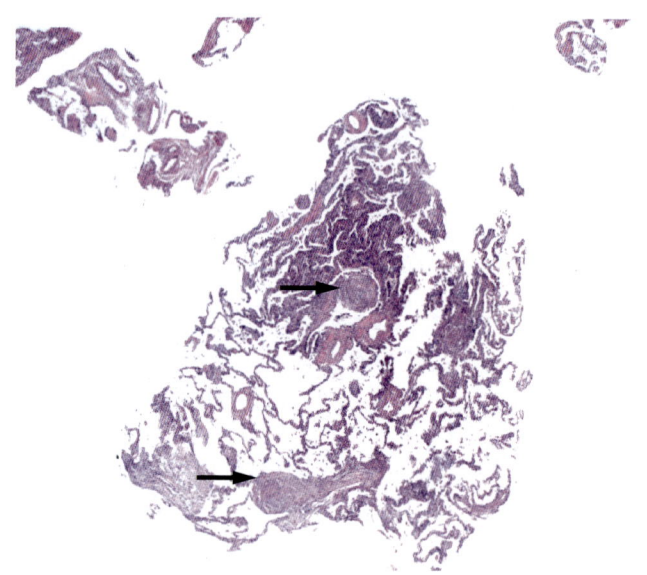

Figure 18.1: Low power of transbronchial biopsy. Arrows indicate scattered plugs of granulation tissue in airspaces, which are shown at higher power in subsequent figures.

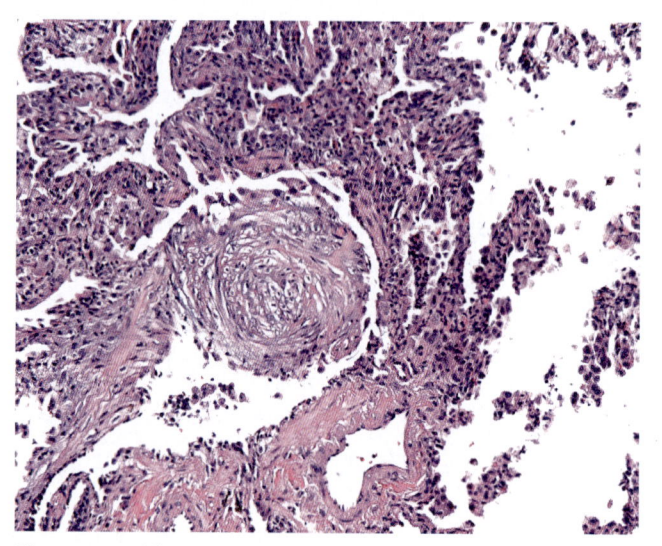

Figure 18.2: High power shows rounded plug of granulation tissue within airspace. This corresponds to tissue indicated by the upper arrow in Figure 18.1.

Chapter 18 • Organizing Pneumonia

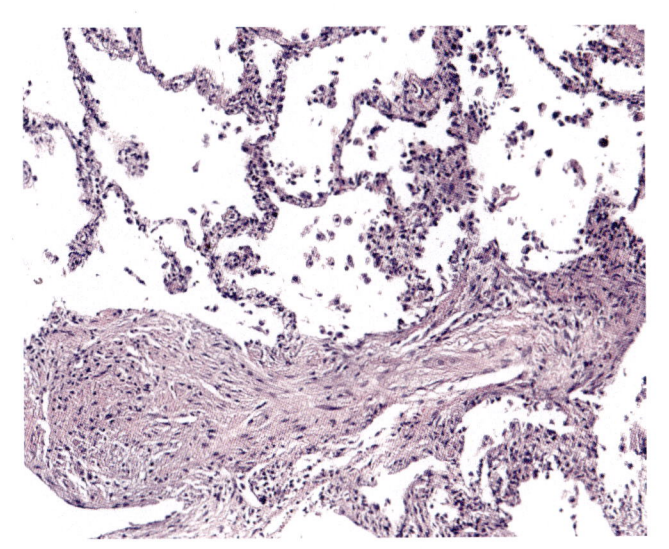

Figure 18.3: High power shows an elongated plug of granulation tissue within an alveolar duct. This corresponds to tissue indicated by the lower arrow in Figure 18.1.

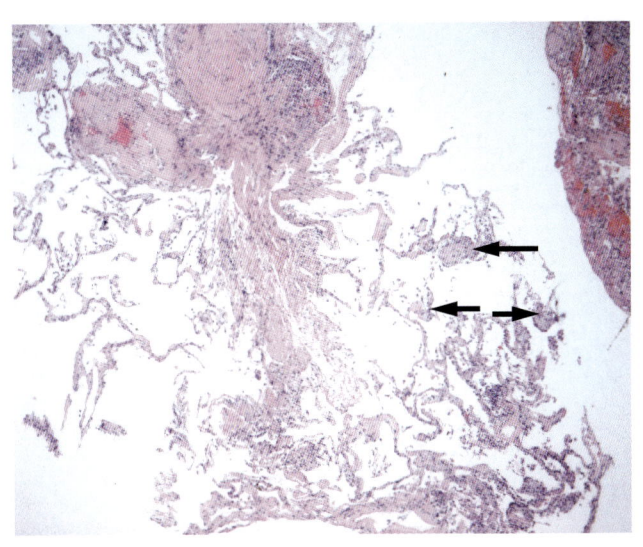

Figure 18.4: Low power of transbronchial biopsy shows smaller, more subtle scattered foci of granulation tissue within airspaces than in Figure 18.1.

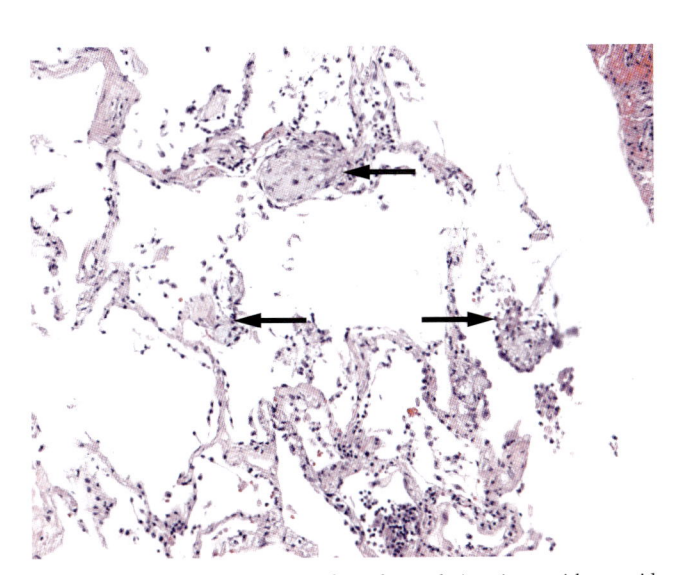

Figure 18.5: Higher power shows foci of granulation tissue with myxoid stroma and fibroblast nuclei that are less conspicuous than those in Figures 18.1, 18.2, and 18.3.

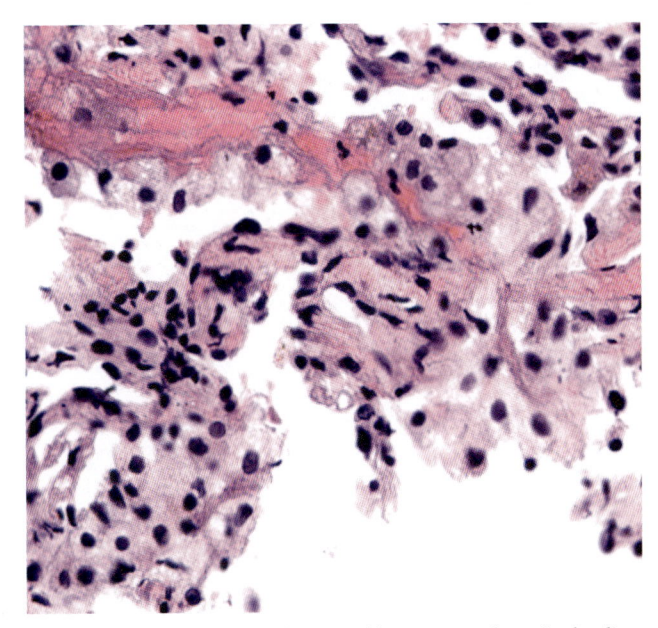

Figure 18.6: High power of collections of foamy macrophages in alveoli at edge of transbronchial biopsy is evidence of small airway obstruction due to organizing pneumonia, although the granulation tissue in the airways was not sampled.

Suggested Readings

Barrios R. Organizing acute pneumonia. In: Cagle PT, ed. *Color Atlas and Text of Pulmonary Pathology.* Philadelphia, Pa: Lippincott Williams & Wilkins; 2004.

Dail HD. Intraalveolar exudates/infiltrates. In: Cagle PT, ed. *Diagnostic Pulmonary Pathology.* New York: Marcel Dekker; 2000.

Leslie KO. Pathology of idiopathic interstitial pneumonias. *Exp Lung Res* 2005;31:S23–40.

Acute Fibrinous and Organizing Pneumonia

19

▶ Anna Sienko, MD

Acute fibrinous and organizing pneumonia, also considered a form of acute lung injury, shares similar clinical presentation, causes, and some histologic features with diffuse alveolar damage. No hyaline membranes are seen in acute fibrinous and organizing pneumonia. The intra-alveolar spaces show a patchy distribution of aggregates of fibrinous material, often as rounded balls, with features of organization of the fibrin by loose fibroblastic tissue. These features may be sampled on transbronchial biopsy. It is currently thought that acute fibrinous and organizing pneumonia may represent a variant of diffuse alveolar damage.

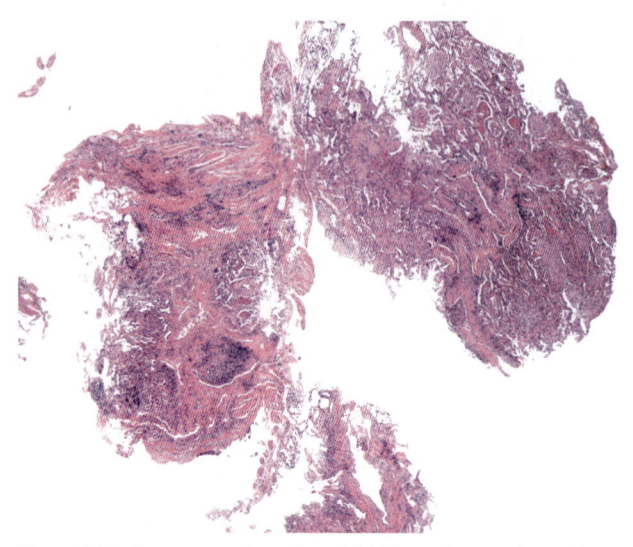

Figure 19.1: Low power of transbronchial biopsy from patient with acute fibrinous and organizing pneumonia shows dense nodular areas with fibrin and granulation tissue.

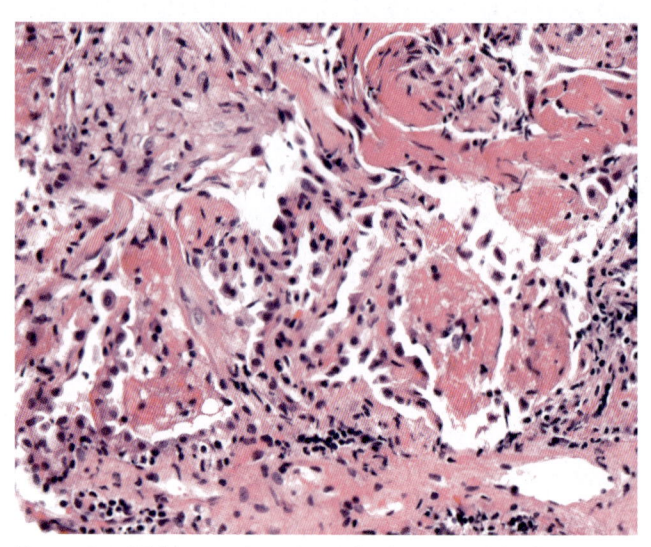

Figure 19.2: High power shows intra-alveolar eosinophilic fibrinous exudates and organizing fibroblastic granulation tissue in acute fibrinous and organizing pneumonia.

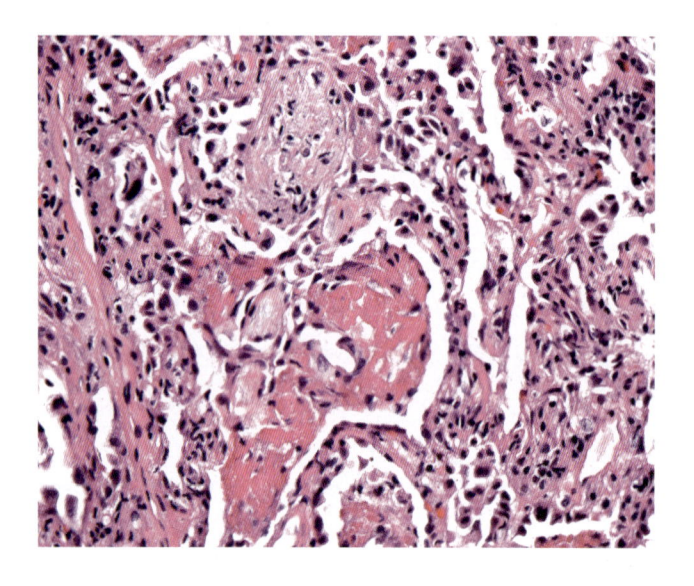

Figure 19.3: Intra-alveolar eosinophilic fibrinous exudate and a rounded ball of fibroblastic granulation tissue are seen at high power in acute fibrinous and organizing pneumonia.

Suggested Reading

Beasley MB, Franks TJ, Galvin JR, et al. Acute fibrinous and organizing pneumonia: a histological pattern of lung injury and possible variant of diffuse alveolar damage. *Arch Pathol Lab Med* 2002;126:1064–1070.

Aspiration Pneumonia

20

- Timothy C. Allen, MD, JD
- Roberto Barrios, MD
- Abida Haque, MD
- Philip T. Cagle, MD

Aspiration pneumonia in adults occurs generally from the aspiration of particulate gastric contents in elderly or disabled patients, the perioperative aspiration of gastric contents, and the aspiration of enteric solutions or other inhaled or locally applied oils (lipoid pneumonia, also termed *exogenous lipid pneumonia*). Aspiration pneumonia in children often involves foreign body aspiration or aspiration of oils or similar materials such as milk, resulting in lipoid pneumonia. Occasionally, aspiration of charcoal or barium solution occurs. Aspiration pneumonia may also be a complication of radiotherapy or chemotherapy to the head and neck or, in patients with diabetes mellitus, as a complication of diabetic gastroparesis.

Histologically, aspiration pneumonia acutely consists of pulmonary edema and congestion, atelectasis, and alveolar epithelial cell necrosis, with an intense neutrophilic infiltrate occurring in 4 to 5 hours. Hyaline membrane formation occurs within 1 to 2 days, and transbronchial biopsy may be performed during this period, suggesting diffuse alveolar damage. A limited transbronchial biopsy may contain any mixture of these features and may be nonspecific. Depending on the circumstances, bacterial clusters, foreign body macrophages, granuloma formation, or foreign material may be present on the transbronchial biopsy. Lipoid pneumonia typically shows collections of foamy, lipid-laden macrophages lying within the alveolar spaces as well as within alveolar septa. In patients with ongoing chronic aspiration, septal fibrosis may be present.

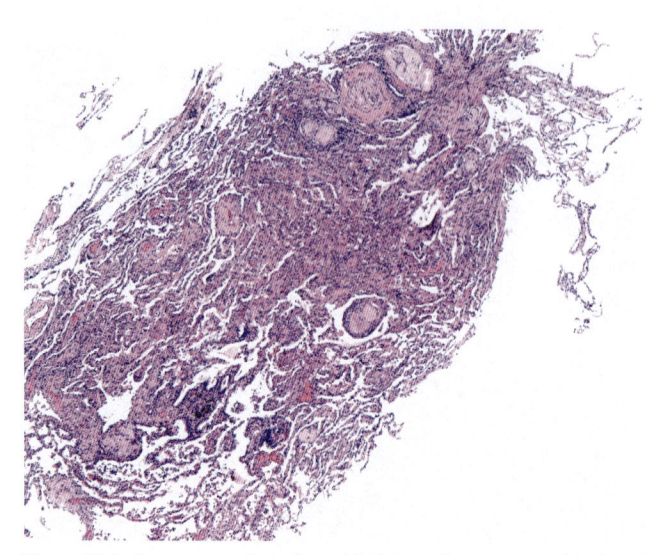

Figure 20.1: Low power of transbronchial biopsy from patient with chronic aspiration shows areas of interstitial pneumonia with fibrosis and chronic inflammation around fragments of foreign material.

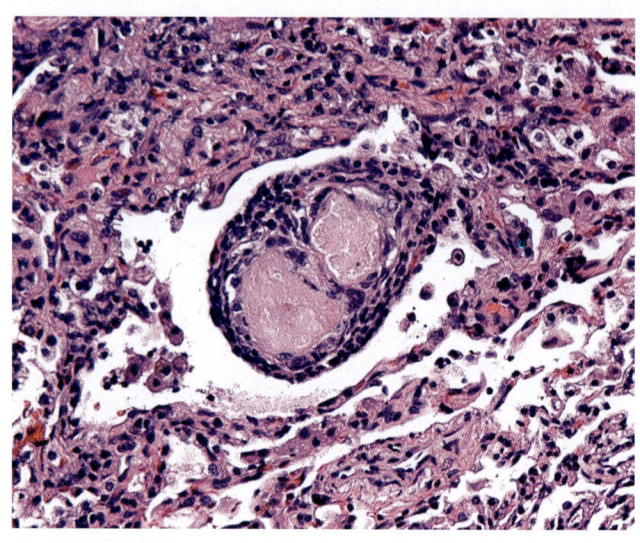

Figure 20.2: High power shows aspirated foreign material surrounded by mononuclear cells.

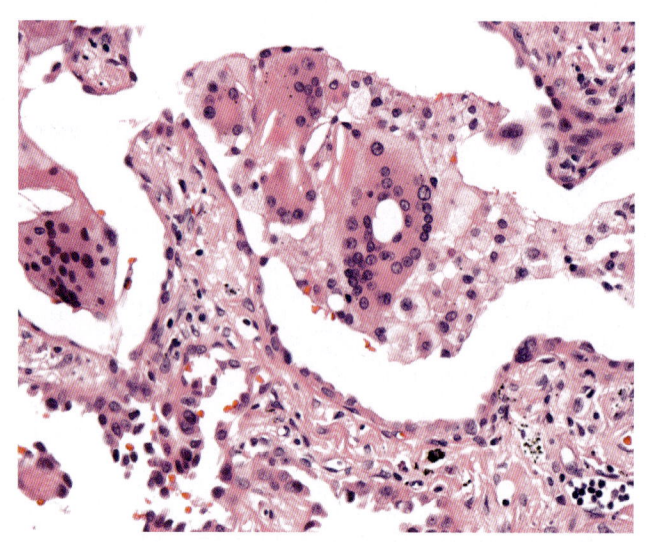

Figure 20.3: High power shows an alveolar space containing foreign body multinucleated giant cells with cholesterol clefts and foamy macrophages consistent with aspiration.

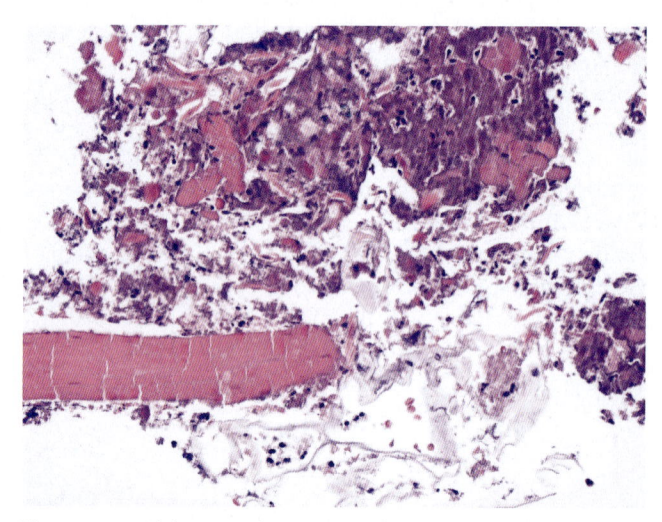

Figure 20.4: High power shows aspirated material consisting of partially digested skeletal muscle and a few yeast.

Suggested Readings

Barrios R. Lipoid pneumonia. In: Cagle PT, ed. *Color Atlas and Text of Pulmonary Pathology.* Philadelphia, Pa: Lippincott Williams & Wilkins; 2004.

Dail DH. Intraalveolar exudates/infiltrates. In: Cagle PT, ed. *Diagnostic Pulmonary Pathology.* New York: Marcel Dekker; 2000.

Hansen LA, Prakash UB, Colby TV. Pulmonary complications of diabetes mellitus. *Mayo Clin Proc* 1989;64:791–799.

Haque A. Aspiration pneumonia. In: Cagle PT, ed. *Color Atlas and Text of Pulmonary Pathology.* Philadelphia, Pa: Lippincott Williams & Wilkins; 2004.

Mukhopadhyay S, Katzenstein AL. Pulmonary disease due to aspiration of food and other particulate matter: a clinicopathologic study of 59 cases diagnosed on biopsy or resection specimens. *Am J Surg Pathol* 2007;31:752–759.

Petroianni A, Ceccarelli D, Conti V, et al. Aspiration pneumonia. Pathophysiological aspects, prevention and management. A review. *Panminerva Med* 2006;48:231–239.

Rosenthal DI, Lewin JS, Eisbruch A. Prevention and treatment of dysphagia and aspiration after chemoradiation for head and neck cancer. *J Clin Oncol* 2006;24:2636–2643.

Shigemitsu H, Afshar K. Aspiration pneumonias: under-diagnosed and under-treated. *Curr Opin Pulm Med* 2007;13:192–198.

Umuroglu T, Takil A, Irmak P, et al. Effects of multiple pulmonary aspirations of enteral solutions on lung tissue damage. *Clin Nutr* 2006;25:45–50.

van der Hoven B, Stiegelis WF, van der Linden AN, et al. Lipoid pneumonitis complicating treatment of Hodgkin's disease. *Neth J Med* 1993;43:183–186.

Intra-alveolar Hemorrhage

▶ Timothy C. Allen, MD, JD
▶ Jaishree Jagirdar, MD
▶ Philip T. Cagle, MD

Etiologies of intra-alveolar hemorrhage are often divided into diseases causing intra-alveolar hemorrhage associated with vasculitis, including capillaritis, and diseases causing intra-alveolar hemorrhage unassociated with vasculitis. Diseases causing intra-alveolar hemorrhage associated with vasculitis/capillaritis include Churg-Strauss syndrome, microscopic polyarteritis, Goodpasture syndrome, Wegener granulomatosis, and connective tissue diseases including rheumatoid arthritis, scleroderma, and polymyositis/dermatomyositis, among many others. Goodpasture syndrome may be diagnosed by the presence of circulating antibodies alone or with immunofluorescent staining of kidney or lung biopsies. Intra-alveolar hemorrhage may occur in patients with systemic lupus erythematosus, and it is associated with reduced serum complement levels and the presence of serum antinuclear antibodies. Wegener granulomatosis is associated with the presence of C-antineutrophil cytoplasmic antibodies and characterized by necrotizing granulomatous vasculitis that may also involve the kidneys and/or the upper respiratory tract.

Diseases causing intra-alveolar hemorrhage unassociated with capillaritis include diffuse alveolar damage, pulmonary hypertension, infections, mitral stenosis, aspiration, and idiopathic pulmonary hemosiderosis, among others. Intra-alveolar hemorrhage may be caused by a large number of drugs and toxins as well, including warfarin, sulfonamides, cocaine, estrogens, and many others. Intra-alveolar hemorrhage may occur in autologous or allogenic bone marrow transplant patients, generally in older patients with preexisting lung disease, and may be fatal. Intra-alveolar hemorrhage may also occur in patients with HIV infection, associated with opportunistic infections (Table 21-1).

Intra-alveolar hemorrhage typically manifests itself as hemoptysis. Chest radiograph and computed tomography scan may demonstrate alveolar consolidation, and laboratory testing may disclose anemia, including an anemia of chronic disease-like pattern if intra-pulmonary blood loss is subtle and longstanding. Bronchoalveolar lavage may or may not be frankly bloody, and although the presence of hemosiderin-laden macrophages assists in the diagnosis of pulmonary hemorrhage, their presence is nonspecific. Hemosiderin-laden macrophages may be found in bronchoalveolar lavage fluid in a large number of disease states, with or without intra-alveolar hemorrhage. Hemosiderin-laden macrophages identified in a lung biopsy may be confirmed with an iron stain such as Prussian blue stain; however, care must be taken not to overdiagnose macrophages containing smoker's pigment as hemosiderin-laden macrophages. Iron deposition in macrophages containing smoker's pigment generally occurs in a fine stippled pattern rather than the larger, coarser deposition of iron found in hemosiderin-laden macrophages. Also, macrophages containing smoker's pigment may additionally contain granular carbonaceous particles.

Transbronchial biopsy may allow the diagnosis of intra-alveolar hemorrhage and may sometimes assist in the identification of the etiology. The most frequent cause of fresh hemorrhage in a transbronchial biopsy is the biopsy procedure itself. Features that suggest hemorrhage in a transbronchial biopsy is not related to the procedure include the presence of hemosiderin-laden macrophages consistent with ongoing previous hemorrhage, fibroblastic organization of the hemorrhage (which indicates the hemorrhage has been present long enough for organization to occur), and findings of a specific cause such as capillaritis.

Table 21-1 Causes of Pulmonary Hemorrhage

1. Localized hemorrhage

Neoplasms
- Angiosarcoma
- Kaposi sarcoma
- Epithelioid hemangioendothelioma
- Diffuse pulmonary lymphangiomatosis

Infection
- *Serratia marcescens* pneumonia
- Leptospirosis
- *Trichosporon beigelii*

Other
- Arteriovenous malformation
- Bronchiectasis
- Bronchitis
- Pulmonary infarction
- Amyloidosis
- Mechanical ventilation
- Thoracic injury
- Cystic fibrosis

2. Diffuse alveolar hemorrhage

Churg-Strauss syndrome
Goodpasture syndrome
Wegener granulomatosis
Idiopathic vasculitides
Microscopic polyarteritis
Behçet disease
Henoch-Schönlein purpura
Essential mixed cryoglobulinemia

Connective tissue diseases
- Rheumatoid arthritis
- Scleroderma
- Systemic lupus erythematosus
- Mixed connective tissue disease
- Polymyositis

Chemical and Drug Related
- Cocaine
- D-penicillamine
- Trimellitic anhydride
- Lymphangiogram-associated
- Streptokinase
- Anticoagulants
- Paraquat

Other
- Idiopathic pulmonary hemosiderosis
- Bone marrow transplantation
- IgA nephropathy
- Idiopathic glomerulonephritis
- Autoimmune hemolytic anemia
- Fat embolism

Chapter 21 • Intra-alveolar Hemorrhage

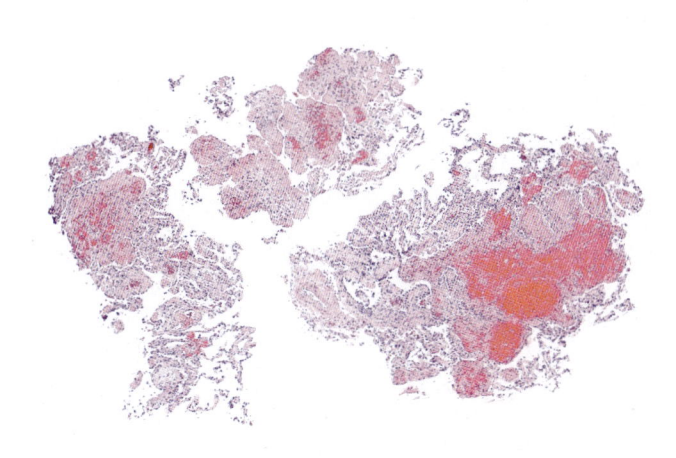

Figure 21.1: Transbronchial biopsy containing bright red blood as a result of the biopsy procedure.

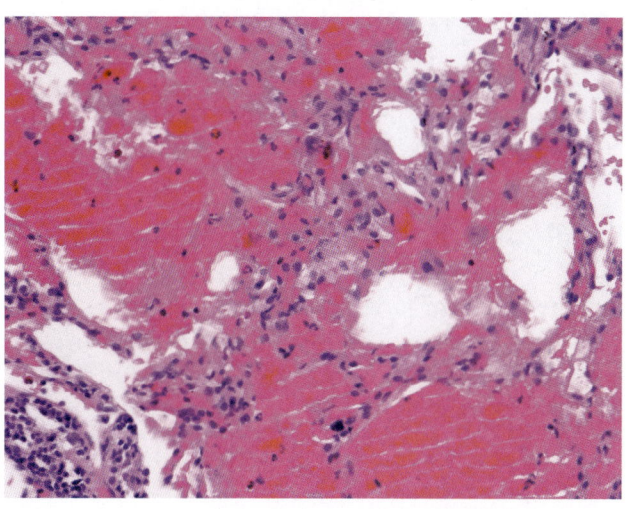

Figure 21.2: High power shows alveolar spaces filled with red blood cells and lesser numbers of white blood cells as a result of the transbronchial biopsy procedure.

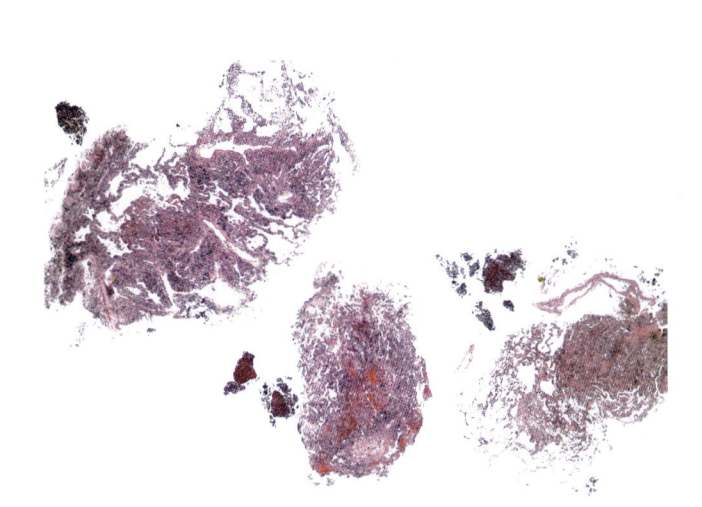

Figure 21.3: Areas of intra-alveolar hemorrhage and perivascular interstitial cellular infiltrates can be seen at low power of this transbronchial biopsy from a patient with Churg-Strauss syndrome.

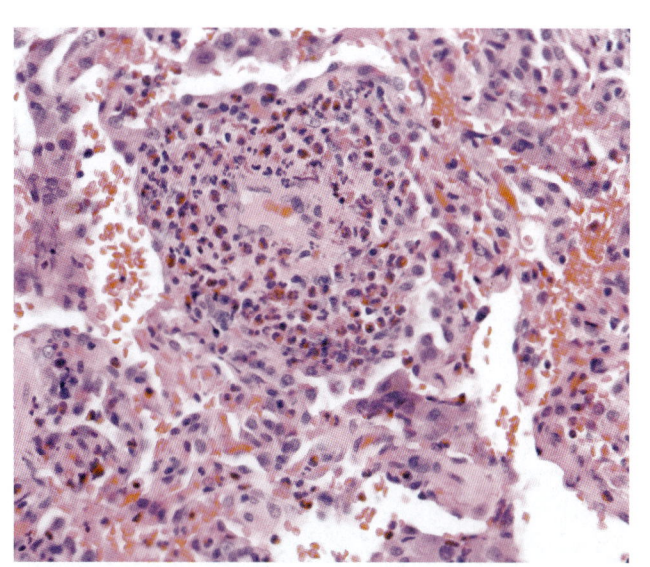

Figure 21.4: Higher power shows eosinophilic vasculitis with surrounding intra-alveolar hemorrhage consistent with alveolar hemorrhage due to Churg-Strauss syndrome.

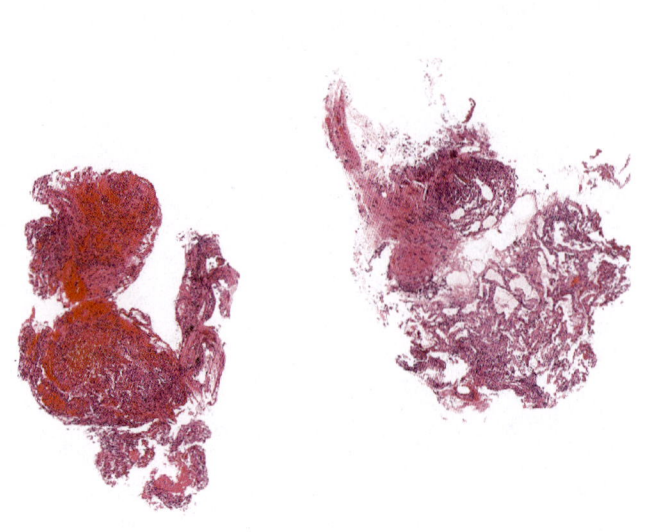

Figure 21.5: Bright red blood is present in this transbronchial biopsy from a patient with systemic lupus erythematosus.

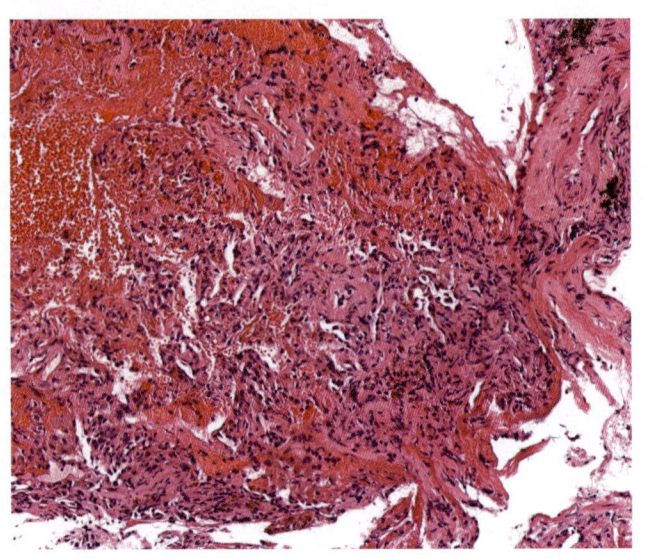

Figure 21.6: Higher power shows diffuse alveolar hemorrhage in this transbronchial biopsy from a patient with systemic lupus erythematosus.

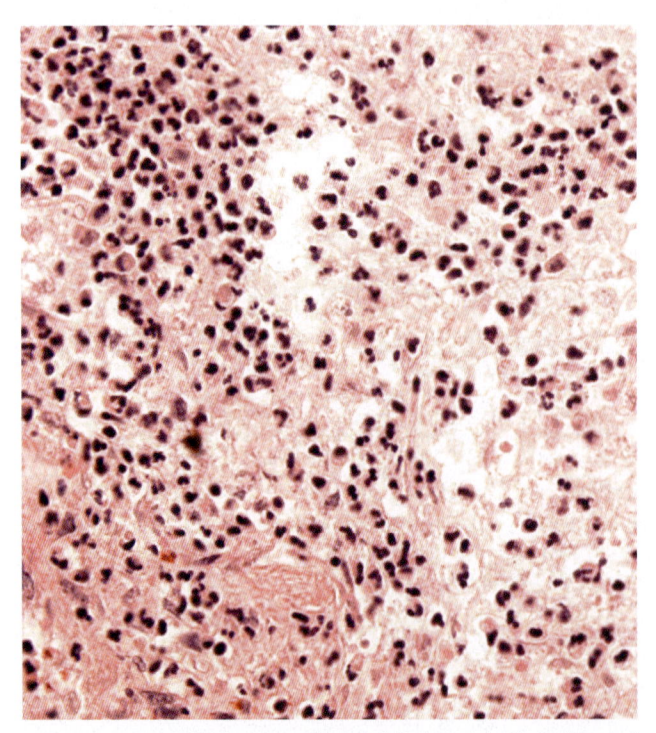

Figure 21.7: Intra-alveolar hemorrhage and fibrin seen in the background of this case of acute bacterial pneumonia.

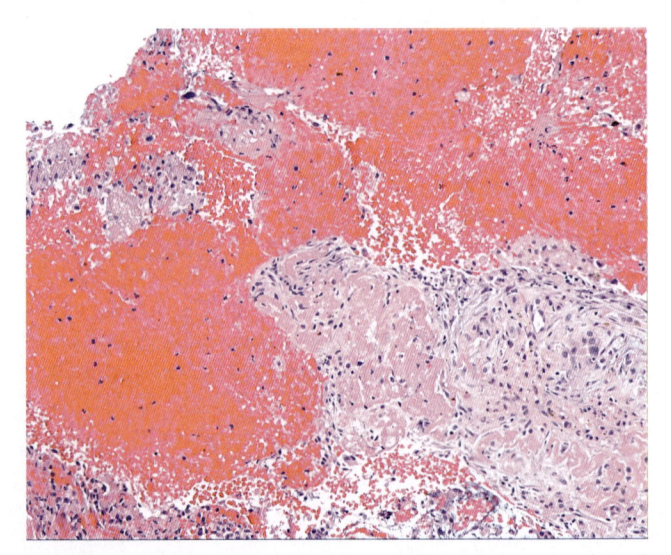

Figure 21.8: Medium power of transbronchial biopsy shows intra-alveolar hemorrhage with early organization of the fibrin by fibroblasts.

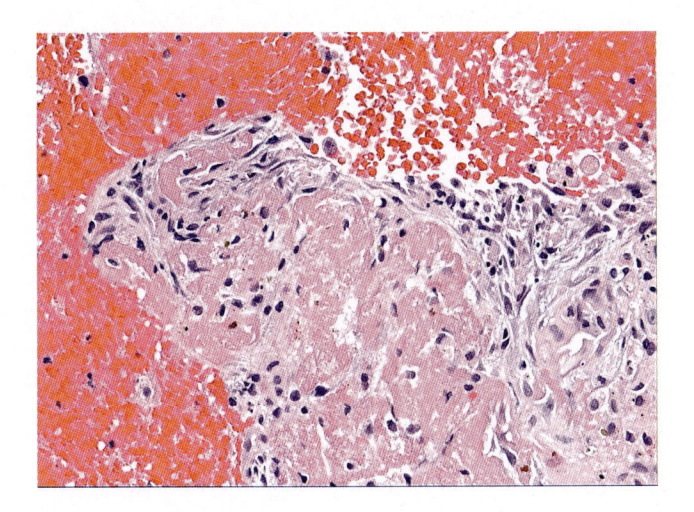

Figure 21.9: Ingrowth of fibroblasts into the fibrin in this intra-alveolar hemorrhage seen in a transbronchial biopsy indicates that the hemorrhage has been present long enough for organization to begin.

Suggested Readings

Santos-Ocampo AS, Mandel BF, Fessler BJ. Alveolar hemorrhage in systemic lupus erythematosus: presentation and management. *Chest* 2000;118:1083–1090.

Specks U. Diffuse alveolar hemorrhage syndromes. *Curr Opin Rheumatol* 2001;13:12–17.

Zimmerman LH. Clinical diagnosis of intraalveolar infiltrates and exudates. In: Cagle PT, ed. *Diagnostic Pulmonary Pathology.* New York: Marcel Dekker; 2000.

Eosinophilic Pneumonia

▶ Roberto Barrios, MD
▶ Keith M. Kerr, FRCPath

Hypereosinophilic syndromes with pulmonary involvement can be idiopathic or associated with a number of conditions such as parasitic infections, drug reactions, and so on. In addition, they can also be acute or chronic depending on the clinical course. It is important to realize that eosinophils are not seen in lungs of normal individuals, so their presence in transbronchial biopsies should alert the pathologist to the possibility of eosinophilic pneumonia or other eosinophil-associated lesions. Pulmonary eosinophilia may be seen in the absence of peripheral blood eosinophilia. The transbronchial biopsy may show a constellation of findings including intra-alveolar eosinophils, macrophages, and an amorphous proteinaceous exudate. When fibrin accompanies the eosinophils, the possibility of acute eosinophilic pneumonia should be considered. As is common in dense eosinophilic infiltrates, Charcot-Leyden crystals may be found. Eosinophils infiltrate the interstitium in about 80% of the cases, and foci of organizing pneumonia may be present. Eosinophilic abscesses with foci of necrosis and palisading of histiocytes are classically described in chronic eosinophilic pneumonia; however, a transbronchial biopsy may not show all of the described features. Although the presence of vasculitis has been described in eosinophilic pneumonias, the pathologist should document this finding, and the possibility of Churg-Strauss vasculitis should be ruled out clinically. Prior treatment with steroids may mask the eosinophilia, and the biopsy may only show accumulation of intra-alveolar macrophages. Some series have reported diagnostic changes of eosinophilic pneumonia by transbronchial biopsy in 64% of patients with peripheral eosinophilia and pulmonary infiltrates.

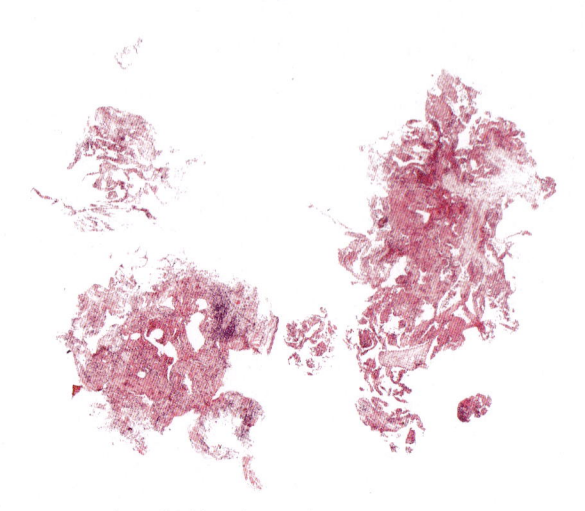

Figure 22.1: Transbronchial lung biopsy from a patient with eosinophilic pneumonia. At low magnification, fibroblastic plugs suggesting organizing pneumonia can be seen. In addition, the cellularity is suggestive of an eosinophilic infiltrate.

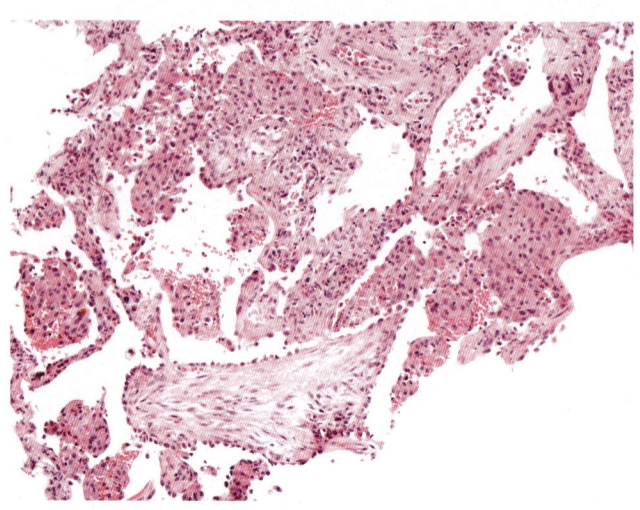

Figure 22.2: At higher power these fragments of lung show both interstitial infiltration and alveolar filling by a mixed cell population. In addition, foci of organizing pneumonia are clearly seen.

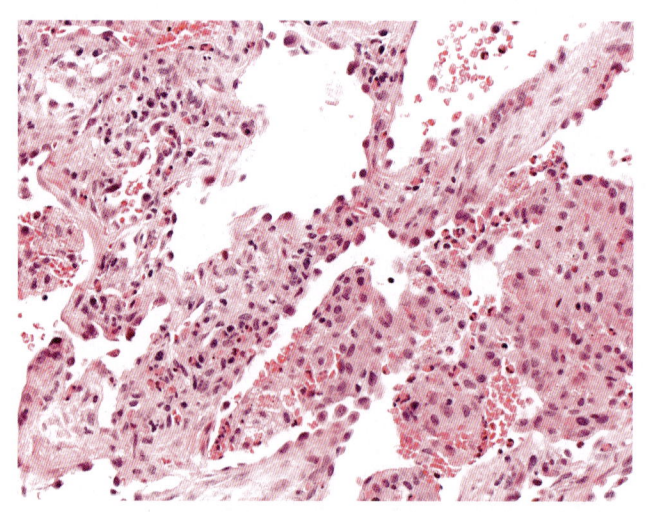

Figure 22.3: The interstitial and the alveolar cellular infiltrates consist of a variable mixture of eosinophils and macrophages together with red blood cells. Most eosinophilic pneumonias include this mixture of cells. In some cases, eosinophils may even be scanty.

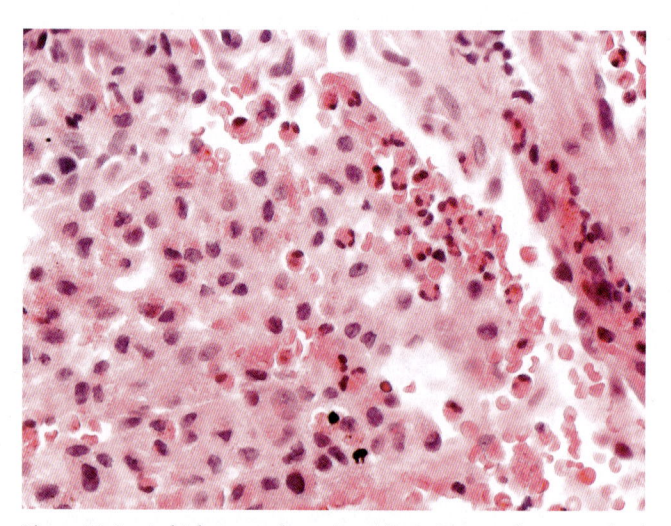

Figure 22.4: At high power the eosinophils and macrophages are clearly seen. Some partially degranulated eosinophils are also present, as are some foamy histiocytes.

Suggested Readings

Miyagawa Y, Nagata N, Shigematsu N. Clinicopathological study of migratory lung infiltrates. *Thorax* 1991;46:233–238.

Silva CI, Muller NL, Fujimoto K, et al. Churg-Strauss syndrome: high resolution CT and pathologic findings. *J Thorac Imaging* 2005;20:74–80.

Tsunemi K, Kanayama I, Kondo T, et al. Acute eosinophilic pneumonia evaluated with high-resolution computed tomography. *Intern Med* 1993;32:891–894.

Lipid Pneumonia

▶ Timothy C. Allen, MD, JD
▶ Roberto Barrios, MD

Lipid pneumonia, also termed endogenous lipoid pneumonia, postobstructive pneumonia, or "golden pneumonia," occurs due to the escape of normally occurring lipids from lung tissue damage from a supparative process or from destroyed alveolar cell walls distal to an obstructing lesion such as lung cancer. It is termed "golden pneumonia" because affected lungs grossly have a golden or yellow-tan color because of the accumulation of lipid. Although large obstructions due to tumors are frequent, obstruction leading to lipid pneumonia may be so small as to involve only a small terminal or respiratory bronchiole. It is hypothesized that transbronchial dissemination of breakdown products from tumor cells, including mucin, may contribute to its spread in lung parenchyma.

Histologically, there is accumulation of fine fat droplets in alveolar macrophages, with occasional associated giant cells and occasional cholesterol crystals. Scattered lymphocytes and plasma cells may be present and reactive type II pneumocyte hyperplasia. There is variable but generally mild interstitial widening with scattered chronic inflammatory cells and occasional interstitial foamy macrophages.

Differential diagnosis includes lipid storage diseases such as Gaucher disease and Niemann-Pick disease, lung reaction to amiodarone therapy, and lipoid pneumonia, also termed exogenous lipid pneumonia.

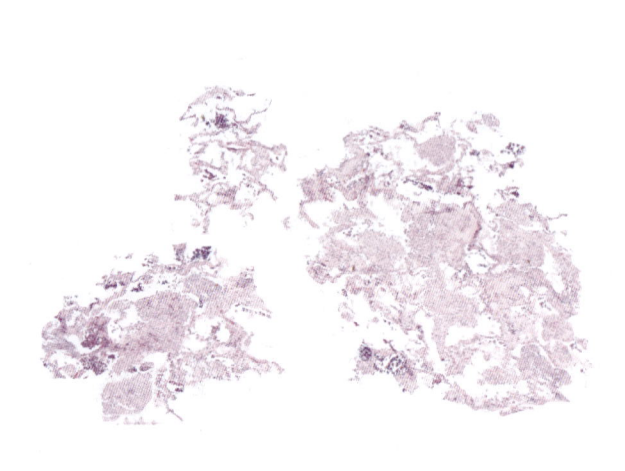

Figure 23.1: Low power of transbronchial biopsy shows nodular aggregates of foamy cells consistent with lipid pneumonia.

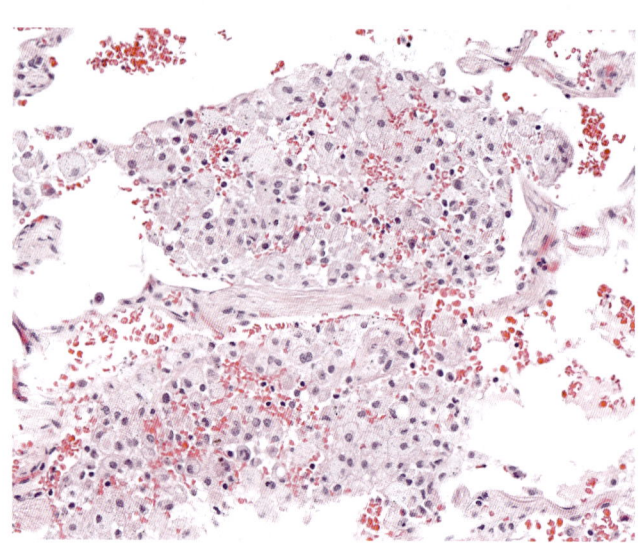

Figure 23.2: Medium power shows collections of lipid-laden, foamy macrophages in lipid pneumonia.

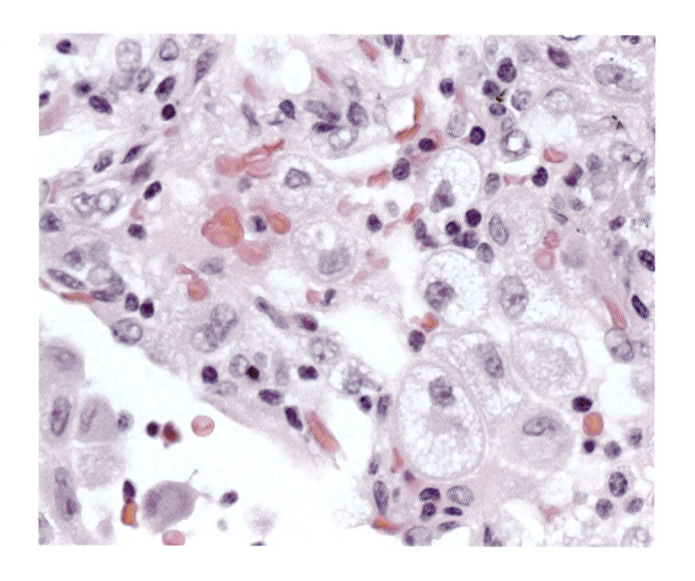

Figure 23.3: High power shows that the cytoplasm of most macrophages is foamy appearing due to lipid material in this transbronchial biopsy of lipid pneumonia.

Suggested Readings

Barrios R. Lipoid pneumonia. In: Cagle PT, ed. *Color Atlas and Text of Pulmonary Pathology*. Philadelphia, Pa: Lippincott Williams & Wilkins; 2004.

Barta Z, Szabo GG, Bruckner G, et al. Endogenous lipoid pneumonia associated with undifferentiated connective tissue disease (UCTD). *Med Sci Monit* 2001;7:134–136.

Berghaus TM, Haeckel T, Wagner T, et al. Endogenous lipoid pneumonia associated with primary sclerosing cholangitis. *Lancet* 2007;369:1140.

Dail DH. Intraalveolar exudates/infiltrates. In: Cagle PT, ed. *Diagnostic Pulmonary Pathology*. New York: Marcel Dekker; 2000.

Sulkowska M, Sulkowski S. Endogenous lipid pneumonia- and alveolar proteinosis-type changes in the vicinity of non-small cell lung cancer: histopathologic, immunohistochemical, and ultrastructural evaluation. *Ultrastruct Pathol* 1998;22:109–119.

Tamura A, Hebisawa A, Fukushima K, et al. Lipoid pneumonia in lung cancer: radiographic and pathological features. *Jpn J Clin Oncol* 1998;28:492–496.

Pulmonary Alveolar Proteinosis

▶ Anna Sienko, MD
▶ Philip T. Cagle, MD

Pulmonary alveolar proteinosis, also termed *alveolar lipoproteinosis*, represents an autoimmune defect of the alveolar macrophages to remove surfactant with the development of autoantibodies that impair macrophage function by neutralizing granulocyte simulating factor. Alveolar proteinosis is most often seen in middle-age patients and more often in men than women. It has also been reported in children with underlying enzyme defects, patients exposed to heavy dust, and in patients with underlying malignancies such as leukemia or lymphoma or in immunodeficiency states. Treatment is most usually by bronchiolar lavage; however, spontaneous remission can also occur. On a transbronchial biopsy, alveolar proteinosis is seen as a uniform expansion of the intra-alveolar spaces with an eosinophilic slightly granular amorphous material often also containing globular clumps of eosinophilic material. Typically, scattered macrophages and scattered cholesterol clefts are also present. No inflammatory component or red blood cells are seen within the material. The interstitium is not expanded and shows no inflammation, although long-standing chronic cases may develop interstitial fibrosis and inflammation. Periodic acid-Schiff (PAS) with diastase stains positive, confirming the presence of surfactant apoprotein that contains glycogen. Pulmonary alveolar proteinosis may be associated with infections including *Nocardia*, mycobacteria, fungus, or virus.

The main differential includes pulmonary edema and *Pneumocystis* infection. Pulmonary edema is usually more uniformly amorphous rather than granular. It is patchy and lacks the cholesterol clefts. *Pneumocystis* infection shows more rounded granular intra-alveolar material that usually does not fill the entire intra-alveolar space and is associated with features of pneumonia. GMS stain is positive in *Pneumocystis* infection. PAS with diastase is negative in both pulmonary edema and *Pneumocystis* pneumonia.

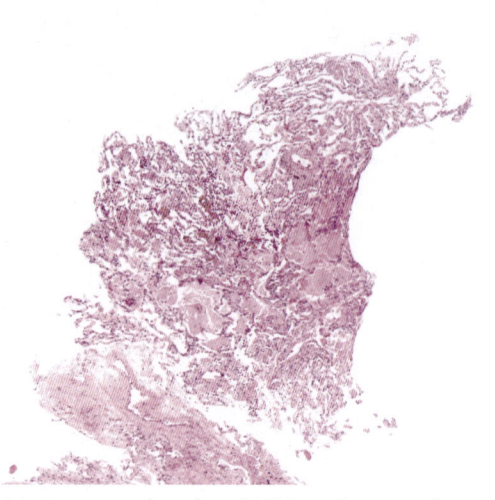

Figure 24.1: Low power of transbronchial biopsy shows granular eosinophilic material filling a portion of the alveolar spaces in this example of pulmonary alveolar proteinosis.

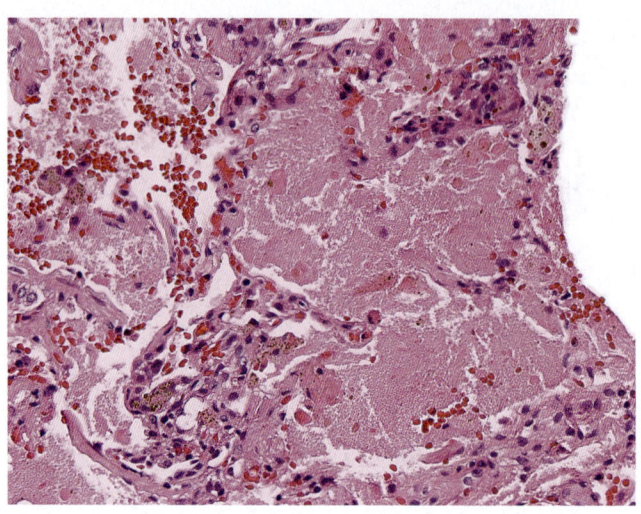

Figure 24.2: High power shows filling of alveolar spaces by granular eosinophilic material with scattered globular clumps of darker eosinophilic material consistent with pulmonary alveolar proteinosis.

Suggested Readings

Barrios R, Bedrossian C. Pulmonary alveolar proteinosis. In: Cagle PT, ed. *Color Atlas and Text of Pulmonary Pathology.* Philadelphia, Pa: Lippincott Williams & Wilkins; 2004.

De Mello DE, Lin Z. Pulmonary alveolar proteinosis: a review. *Pediatr Pathol Mol Med* 2001;20:413–432.

Seymour JF, Presneill JJ. Pulmonary alveolar proteinosis: progress in the first 44 years. *Am J Respir Crit Care Med* 2002;166:215–235.

Sarcoidosis

▶ Armando E. Fraire, MD

Sarcoidosis, a systemic disease of unknown etiology often affecting the lungs and mediastinal lymph nodes, is characterized histopathologically by granulomas that are found distinctively along the path of the bronchovascular bundles. The cardinal diagnostic feature of sarcoidosis in the lung, as in other anatomic sites, is the nonnecrotizing granuloma. This granuloma is made up of tight conglomerates of epithelioid histiocytes and multinucleated giant cells of the Langerhans type, surrounded by a peripheral rim of fibroblasts. Typically, the granulomas are often naked, that is, devoid of a peripheral rim of lymphocytes, a feature that can be seen in nonsarcoidal granulomas. A variety of cytoplasmic inclusions can be seen within the multinucleated giant cells, including asteroid bodies, conchoid bodies, and colorless birefringent particles. None of these inclusions are diagnostic, but their presence may alert the pathologist to the possibility of sarcoid. Rarely, the granulomas may involve the vascular walls or become confluent, leading to conditions known as *sarcoid vasculitis* or *confluent sarcoid,* respectively. Transbronchial lung biopsy is very useful in the diagnosis of sarcoidosis, allowing a diagnosis to be made in ≥70% of the cases. However, endobronchial biopsies are also useful. The actual yield of these two diagnostic modalities varies primarily on account of the stage of the disease. The diagnostic yield in either type of biopsy can be increased by step sectioning of the tissue blocks.

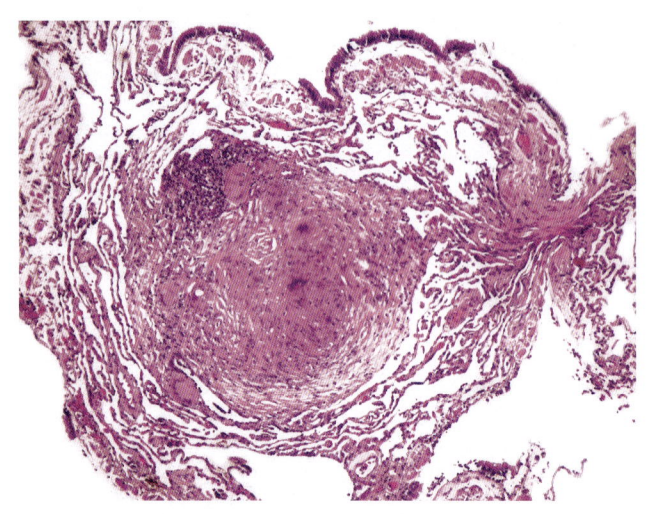

Figure 25.1: A discrete nonnecrotizing granuloma is seen at low power in this transbronchial biopsy from a patient with sarcoidosis.

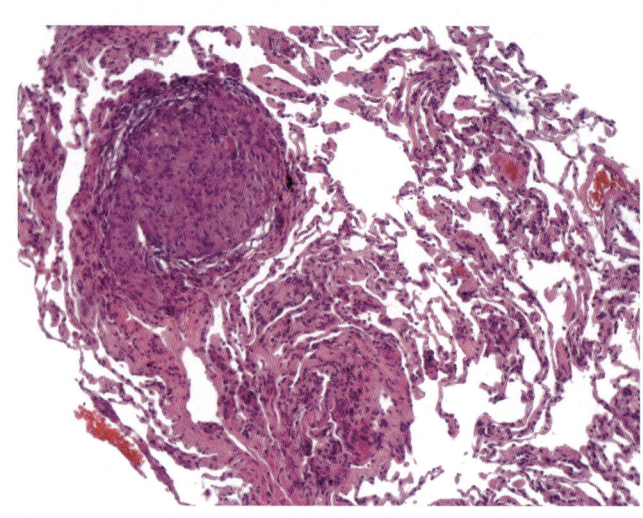

Figure 25.2: Another sample of tissue from the same transbronchial biopsy procedure shows well-formed nonnecrotizing granuloma in association with blood vessels in this case of sarcoidosis.

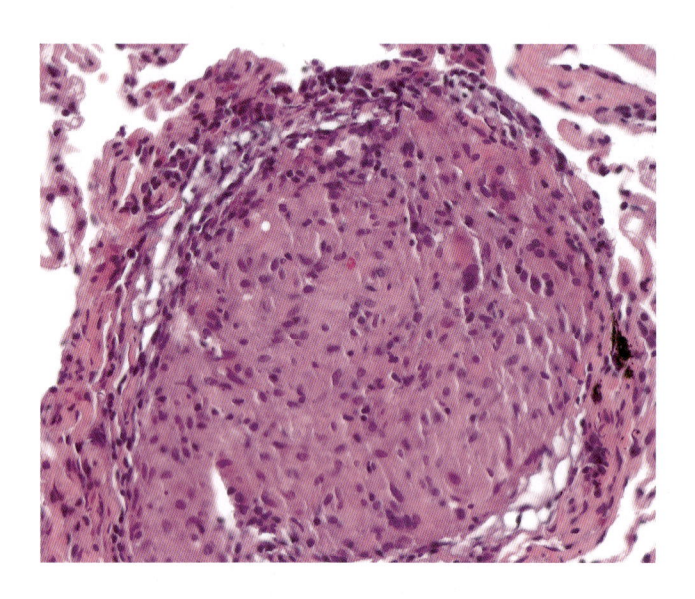

Figure 25.3: High power view of the sarcoid granulomas shown in Figure 25.2. Note a well-formed granuloma made almost entirely of epithelioid histiocytes and the absence of necrosis.

Suggested Readings

Bjermer L, Thunell M, Rosenhall L, et al. Endobronchial biopsy positive sarcoidosis: relation to bronchoalveolar lavage and course of disease. *Respir Med* 1991;85:229.

Mitchell DM, Mitchell DN, Collins JV, et al. Transbronchial lung biopsy through fibreoptic bronchoscope in diagnosis of sarcoidosis. *BMJ* 1980;280:679.

Mohan H, ed. Inflammation and healing. *Textbook of Pathology*. New Delhi, Anshan, and Tunbridge Wells: Jaypee Medical; 2005:133–179.

Popper HH. Granulomas and granulomatous inflammation. In: Cagle PT, ed. *Diagnostic Pulmonary Pathology*. New York: Marcel Dekker; 2000:287–329.

Roethe RA, Fuller PB, Byrd RB, et al. Transbronchoscopic lung biopsy in sarcoidosis: Optimal number and sites for diagnosis. *Chest* 1980;77:400.

Takayama K, Nagata N, Miyagawa Y, et al. The usefulness of step sectioning of transbronchial lung biopsy specimen in diagnosing sarcoidosis. *Chest* 1992;102:1441.

Hypersensitivity Pneumonitis

▶ Armando E. Fraire, MD
▶ Philip T. Cagle, MD

Broadly defined as a state of exaggerated immune response to a wide variety of antigenic substances, hypersensitivity pneumonitis refers to an inflammatory condition clinically characterized by a flulike illness and histologically typified by a triad of peribronchiolar chronic interstitial pneumonitis, organizing pneumonia, and the formation of loose incomplete granulomas. However, this hypersensitivity pneumonitis triad is seen in only 70% to 80% of the cases. Often only two of the three elements of the triad are seen in biopsy material. Three stages of the disease are recognized both clinically and histopathologically: acute; subacute, the most prevalent; and chronic. The discussion here primarily applies to this subacute form. A variant of hypersensitivity pneumonitis occurring in association with hot tub usage has been termed *hot tub lung*.

Endobronchial lung biopsies are not useful in the diagnosis of hypersensitivity pneumonitis because they will miss most if not all of the elements of the histopathologic triad just described. Transbronchial lung biopsies, however, are much more helpful. The bronchiolitis or peribronchiolitis of hypersensitivity pneumonitis is chiefly mononuclear, lymphocytic, and not associated with necrosis of the bronchial epithelium. The chronic interstitial inflammation is bronchiolocentric, in continuity with the peribronchial inflammation, and characterized by lymphocytic or lymphoplasmacytic infiltrates. The granulomas of hypersensitivity pneumonitis are poorly formed, often referred to as incomplete, and they are, by definition, nonnecrotizing. Isolated giant cells with or without cholesterol clefts or Schaumann bodies may constitute the only evidence of a granulomatous response. These granulomas of hypersensitivity pneumonitis are really granulomatoid aggregates of multinucleated histiocytes, lymphocytes, and/or plasma cells and blend into the surrounding interstitial inflammatory infiltrate, a feature that assists in differentiating these granulomas from other granulomatous conditions. Granulomas can also be found in the chronic stage of the disease.

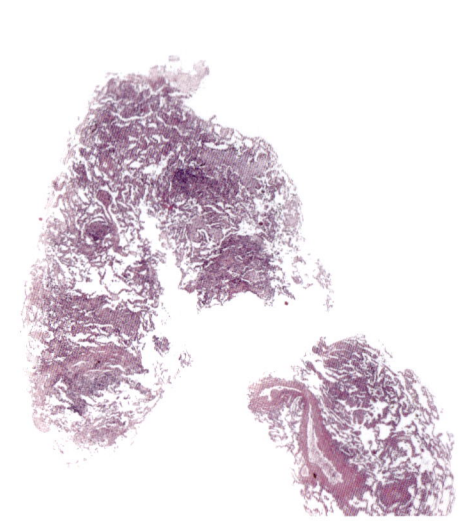

Figure 26.1: At low power, this transbronchial biopsy from a patient with hypersensitivity pneumonitis shows cellular areas consistent with interstitial pneumonia and plugs of granulation tissue consistent with an organizing pneumonia.

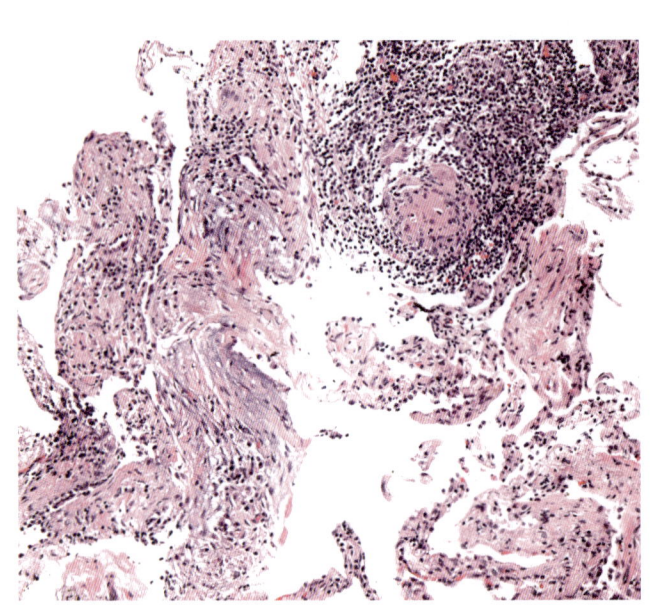

Figure 26.2: Medium power of the transbronchial biopsy shows interstitial lymphocytic infiltrates (interstitial pneumonia), intra-alveolar granulation tissue (organizing pneumonia), and a multinucleated giant cell.

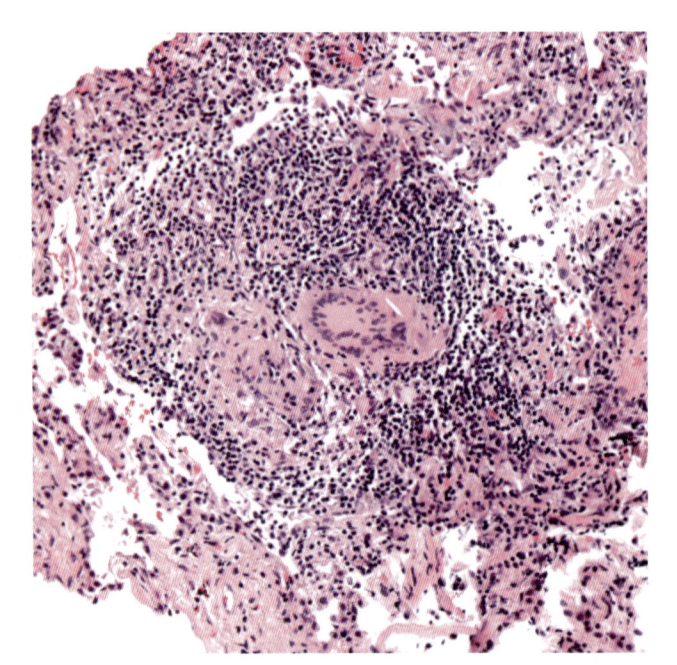

Figure 26.3: High power shows two multinucleated giant cells in a loose, poorly formed granuloma typical of hypersensitivity pneumonitis.

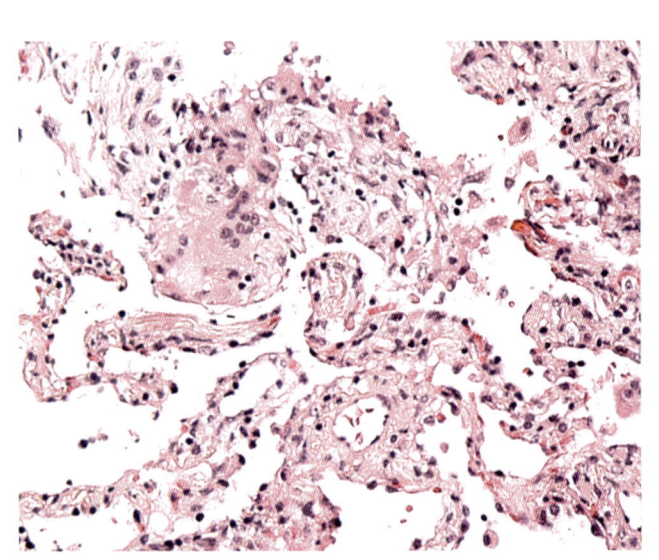

Figure 26.4: High power from a transbronchial biopsy in a case of hypersensitivity pneumonitis shows a multinucleated giant cell in the interstitium that is subtle and could be overlooked at low power.

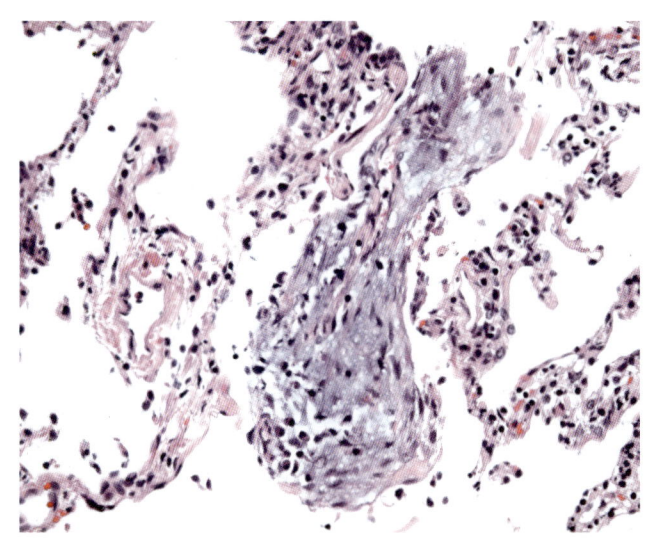

Figure 26.5: High power of myxoid, fibroblastic granulation tissue within an alveolar duct in a transbronchial biopsy from a patient with hypersensitivity pneumonitis.

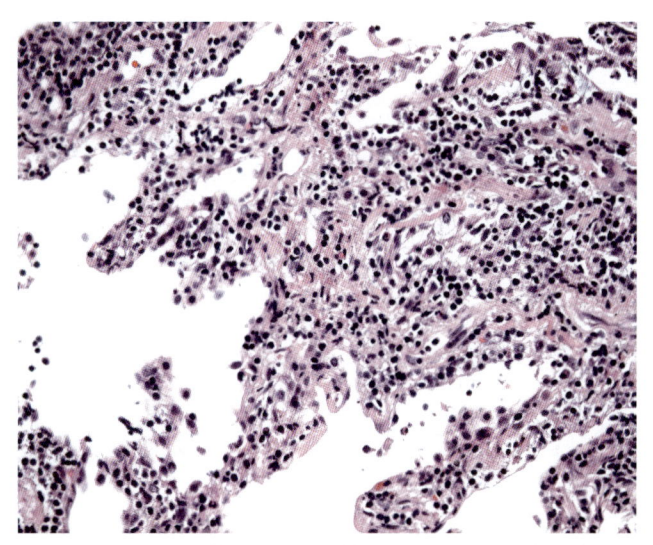

Figure 26.6: Interstitial lymphocytic infiltrates are seen on medium power in this transbronchial biopsy from a patient with hypersensitivity pneumonitis.

Suggested Readings

Cappelluti E, Fraire AE, Schaefer OP. A case of "hot tub lung" due to *Mycobacterium avium* complex in an immunocompetent host. *Arch Intern Med* 2003;163:845–848.

Cheung OY, Muhm JR, Helmers RA, et al. Surgical pathology of granulomatous interstitial pneumonia. *Ann Diagn Pathol* 2003;7:127–138.

Churg A, Muller NL, Flint J, et al. Chronic hypersensitivity pneumonitis. *Am J Surg Pathol* 2006;30:201–208.

Reyes CN, Wenzel FJ, Lawton BR, et al. The pulmonary pathology of farmer's lung disease. *Chest* 1982;81:152–156.

Richerson HB. Hypersensitivity pneumonitis—pathology and pathogenesis. *Clin Rev Allergy* 1983;1:469–486.

Collagen Vascular Diseases

▶ Timothy C. Allen, MD, JD
▶ Jaishree Jagirdar, MD
▶ Philip T. Cagle, MD

Collagen vascular diseases that may involve the lungs include rheumatoid arthritis, systemic lupus erythematosus, progressive systemic sclerosis, Sjögren syndrome, and polymyositis/dermatomyositis. Lung disease may occasionally precede the diagnosis of systemic disease, especially in patients with rheumatoid arthritis or polymyositis, but in most cases the patient has already been diagnosed with collagen vascular disease before lung involvement becomes manifest. Serologic changes diagnostic of collagen vascular disease may sometimes be absent in those patients whose initial presentation is lung involvement.

Pulmonary manifestations of collagen vascular disease include diffuse abnormalities—usual interstitial pneumonia, lymphoid interstitial pneumonia, and nonspecific interstitial pneumonia—and patchy or focal lesions—organizing pneumonia and rheumatoid nodules. Pulmonary hypertension, vasculitis, including capillaritis, and intra-alveolar hemorrhage may also be found, as well as pleural disease including fibrous and fibrinous pleuritis, pleural effusions, and rheumatoid nodules. Bronchial and bronchiolar lesions such as follicular bronchitis or bronchiolitis, bronchiectasis, and constrictive bronchitis may occur. Immunosuppressive and cytotoxic treatment may also cause lung disease in these patients, including drug reactions (diffuse alveolar damage, hypersensitivity pneumonitis, etc.) as well as histopathology related to opportunistic infections (interstitial pneumonia, organizing pneumonia, diffuse alveolar damage, etc.).

The various pulmonary findings in collagen vascular disease just listed overlap considerably with the findings in many other lung diseases. There are many different causes of interstitial pneumonia, for example, besides collagen vascular disease. Only the sampling of a rheumatoid nodule can be considered specific for a collagen vascular disease diagnosis. Therefore, the findings on a transbronchial biopsy may include direct manifestation of a collagen vascular disease in the differential diagnosis, but, by themselves, these histopathologic findings are not definitively diagnostic of collagen vascular disease. Clinical correlation and perhaps additional studies are needed to determine whether or not a finding is most likely a direct manifestation of a collagen vascular disease. In particular, these patients are subject to opportunistic infections and drug reactions because of their therapy. Because the histologic findings of an infection or drug reaction are similar to many of the direct manifestations of collagen vascular disease in the lung, the pathologist should also typically consider them in the differential diagnosis. Although the transbronchial biopsy may not permit a definitive diagnosis of collagen vascular disease, note that the information conveyed to the clinician about the pulmonary histopathology is of considerable value in diagnosing and managing the patient in conjunction with the clinical, imaging, and ancillary study findings.

Depending on the amount of clinical and ancillary information that is available and any additional histologic findings such as rheumatoid nodules or viral inclusions, we recommend giving a descriptive diagnosis of the histologic findings and including collagen vascular disease in the differential diagnosis in the comment. If communication with the clinician favors direct pulmonary manifestation of collagen vascular disease, this can be conveyed in the comment, or the diagnosis may suggest that the findings are "compatible with" or "consistent with" collagen vascular disease. Nevertheless, in virtually all cases, a definitive diagnosis of collagen vascular disease cannot be made on the basis of the transbronchial biopsy alone.

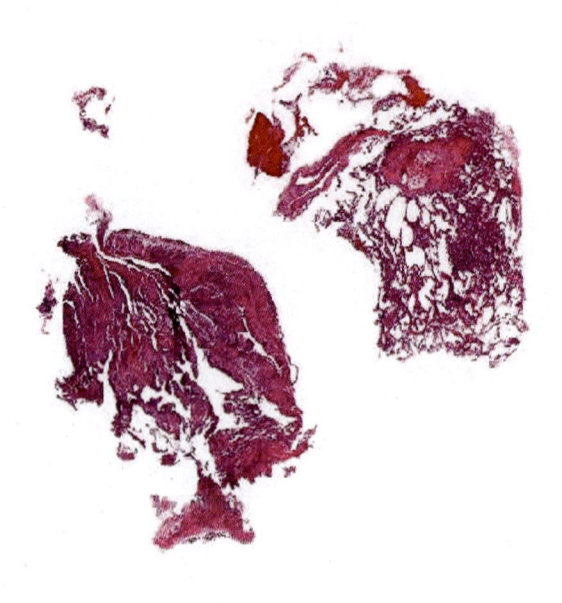

Figure 27.1: Transbronchial biopsy from a patient with clinical diagnoses of scleroderma and interstitial lung disease shows two fragments of lung parenchyma, one with chronic inflammation and the other with fibrosis.

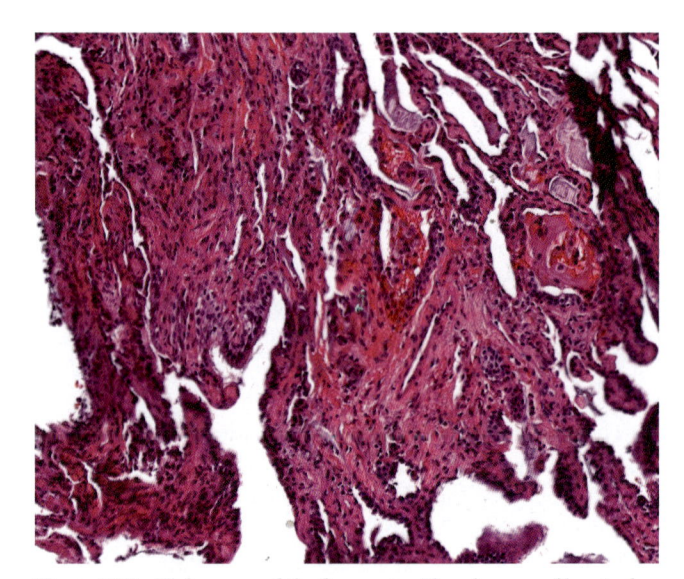

Figure 27.2: High power of the fragment with pulmonary fibrosis shows extensive interstitial mature collagen in this limited sample. The findings are compatible with pulmonary involvement with scleroderma but are not specific and not diagnostic of scleroderma. Features diagnostic of pulmonary infection or other specific diseases are not observed on this limited sample and thus do not provide a basis for withholding immunosuppressive therapy. The patient was subsequently treated with Cytoxan and prednisone.

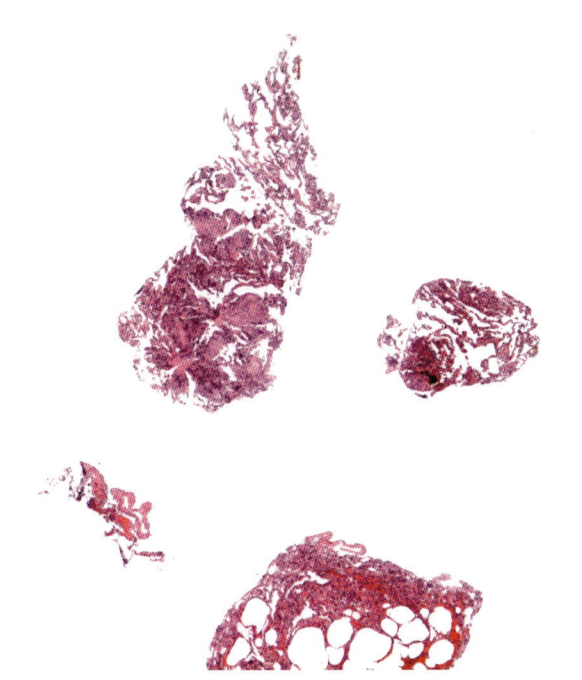

Figure 27.3: Nodules of organizing pneumonia can be seen at low power in this transbronchial biopsy from a patient with rheumatoid arthritis.

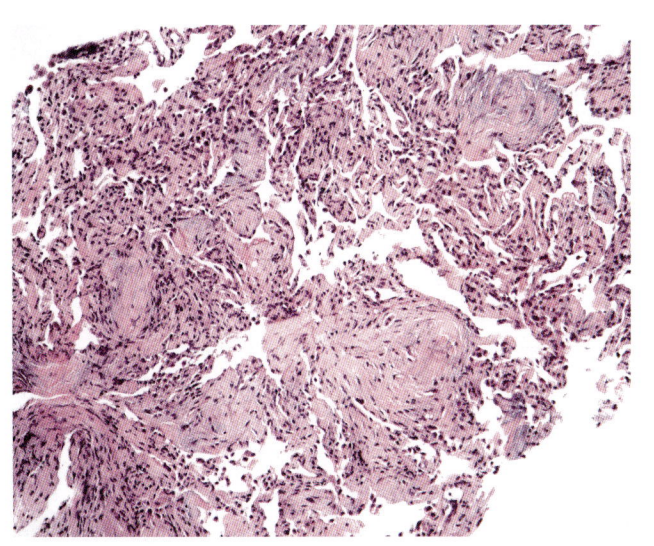

Figure 27.4: High power of the transbronchial biopsy shows granulation tissue of organizing pneumonia and interstitial lymphocytic infiltrates. These findings could be a direct manifestation of lung involvement by the patient's rheumatoid arthritis or could be the result of a hypersensitivity pneumonitis-like reaction to methotrexate or an opportunistic infection. The pathologist diagnosed "organizing pneumonia and interstitial pneumonia" and recommended clinical correlation. If no clinical history had been available for this patient, the findings of "organizing pneumonia and interstitial pneumonia" would suggest a much larger differential diagnosis that still would have potentially included infection, collagen vascular disease, hypersensitivity pneumonitis, and drug reaction.

Suggested Readings

Dawson J, Fewins H, Desmond J, et al. Fibrosing alveolitis in patients with rheumatoid arthritis as assessed by high resolution computed tomography, chest radiography, and pulmonary function tests. *Thorax* 2001;56:622–627.

Flint JDA. Vasculitis. In: Cagle PT, ed. *Diagnostic Pulmonary Pathology.* New York: Marcel Dekker; 2000.

Katzenstein AL. Idiopathic interstitial pneumonia: classification and diagnosis. *Monogr Pathol* 1993;36:1–31.

King TE. Diagnosis of interstitial infiltrates. In: Cagle PT, ed. *Diagnostic Pulmonary Pathology.* New York: Marcel Dekker; 2000.

White ES, Tazelaar HD, Lynch JP 3d. Bronchiolar complications of connective tissue diseases. *Semin Respir Crit Care Med* 2003;24:543–566.

Yousem S, Colby T, Carrington C. Lung biopsy in rheumatoid arthritis. *Am Rev Respir Dis* 1985;131:770–777.

28 Drug Reactions

▶ Timothy C. Allen, MD, JD
▶ Jaishree Jagirdar, MD
▶ Philip T. Cagle, MD

Pulmonary reactions to drugs may be idiosyncratic or dose related and include diffuse alveolar damage, intra-alveolar hemorrhage, nonspecific interstitial pneumonia, usual interstitial pneumonia, organizing pneumonia, lymphocytic interstitial pneumonia, giant cell interstitial pneumonia, pulmonary edema, granulomatous interstitial pneumonia, pulmonary hypertension, and eosinophilic pneumonia. Transbronchial biopsy may be sufficient to diagnose many of these patterns, but because these patterns are nonspecific and may be caused by many other etiologies, a definitive diagnosis of drug reaction is not possible from the biopsy findings alone in most cases. Clinical history is of great importance in suggesting that the features on transbronchial biopsy are drug related. Table 28.1 lists the drugs that are well established as causes of pulmonary reactions. This list is not exhaustive, and it continues to grow as new drugs come to market or reactions to previously marketed drugs are documented.

Table 28.2 lists pulmonary histopathologic manifestations of drug reactions. Diffuse alveolar damage is the most common manifestation of drug reactions. A few drugs produce relatively distinct histologic features that may be identified on transbronchial biopsy; for example, amiodarone-induced diffuse alveolar damage may be associated with finely vacuolated foamy macrophages and finely vacuolated epithelial cells.

Other than a few examples such as amiodarone, because the histopathologic patterns in drug reactions are nonspecific and potentially have other etiologies, we recommend diagnosing the histologic pattern (e.g., diffuse alveolar damage) and including drug reaction in the differential diagnosis in a comment, particularly when no clinical history is available. If the clinician communicates a clinical suspicion of a specific drug reaction, this can be reflected in the comment, or the diagnosis may suggest that the findings are "compatible with" or "consistent with" the specific drug reaction. Although, with a few exceptions, a definitive diagnosis of drug reaction cannot be made by transbronchial biopsy, the information that a pattern is compatible with a drug reaction is very helpful information to the clinician, who can interpret this finding within the clinical and radiologic context.

Table 28-1	Drugs Causing Lung Disease

Anticoagulants
    Amiodarone
    Fibrinolytic agents
    Protamine
    Tocainide
Antibiotics
    Nitrofurantoin
    Sulfasalazine
    Sulfonamides
    Amphotericin B
Chemotherapeutic: Cytotoxic
    Chlorambucil
    Azathioprine
    Busulfan
    Procarbazine
    Vinblastine
    Bleomycin
    Cyclophosphamide
    Melphalan
    Nitrosoureas
    Mitomycin
Chemotherapeutic: Noncytotoxic
    Methotrexate
    Cytarabine
    Procarbazine
Intravenous
    Talc
    Morrhuate sodium
    Blood
    L-tryptophan
Analgesic
    Naloxone
    Heroin
    Methadone
    Salicylates
    Propoxyphene
Anti-inflammatory
    Nonsteroidal anti-inflammatory agents
    Acetylsalicylic acid
    Penicillamine
    Gold
    Methotrexate

Table 28-2	Histologic Patterns in Lung in Drug Reactions

Diffuse alveolar damage
Intra-alveolar hemorrhage
Nonspecific interstitial pneumonia
Usual interstitial pneumonia
Organizing pneumonia
Lymphocytic interstitial pneumonia
Giant cell interstitial pneumonia
Pulmonary edema
Granulomatous interstitial pneumonia
Pulmonary hypertension
Eosinophilic pneumonia

Chapter 28 • Drug Reactions

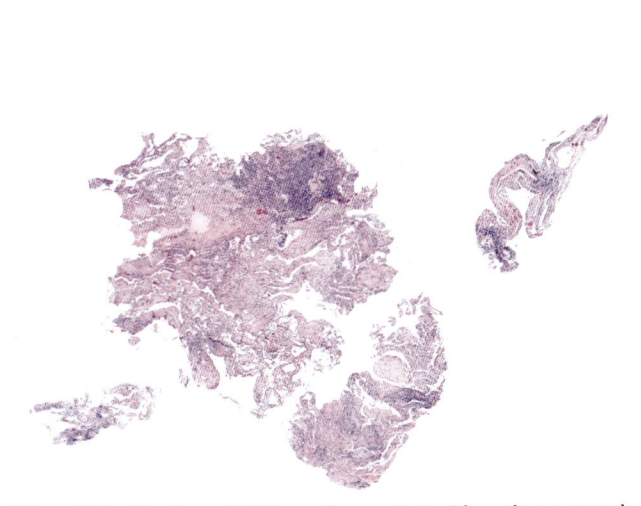

Figure 28.1: Transbronchial biopsy from patient with methotrexate pulmonary toxicity shows interstitial lymphocytic infiltrates and organizing pneumonia recognizable at low power.

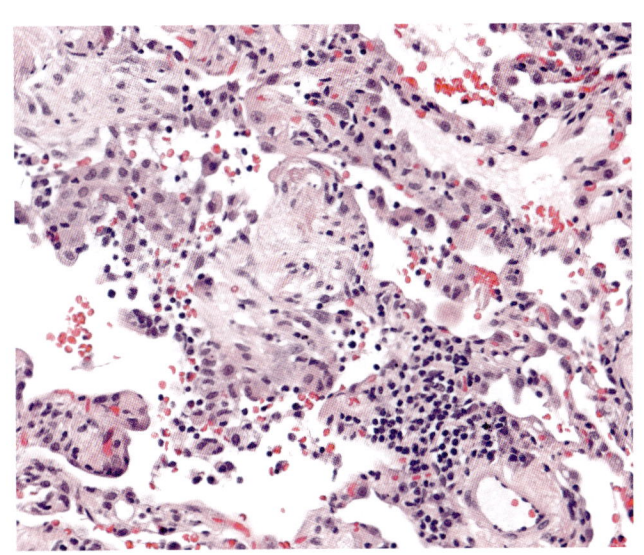

Figure 28.2: High power of methotrexate pulmonary toxicity shows granulation tissue of organizing pneumonia and interstitial lymphocytic infiltrates compatible with a hypersensitivity pneumonitis-like reaction to methotrexate. Although compatible with the clinical history of methotrexate reaction, the findings are not specific and could be due to infection or other etiology. Therefore, clinical correlation is recommended.

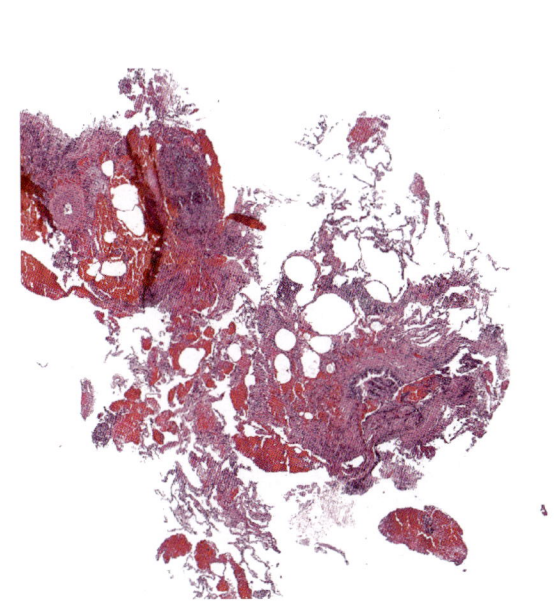

Figure 28.3: This transbronchial biopsy was performed to rule out infection in a bone marrow transplant patient who received sirolimus (rapamycin) and developed bilateral interstitial infiltrates. The biopsy shows interstitial lymphocytic infiltrates and organizing pneumonia at low power. Special stains, cytology specimens, and microbiologic cultures were negative for infectious organisms.

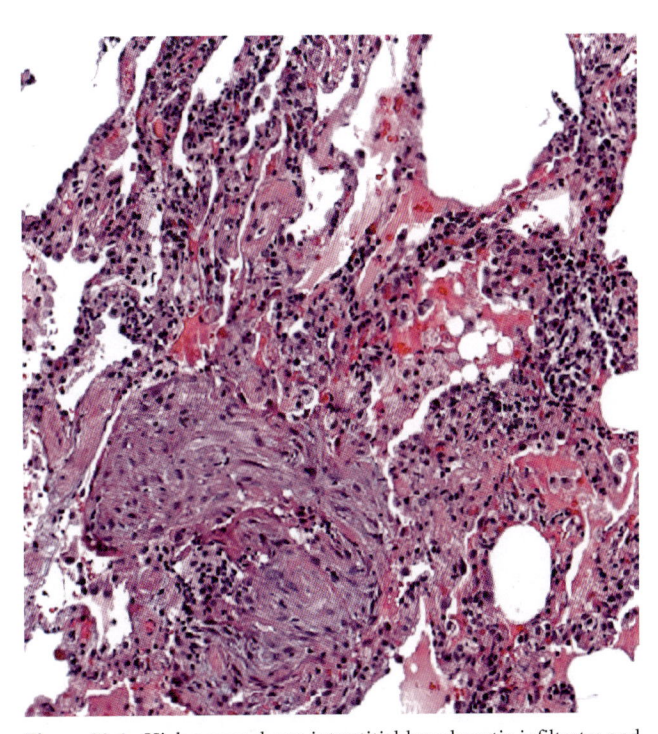

Figure 28.4: High power shows interstitial lymphocytic infiltrates and granulation tissue of organizing pneumonia compatible with sirolimus (rapamycin) pulmonary toxicity. Several patterns of pulmonary toxicity are associated with sirolimus including interstitial pneumonia, organizing pneumonia, alveolar hemorrhage, and pulmonary alveolar proteinosis.

Suggested Readings

Barrios R, Cermik H. Amiodarone. In: Cagle PT, ed. *Color Atlas and Text of Pulmonary Pathology.* Philadelphia, Pa: Lippincott Williams & Wilkins; 2004.

Barrios R, Laga AC, Ostrowski M, et al. Other drugs. In: Cagle PT, ed. *Color Atlas and Text of Pulmonary Pathology.* Philadelphia, Pa: Lippincott Williams & Wilkins; 2004.

Rosenow EC, Myers JL, Swensen SJ, et al. Drug-induced pulmonary disease: an update. *Chest* 1992;102:239–250.

Sharma A. Interstitial lymphocytic infiltrates. In: Cagle PT, ed. *Diagnostic Pulmonary Pathology.* New York: Marcel Dekker; 2000.

Inflammatory Bowel Disease

29

▶ Anna Sienko, MD

Pulmonary manifestations in inflammatory bowel disease, both in Crohn disease and ulcerative colitis, are well documented. Best characterized and seen more often in Crohn disease than in ulcerative colitis, pulmonary manifestations can include bronchitis, bronchiectasis, bronchiolitis obliterans, organizing pneumonia, nodular suppuration, pulmonary vasculitis, and noninfectious granulomatous inflammation. Granulomatous inflammation in patients with ulcerative colitis has also been reported associated with azathioprine treatment. On biopsy, granulomas of various sizes can be seen in random distribution both within the interstitium as well as near or around bronchioles. The granulomas tend to be fairly well formed, surrounded by multinucleated giant cells and without central necrosis. The differential diagnosis of granulomatous inflammation can be extensive and includes infection, drugs, sarcoidosis, and hypersensitivity pneumonia. If there is an associated organizing pneumonia present or features of vasculitis, the diagnosis of pulmonary manifestation of inflammatory bowel disease can be difficult on a biopsy. Rarely in patients with inflammatory bowel disease, coexistence of sarcoidosis or a "true" vasculitis, such as Churg-Strauss syndrome, Wegener granulomatosis, and microscopic polyangiitis, have been reported. Good clinical history and correlation with the pathologic findings are key to the diagnosis. Microbiologic cultures, special stains for organisms, serum antineutrophil cytoplasmic antibody (ANCA), and angiotensin-converting enzyme (ACE) studies are recommended to aid in the differential diagnosis.

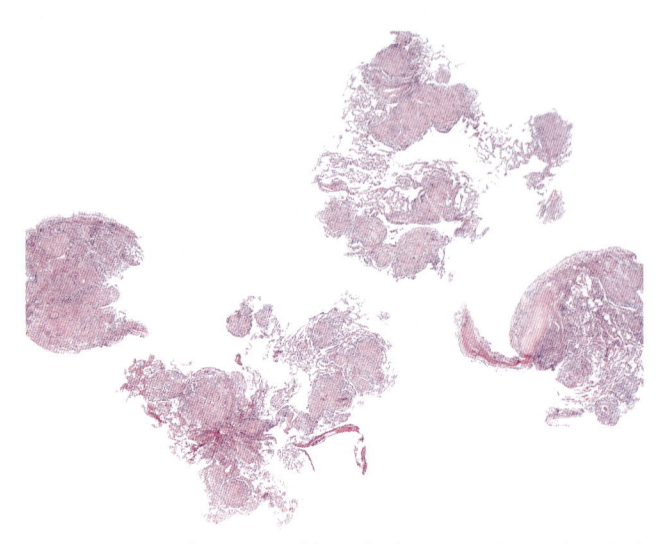

Figure 29.1: Granulomas are visible on this low power of a transbronchial biopsy from a patient with Crohn disease.

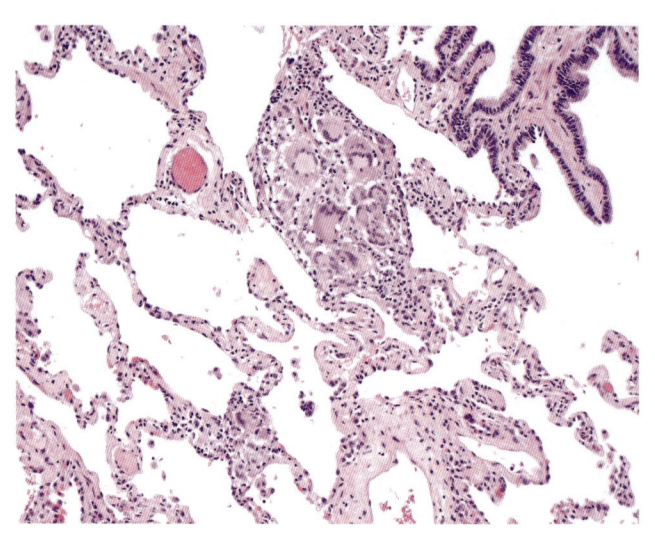

Figure 29.2: High power shows non-necrotizing granuloma in a patient with Crohn disease. Special stains for organisms, microbiologic cultures and other studies ruled out granulomatous infection. Sarcoidosis and hypersensitivity pneumonitis were also ruled out clinically and serologically.

Suggested Readings

Black H, Mendoza M, Murin S. Thoracic manifestations of inflammatory bowel disease. *Chest* 2007;131:524–532.

Casey MB, Tazelaar HD, Myers JL, et al. Noninfectious lung pathology in patients with Crohn's disease. *Am J Surg Pathol* 2003;27:213–219.

Lucero PF, Frey WC, Shaffer RT, et al. Granulomatous lung masses in an elderly patient with inactive Crohn's disease. *Inflamm Bowel Dis* 2001;7:256–259.

Nagy F, Molnar T, Makula E, et al. A case of interstitial pneumonitis in a patient with ulcerative colitis treated with azathioprine. *World Gastroenterol* 2007;13:316–319.

Pneumoconioses

▶ Timothy C. Allen, MD, JD
▶ Philip T. Cagle, MD

The pneumoconioses are a group of diseases characterized by lung parenchymal changes due to inhalation of inorganic dusts. The exposures causing these diseases most frequently occur in occupational settings. Included among the pneumoconioses are asbestosis, silicosis, silicatosis, mixed pneumoconiosis, mixed dust pneumoconiosis, coal worker's pneumoconiosis, siderosis, aluminosis, and giant cell interstitial pneumonia/hard metal pneumoconiosis. Detailed discussions of these entities are beyond the scope of this book.

Many more individuals are exposed to inorganic dusts than develop disease from the exposure, and all of these individuals are potentially susceptible to other types of unrelated lung disease. Therefore, the gold standard for the diagnosis of a pneumoconiosis is a tissue sample that is sufficiently large enough to avoid the sample restrictions of a limited transbronchial biopsy. However, transbronchial biopsies may provide potentially useful evidence of a particular exposure without providing sufficient material by themselves for the diagnosis of disease: Asbestos bodies indicate exposure to asbestos, but there is insufficient tissue in a transbronchial biopsy to quantify the exposure or assess the presence of diffuse interstitial fibrosis characteristic of the disease asbestosis. Other findings that may be seen on transbronchial biopsy that indicate an exposure but do not permit definitive diagnosis of a pneumoconiosis by themselves include coal dust macules, multinucleated giant cells within alveolar spaces (hard metal pneumoconiosis), and early silicotic nodule with dust-laden macrophages and tiny, weakly birefringent silica particles on polarization. Although the transbronchial biopsy can potentially convey some information about exposure, it is simply too small a sample to provide a definitive diagnosis of a pneumoconiosis or to rule out a pneumoconiosis if apparently negative. Correlation of findings on a transbronchial biopsy with clinical and radiologic findings may be helpful, if a larger biopsy is not clinically indicated.

Although mature interstitial fibrosis may be seen in a transbronchial biopsy, its extent and distribution cannot be determined on such a limited biopsy. Fibrosis may be focal and fortuitously sampled by the transbronchial biopsy or may be the result of potential causes such as previous infections that can no longer be identified as an etiology. Therefore, the pathologist should not make a definitive diagnosis for certain fibrotic diseases such as pneumoconioses on the basis of a transbronchial biopsy alone.

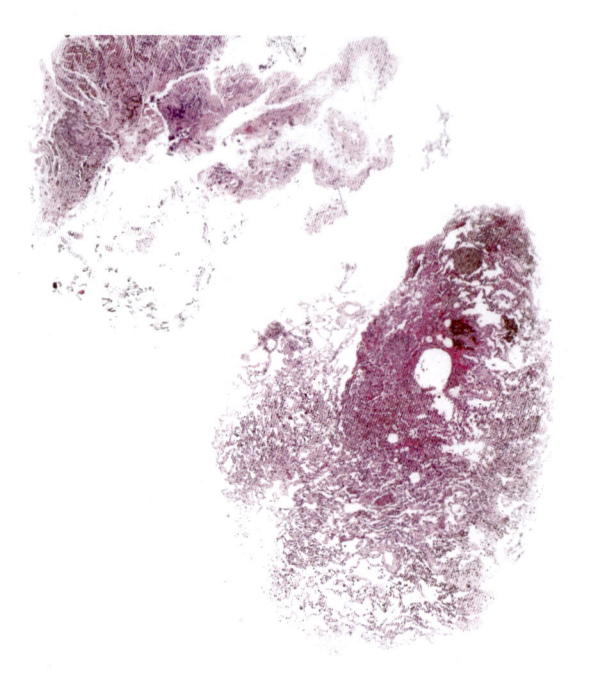

Figure 30.1: A small round nodule of pigmented macrophages is seen in this low power of a transbronchial biopsy. The biopsy was performed to rule out malignancy for clinical reasons.

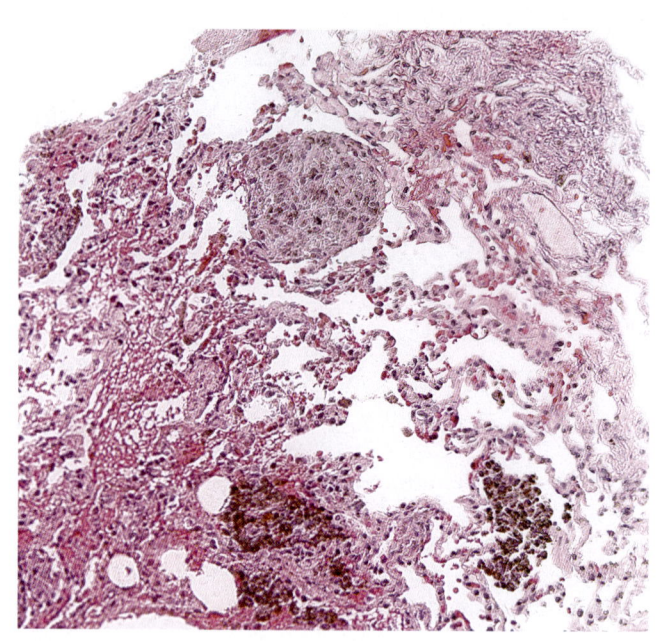

Figure 30.2: High power shows a tiny early silicotic nodule composed of pigmented macrophages. This nodule indicates that the patient has had an exposure to silica, but this one tiny nodule is insufficient to cause disease by itself, and the amount of tissue sampled on this biopsy does not permit assessment of whether or not there are more extensive silicotic nodules elsewhere in the lungs.

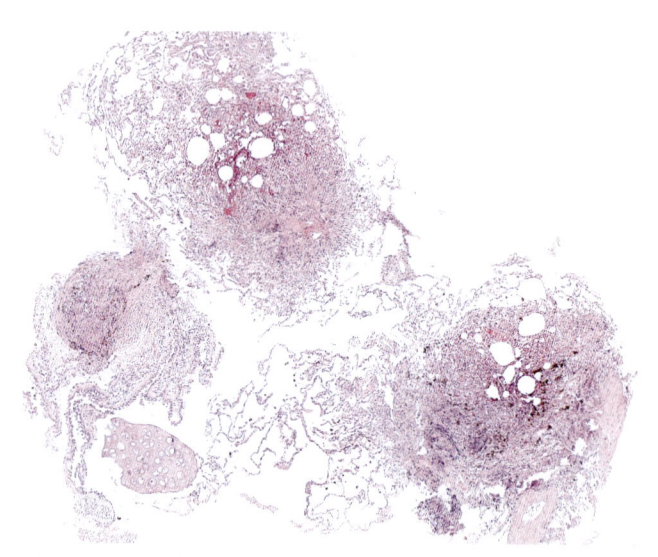

Figure 30.3: Low power shows transbronchial biopsy containing nodules composed of pigmented macrophages in a patient with exposure to mixed dusts in a foundry.

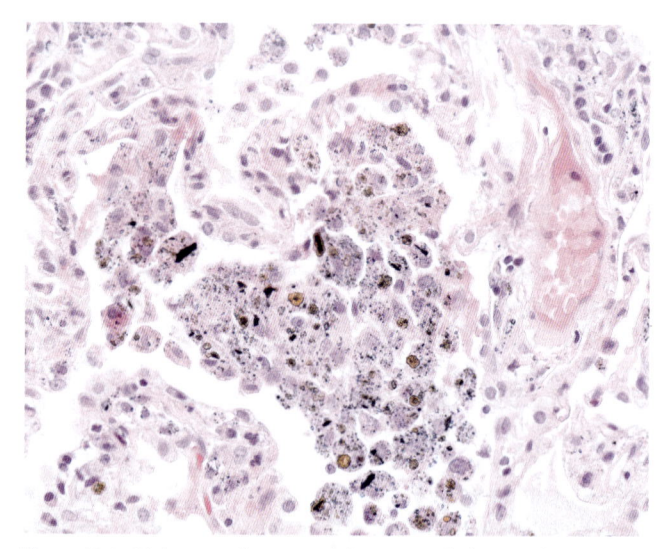

Figure 30.4: High power shows a nodule composed of macrophages containing anthracotic pigment. There are round iron-coated (ferruginous) bodies with round black centers consistent with iron or coal fly ash. These findings indicate exposure to carbon (coal) and iron.

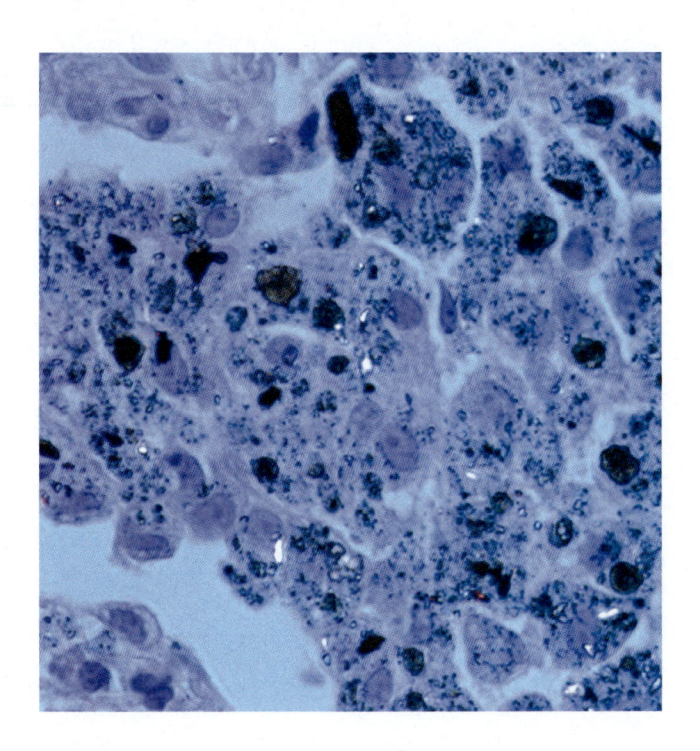

Figure 30.5: On polarized light, the pigmented macrophages in the same nodule contain tiny, weakly birefringent particles consistent with silica and larger, brighter birefringent particles consistent with silicates. These findings indicate that the individual has had exposure to multiple types of particles, including silica and silicates as well as coal and iron.

Suggested Readings

Cagle PT. Endobronchial and transbronchial biopsies. In: Cagle PT, ed. *Diagnostic Pulmonary Pathology.* New York: Marcel Dekker; 2000.

Churg AM, Green FHY. Occupational lung disease. In: Churg AM, Myers JL, Tazelaar HD, et al., eds. *Thurlbeck's Pathology of the Lung.* 3rd ed. New York: Thieme; 2005.

Pneumoconioses. In: Cagle PT, ed. *Color Atlas and Text of Pulmonary Pathology.* Philadelphia, Pa: Lippincott Williams & Wilkins; 2004.

Idiopathic Interstitial Pneumonias

31

▶ Timothy C. Allen, MD, JD
▶ Philip T. Cagle, MD

The idiopathic interstitial pneumonias include usual interstitial pneumonia (UIP, the pathologic correlate of idiopathic pulmonary fibrosis, or IPF), nonspecific interstitial pneumonia (NSIP), respiratory bronchiolitis-associated interstitial lung disease (RBILD), desquamative interstitial pneumonia (DIP), cryptogenic organizing pneumonia (COP), and acute interstitial pneumonia (AIP). Although several of the idiopathic interstitial pneumonias (UIP, RBILD, DIP) have a very strong association with tobacco smoking, the idiopathic interstitial pneumonias are traditionally considered to be of unknown etiology. A review of the clinical and pathologic features of each disease is beyond the scope of this chapter; however, the references to this chapter provide significant information about these diseases. Traditionally, lymphocytic interstitial pneumonia (LIP) and giant cell interstitial pneumonia (GIP) were also considered in the category of idiopathic interstitial pneumonias, but LIP is now recognized to be associated with other conditions in the majority of cases, and GIP is now recognized usually to be a hard metal pneumoconiosis.

The transbronchial biopsy has a role in the diagnosis of the idiopathic interstitial pneumonias primarily in one of two ways. In many cases, the transbronchial biopsy shows a histopathologic pattern for which an idiopathic interstitial pneumonia is a consideration in the differential diagnosis. In other cases, the transbronchial biopsy provides a supportive role for a clinical and radiologic diagnosis because it fails to reveal any histopathologic features that suggest a different diagnosis than the clinically suspected idiopathic interstitial pneumonia. For example, granulomas or hyaline membranes in a transbronchial biopsy indicate that another process besides UIP may be responsible for the clinical and radiologic findings in a suspected case of IPF.

UIP cannot be diagnosed by means of a transbronchial biopsy alone. Transbronchial biopsy may show areas of mature interstitial fibrosis or even fortuitously a fibroblast focus, but provides too small a sample to allow a diagnosis of UIP by itself. Nevertheless, transbronchial biopsy has potential roles in the diagnosis and management of patients with UIP. As already noted, transbronchial biopsy may be used in conjunction with imaging and clinical findings of IPF to help "rule out" other causes of these radiologic and clinical findings and to support a diagnosis of IPF. When patients experience changes in their clinical course, transbronchial biopsy may be used to rule out superimposed infection, diffuse alveolar damage, and so on.

The histopathologic diagnosis of UIP can be rendered on wedge biopsies or larger specimens, although even with wedge biopsies, clinical and radiologic correlation is often important. Currently, patients requiring wedge biopsies for a diagnosis of UIP generally do so because their disease has atypical radiologic or clinical features.

NSIP is most often cellular showing interstitial lymphocytic infiltrates, but it may also be fibrotic or mixed cellular and fibrotic. On transbronchial biopsy, interstitial lymphocytic infiltrates have a long differential diagnosis including infections, hypersensitivity pneumonitis, collagen vascular disease, and drug reactions, among others. The diagnosis of NSIP requires that the findings not have an identifiable etiology and, as with other idiopathic interstitial pneumonias, sample size puts limitations on the diagnosis of NSIP by transbronchial biopsy. Some apparent cases of NSIP are later found to be another condition such as hypersensitivity pneumonitis. If a transbronchial biopsy shows an interstitial lymphocytic infiltrate without specific diagnostic features such as granulomas, viral inclusions, and so on, we recommend giving a descriptive diagnosis of interstitial lymphocytic infiltrates or interstitial pneumonia and providing the differential diagnosis, including NSIP, in the comment. In these situations, clinical and radiologic correlation with appropriate additional studies is often necessary to arrive at the final diagnosis.

Macrophages containing smokers pigment are often seen in transbronchial biopsies from tobacco smokers and serve as an indicator of exposure to tobacco smoke. These macrophages may be a component of defined tobacco-related diseases RBILD and DIP that are traditionally included in the idiopathic interstitial pneumonias. Diagnostic features of RBILD include a mild lymphocytic infiltrate in terminal airways, mild airway fibrosis, metaplastic bronchiolar epithelium extending from terminal airways into alveolar ducts, and associated macrophages containing finely granular brown pigment. Diagnosis of RBILD can be made on transbronchial biopsy with appropriate clinical and radiologic correlation if a diagnostic area is sampled. The features of DIP (diffuse mild thickening of alveolar walls by fibrous tissue and the uniform filling of airspaces by pigmented macrophages) may be seen on a transbronchial biopsy, but the sample size is often insufficient to rule out a less extensive process like RBILD or a so-called DIP-like reaction that may be seen in association with other lesions. The transbronchial biopsy may serve to add support to a clinical and radiologic diagnosis by demonstrating compatible features in the absence of other specific diseases.

COP shows features of organizing pneumonia that may be sampled on transbronchial biopsy. The many known causes of organizing pneumonia (see Chapter 18) must be ruled out before a diagnosis of COP can be made. The small size of the transbronchial biopsy may not permit identification of a potential etiology for the organizing pneumonia. Therefore, in most cases with this histopathologic pattern, we recommend diagnosing organizing pneumonia and providing a differential diagnosis in the comment. Clinical and radiologic correlation and additional studies such as microbiologic cultures when appropriate are often necessary to arrive at the final diagnosis.

AIP, referred to clinically as Hamman-Rich syndrome, is a rapidly progressive frequently fatal fibrosing lung disease of unknown etiology that histologically has features of diffuse alveolar damage that may be seen on transbronchial biopsy. Identifiable etiologies for diffuse alveolar damage must be ruled out, including serologic, microbiologic, and special stain evaluation for infectious organisms, before a diagnosis of AIP can be rendered.

Chapter 31 • Idiopathic Interstitial Pneumonias

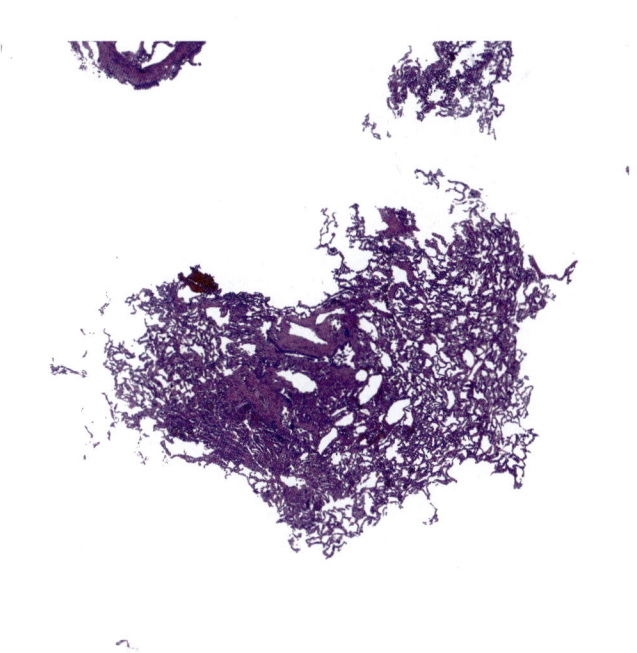

Figure 31.1: Low power of transbronchial biopsy from patient with nonspecific interstitial pneumonia (NSIP) shows relatively uniform interstitial lymphocytic infiltrates. Although this patient was eventually diagnosed with NSIP, the differential diagnosis for the interstitial lymphocytic infiltrates on this biopsy includes many other entities, such as infections, hypersensitivity pneumonitis, and collagen vascular disease.

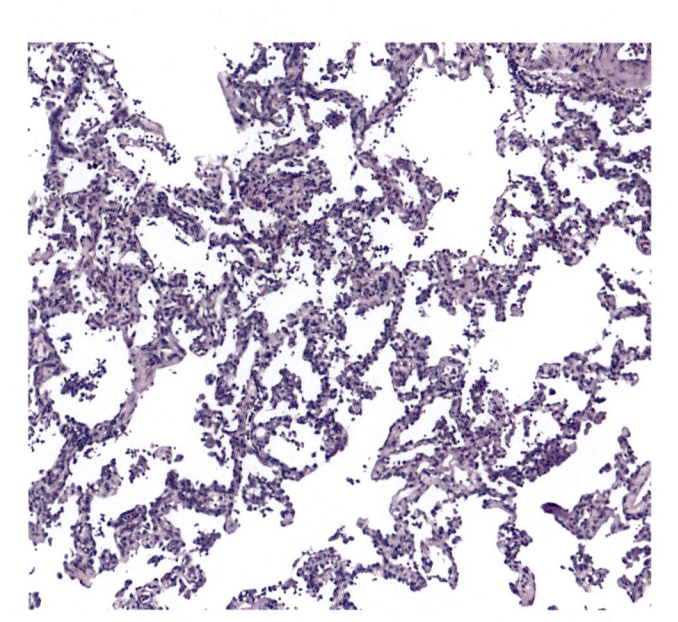

Figure 31.2: High power shows relatively uniform interstitial lymphocytic infiltrates without histopathologic findings diagnostic of a specific disease such as granulomas or viral inclusions. However, although this patient was eventually diagnosed with nonspecific interstitial pneumonia, the biopsy alone does not rule out other causes of interstitial lymphocytic infiltrates.

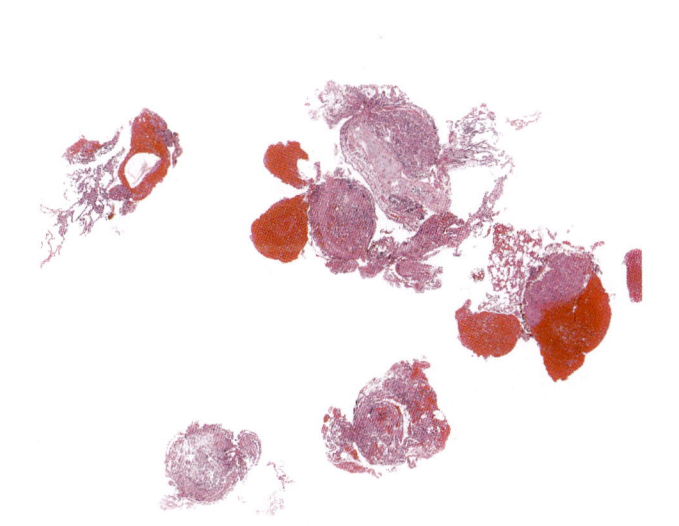

Figure 31.3: Low power of transbronchial biopsy shows differing amounts of fibrosis including focally advanced fibrosis. No features diagnostic of a specific entity such as granulomas, cancer, viral inclusions, hyaline membranes, and so on, are observed. Although this biopsy happens to be from a patient with usual interstitial pneumonia (UIP), a diagnosis of UIP cannot be made on this biopsy alone because it is too small to permit evaluation of the diagnostic features of UIP.

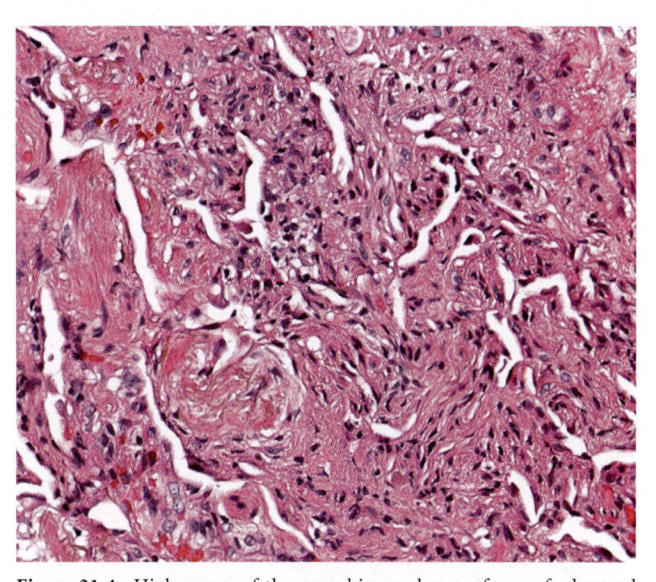

Figure 31.4: High power of the same biopsy shows a focus of advanced fibrosis. This feature might be seen in usual interstitial pneumonia (UIP), but there is no way to determine from this biopsy whether this fibrosis is merely a focal scar, random scarring from a healed infection, and so on. Although nothing is seen that contradicts a diagnosis of UIP, a diagnosis of UIP cannot be made on the basis of this small tissue sample alone.

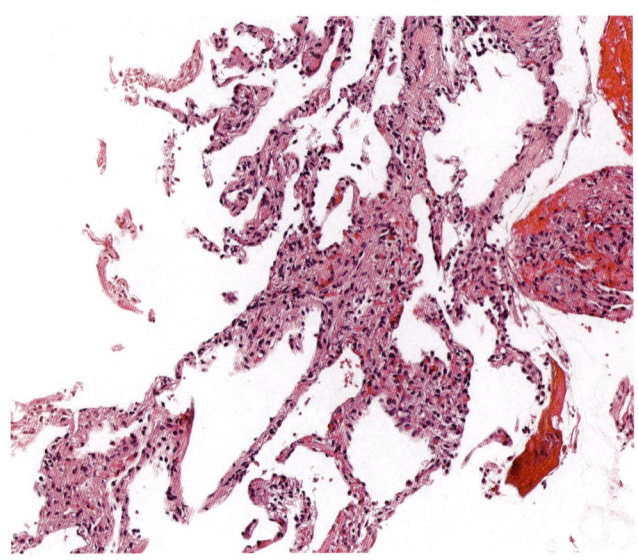

Figure 31.5: From the same biopsy, another focus at high power shows normal septa and a smaller scar. These features might also be seen in usual interstitial pneumonia (UIP), but again there is no way to determine from this biopsy whether this fibrosis is merely a focal scar, random scarring from a healed infection, and so on. Although nothing is seen that contradicts a diagnosis of UIP, a diagnosis of UIP cannot be made on the basis of this small tissue sample alone.

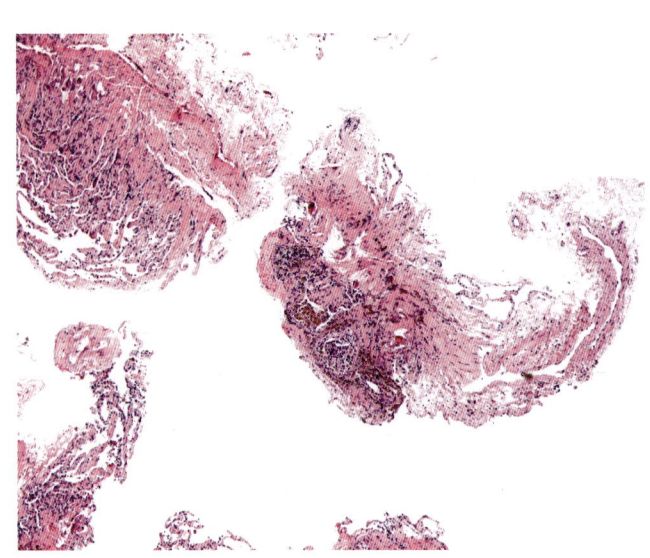

Figure 31.6: Low power of transbronchial biopsy from a tobacco smoker with respiratory bronchiolitis-associated interstitial lung disease shows interstitial fibrosis and focally airspaces containing pigmented macrophages.

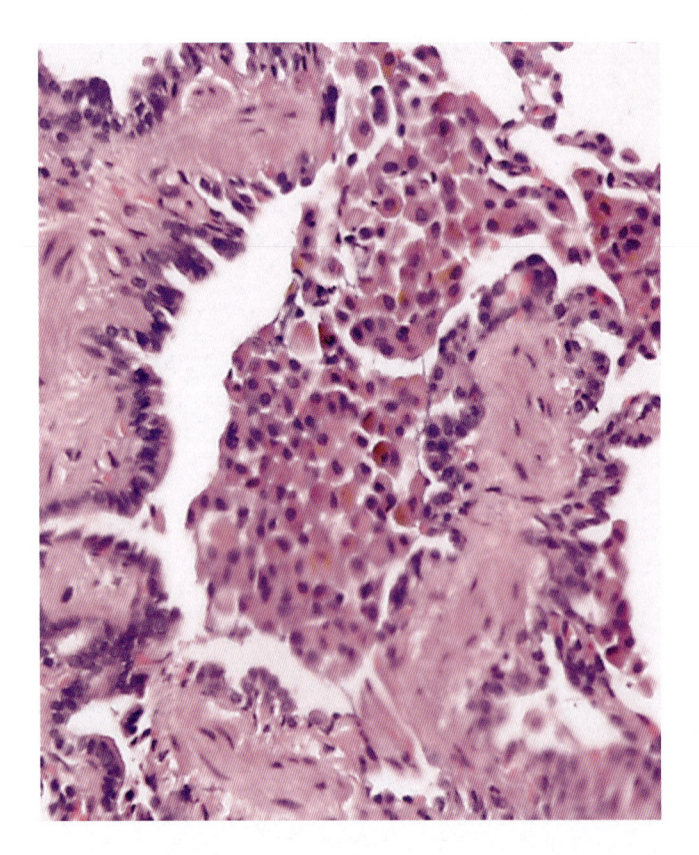

Figure 31.7: High power shows collection of macrophages containing smokers pigment within the lumen of a sampled bronchiole, a finding that is consistent with the diagnosis of respiratory bronchiolitis-associated interstitial lung disease in this patient.

Suggested Readings

Cagle PT. Respiratory bronchiolitis-associated interstitial lung disease/desquamative interstitial pneumonia. In: Cagle PT, ed. *Diagnostic Pulmonary Pathology*. New York: Marcel Dekker; 2000.

Glaspole IN, Wells AU, du Bois RM. Lung biopsy in diffuse parenchymal lung disease. *Monaldi Arch Chest Dis* 2001;56:225–232.

Haque A. Acute interstitial pneumonia. In: Cagle PT, ed. *Diagnostic Pulmonary Pathology*. New York: Marcel Dekker; 2000.

Laga A, Allen T, Cagle PT. Usual interstitial pneumonia. In: Cagle PT, ed. *Diagnostic Pulmonary Pathology*. New York: Marcel Dekker; 2000.

Leslie KO. Pathology of the idiopathic interstitial pneumonias. *Exp Lung Res* 2005;31:S23–40.

Poletti V, Chilosi M, Olivieri D. Diagnostic invasive procedures in diffuse infiltrative lung diseases. *Respiration* 2004;71:107–119.

Lymphangioleiomyomatosis

▶ Timothy C. Allen, MD, JD

Lymphangioleiomyomatosis is a rare disease characteristically found in women of childbearing age, presenting with shortness of breath, cough, recurrent pneumothoraces, and chylothorax. Patients demonstrate accumulation of atypical or immature smooth muscle cells along lung and pleural lymphatics. Lymph nodes in the mediastinum, abdomen, and lower cervical chain may also be involved. Clinical history and radiologic features are typically helpful in the diagnosis. Pathogenesis is unknown, and most patients die due to progressive respiratory failure within 10 years. Similar histologic findings occur in women with tuberous sclerosis, and approximately 30% of tuberous sclerosis patients have lymphangioleiomyomatosis.

Lymphangioleiomyomatosis is most frequently identified on wedge biopsy, but even then the lesions may be subtle and easily overlooked. Occasionally, though, lymphangioleiomyomatosis can be diagnosed on transbronchial biopsy. Characteristic lesions composed of a disorderly proliferation of atypical, spindled, or occasionally epithelioid smooth muscle cells involve alveolar septa, bronchioles, vessels, or lymphatic spaces. The smooth muscle cells may form nodules, with associated air trapping and cyst formation; and blood vessel involvement may cause hemorrhage with associated hemosiderin-laden macrophages. Any of these features may dominate the biopsy findings. When air trapping and cysts predominate and the smooth muscle proliferation is subtle, the findings may suggest emphysema.

If the diagnosis of lymphangioleiomyomatosis is clinically suspected, immunostains may help diagnose lymphangioleiomyomatosis when the transbronchial biopsy is without diagnostic features on hematoxylin and eosin (H&E) stain. HMB-45 selectively stains the abnormal smooth muscle cells but not normally occurring smooth muscle. Estrogen receptor, progesterone receptor, desmin, actin, and MART1 immunopositivity also may occur in the lesions.

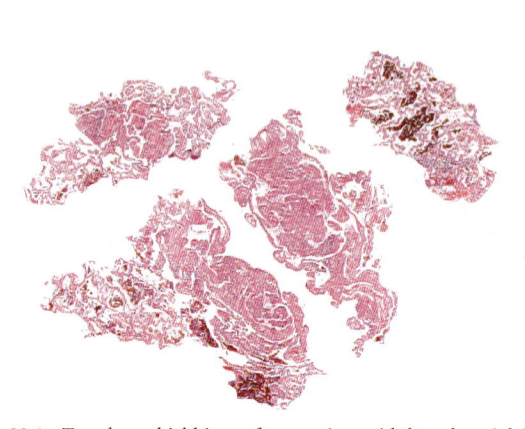

Figure 32.1: Transbronchial biopsy from patient with lymphangioleiomyomatosis at low power shows cyst-like spaces and thickened interstitium that consists of nodules of atypical smooth muscle cells on higher power.

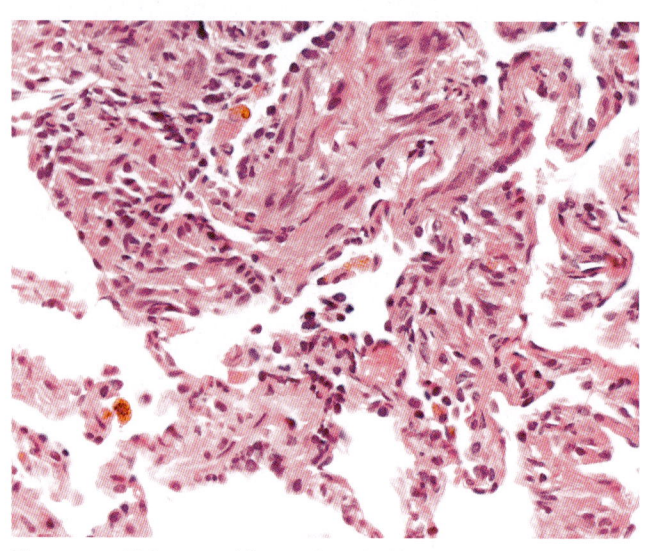

Figure 32.2: High power of the transbronchial biopsy shows atypical spindle cells in the interstitium in this patient with lymphangioleiomyomatosis.

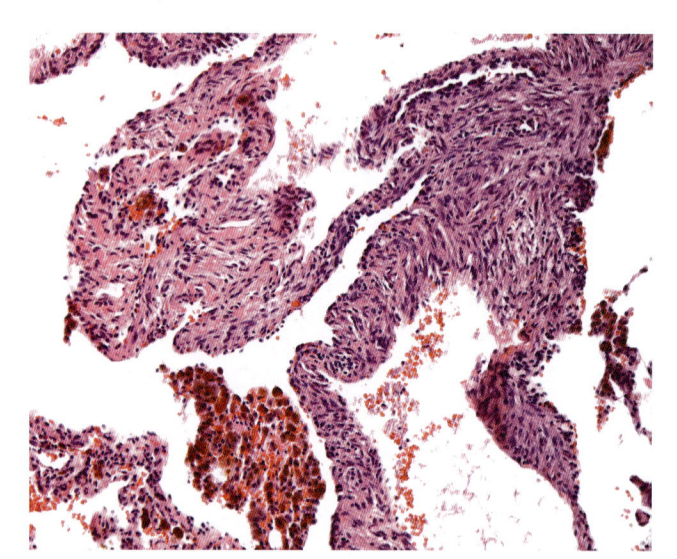

Figure 32.3: Medium high power of another portion of the transbronchial biopsy shows more cellular interstitial nodules of atypical spindle cells in patient with lymphangioleiomyomatosis.

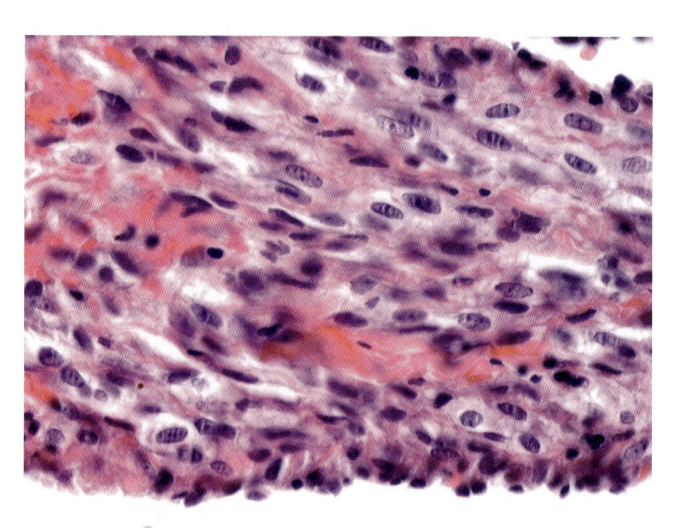

Figure 32.4: High power of a nodule of the atypical smooth muscle spindle cells in the transbronchial biopsy from a patient with lymphangioleiomyomatosis.

Suggested Readings

Delgrange E, Delgrange B, Wallon J, et al. Diagnostic approach to pulmonary lymphangioleiomyomatosis. *J Intern Med* 1994;236:461–464.

Jagirdar J. Lymphangioleiomyomatosis. In: Cagle PT, ed. *Color Atlas and Text of Pulmonary Pathology.* Philadelphia, Pa: Lippincott Williams & Wilkins; 2004.

Khoor A, Tazelaar HD. Pulmonary hemorrhage. In: Cagle PT, ed. *Color Atlas and Text of Pulmonary Pathology.* Philadelphia, Pa: Lippincott Williams & Wilkins; 2004.

Kitaichi M, Izumi T. Lymphangioleiomyomatosis. *Curr Opin Pulm Med* 1995;1:417–424.

Leslie KO, Gruden JF, Parish JM, et al. Transbronchial biopsy interpretation in the patient with diffuse parenchymal lung disease. *Arch Pathol Lab Med* 2007;131:407–423.

Naalsund A, Johansen B, Foerster A, et al. When to suspect and how to diagnose pulmonary lymphangioleiomyomatosis. *Respirology* 1996;1:207–212.

Pinkard NB. Enlarged Airspaces. In: Cagle PT, Ed. *Diagnostic Pulmonary Pathology.* New York: Marcel Dekker; 2000.

Intravenous Drug Abuse

▶ Timothy C. Allen, MD, JD

Intravenous injection of drugs meant for oral administration results in the deposition within lung capillaries, arterioles, or small to medium-size arteries of filler substances or tablet disintegrants, including talc, cornstarch, microcrystalline cellulose, and crospovidone. Talc or other powdery materials used to dilute, or cut, illicit drugs such as heroin can also deposit in the lung vasculature. As a result of the deposit of these foreign materials within the lung vasculature, angiothrombosis or foreign body granulomatous reaction can occur. Pulmonary hypertension is a rare result of long-term drug abuse most likely due to ongoing vascular obstruction.

In transbronchial biopsies from intravenous drug abusers, granulomatous inflammation or foreign body giant cell granulomas may be identified in the lumen and walls of capillaries and arterioles and occasionally in small to medium-size arteries. Granulomas may be found outside of the vasculature, and there may be variable amounts of fibrosis present. Multinucleated giant cells can contain polarizable crystalline foreign material (microcrystalline cellulose); polarizable round particles with a "Maltese cross" pattern (cornstarch); or irregular, platelike, approximately 0.5 to 50 μm polarizable foreign material (talc).

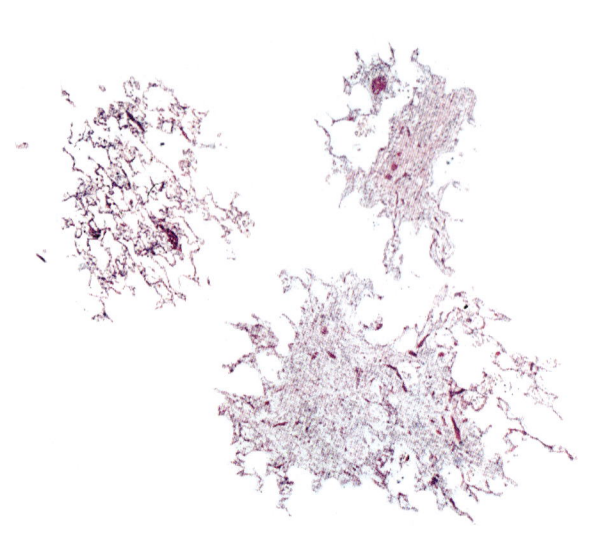

Figure 33.1: Transbronchial biopsy from an intravenous drug abuser shows areas of fibrosis at low power.

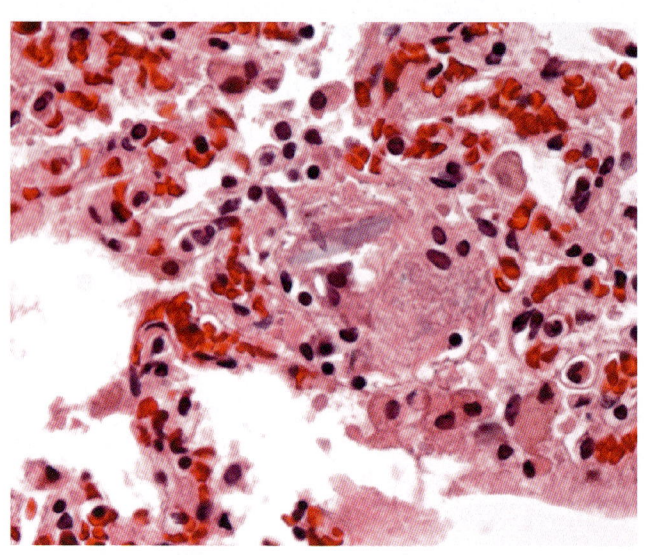

Figure 33.2: Foreign body granuloma containing an elongate platelike crystal and smaller irregular crystalline particles is present in the interstitium in this high power of a transbronchial biopsy from an intravenous drug abuser.

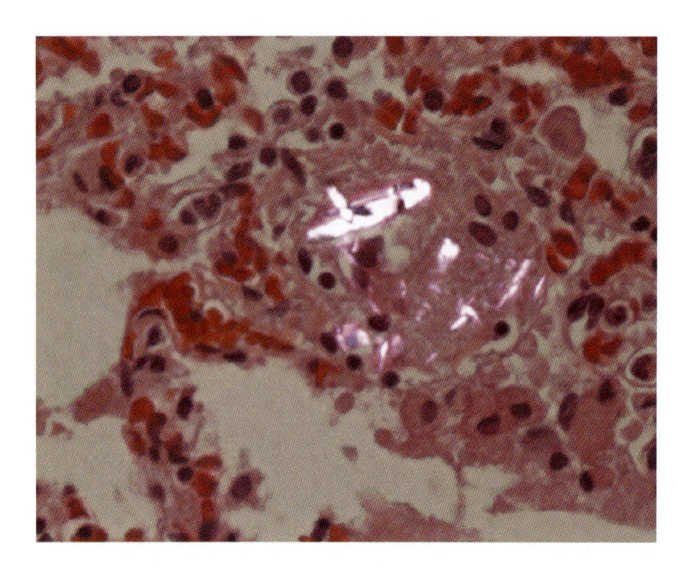

Figure 33.3: On polarized light, the crystalline material is brightly birefringent within the foreign body granuloma, consistent with talc or similar material injected intravenously and deposited in the lungs.

Suggested Readings

English JC. Pulmonary vascular lesions. In: Cagle PT, ed. *Color Atlas and Text of Pulmonary Pathology.* Philadelphia, Pa: Lippincott Williams & Wilkins; 2004.

Haque A, Bedrossian C. Foreign body granulomas. Part 1: Intravenous drug abuse. In: Cagle PT, ed. *Color Atlas and Text of Pulmonary Pathology.* Philadelphia, Pa: Lippincott Williams & Wilkins; 2004.

Laga AC, Allen T, Cagle PT. Intravenous drug abuse. In: Cagle PT, ed. *Color Atlas and Text of Pulmonary Pathology.* Philadelphia, Pa: Lippincott Williams & Wilkins; 2004.

Leslie KO, Gruden JF, Parish JM, et al. Transbronchial biopsy interpretation in the patient with diffuse parenchymal lung disease. *Arch Pathol Lab Med* 2007;131:407–423.

Langerhans Cell Histiocytosis

34

▶ Timothy C. Allen, MD, JD
▶ Philip T. Cagle, MD

More than 90% of cases of pulmonary Langerhans cell histiocytosis occur in cigarette smokers ranging from approximately 20 to 50 years of age. Men and women are about equally affected. The disease is probably underreported because many patients are asymptomatic and undergo spontaneous remission. About two thirds of patients present with symptoms attributable to smoking, such as dry cough, shortness of breath, and occasionally weight loss, fever, or night sweats; about 25% have no symptoms and are identified by abnormal routine chest radiographs; and about 10% to 20% present with spontaneous pneumothorax. Chest radiograph is often diagnostic and most commonly shows a pattern of reticulomicronodular infiltration involving both lungs, predominantly upper and middle lung fields with sparing of the costophrenic angles. Cysts are often identifiable within the infiltrates. With advanced disease, cyst formation is the most prominent radiologic feature. High-resolution computed tomography scan is typically incorporated into the patient's workup and gives additional radiographic detail such as small poorly delimited nodules. Most patients show resolution of disease after smoking cessation; however, a few patients develop widespread honeycombing and ultimately succumb to their disease.

Wedge biopsy is generally employed in diagnosing pulmonary Langerhans cell histiocytosis; however, transbronchial biopsy may be diagnostic, and diagnostic yield has been reported at between 10% and 40% for transbronchial biopsies. Disease begins around small airways with an interstitial infiltrate of Langerhans cells. With disease progression, temporally heterogeneous, roughly symmetrical stellate nodules develop from the smaller infiltrates. The nodules contain varying numbers of eosinophils, fibroblasts, lymphocytes, and Langerhans cells—medium to large cells with convoluted, elongated, or folded pale nuclei with one or several small nucleoli and abundant pale pink cytoplasm. Langerhans cells are characteristically immunopositive with CD1a and S-100 and immunonegative with CD68. A desquamative interstitial pneumonia (DIP)-like accumulation of pigmented macrophages often is present in airspaces adjacent to the nodules. The mixed inflammatory infiltrate may be associated with adjacent pigmented macrophages; however, fragmented biopsies may not be diagnostic. Disease progression causes cyst formation within nodules and central scarring, with loss of Langerhans cells with progression of disease. Older lesions may coalesce, and ultimately emphysematous-like changes and honeycombing result.

The diagnosis of pulmonary Langerhans cell histiocytosis on transbronchial biopsy requires clinical and radiographic correlation. Differential diagnosis includes a cellular neoplasm and organizing pneumonia. Because various inflammatory conditions may contain scattered CD1a-positive Langerhans cells, diagnosis should be based predominantly on the characteristic histologic features, with immunostains performed to support the diagnosis. Advanced lesions consist of less cellular scars, so they will likely have few Langerhans cells, and therefore the immunostains may not be useful in confirming an advanced scarred lesion.

Respiratory bronchiolitis-associated interstitial lung disease and DIP may contain areas of pigmented macrophages and occur in smokers, and caution must be used in differentiating these lesions from pulmonary Langerhans cell histiocytosis. Immunostains in these situations may be particularly helpful.

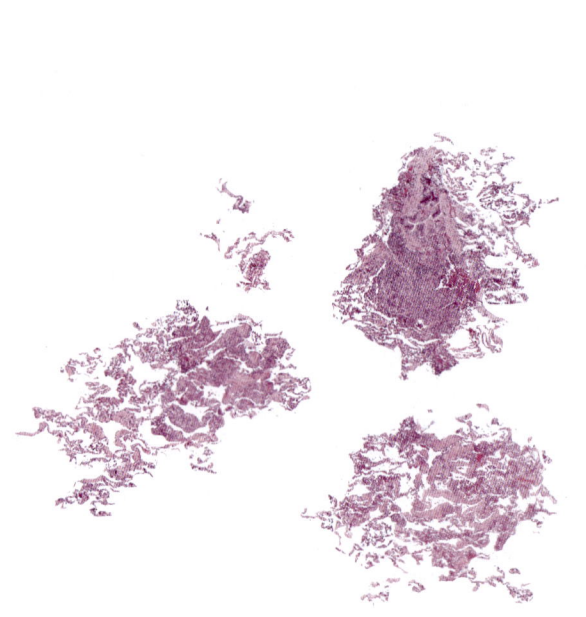

Figure 34.1: Transbronchial biopsy from patient with Langerhans cell histiocytosis shows irregular to stellate cellular nodules at low power.

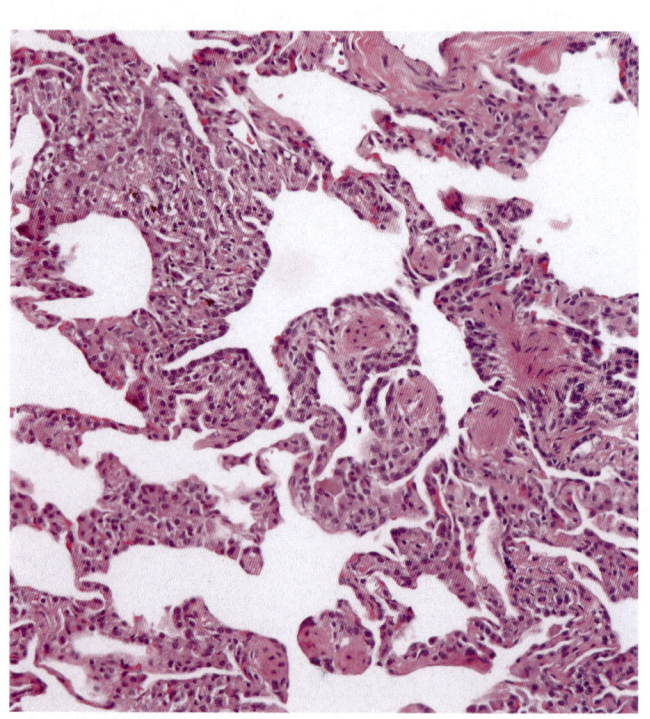

Figure 34.2: Medium power of one of the cellular nodules shows collections of mononuclear inflammatory cells including cells consistent with Langerhans cells surrounding a bronchiole, which can be identified by the focal bronchiolar epithelium and the presence of smooth muscle bundles.

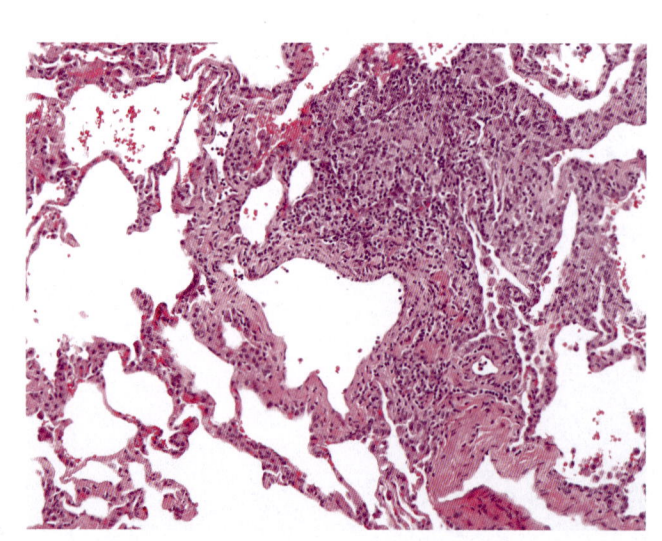

Figure 34.3: Medium power of one of the irregularly stellate cellular nodules composed of lymphocytes, Langerhans cells, fibroblasts, and a few scattered eosinophils.

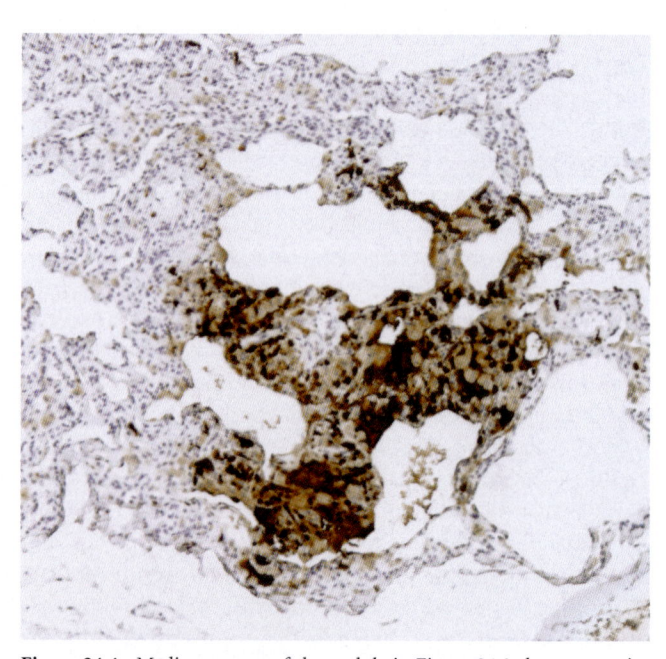

Figure 34.4: Medium power of the nodule in Figure 34.3 shows extensive immunopositivity for S-100 in the Langerhans cells consistent with pulmonary Langerhans cell histiocytosis.

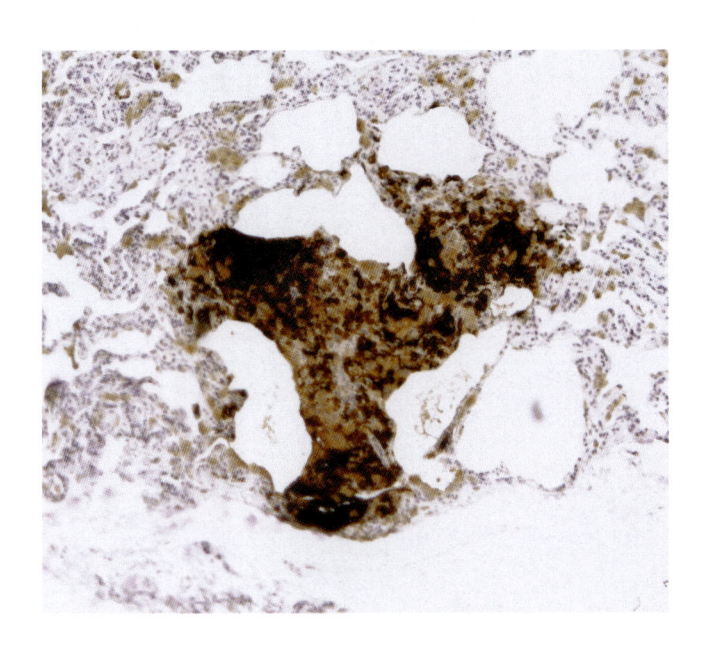

Figure 34.5: Medium power of the nodule in Figures 34.3 and 34.4 shows extensive immunopositivity for Cd1a in the Langerhans cells consistent with pulmonary Langerhans cell histiocytosis. As lesions mature, scarring develops and cellularity decreases, so the number of S-100-positive, Cd1a-positive Langerhans cells decreases and may be markedly decreased in advanced lesions.

Suggested Readings

Allen T, Ostrowski M. Pulmonary Langerhans cell histiocytosis. In: Cagle PT, ed. *Color Atlas and Text of Pulmonary Pathology.* Philadelphia, Pa: Lippincott Williams & Wilkins; 2004.

Guinee DG. Pulmonary eosinophilia. In: Cagle PT, ed. *Color Atlas and Text of Pulmonary Pathology.* Philadelphia, Pa: Lippincott Williams & Wilkins; 2004.

Leslie KO, Gruden JF, Parish JM, et al. Transbronchial biopsy interpretation in the patient with diffuse parenchymal lung disease. *Arch Pathol Lab Med* 2007;131:407–423.

Tazi A. Adult pulmonary Langerhans' cell histiocytosis. *Eur Respir J* 2006;27:1272–1285.

Vassallo R, Ryu JH. Pulmonary Langerhans' cell histiocytosis. *Clin Chest Med* 2004; 25:561–571.

Acute Transplant Rejection

35

▶ Anna Sienko, MD

Transbronchial biopsy is frequently used for evaluation of lung transplant recipients, both for scheduled routine follow-up, for diagnosis when the patient develops functional or radiologic changes, for frank illness, and for assessment of response to therapy. One of the most frequent uses of the transbronchial biopsy in lung transplant recipients is for the diagnosis of acute transplant rejection.

Acute allograft rejection is a cell-mediated process with characteristic perivascular infiltrate composed of T-cell lymphocytes. The classification of acute cellular rejection is based on the revised working formulation scheme. It relies primarily on a numerical grading system that evaluates the presence or absence of perivascular lymphocytic infiltrate in a perivascular distribution of single or multiple vessels and the presence or absence of associated lung parenchymal damage (A grade; graded depending on increasing severity of the lymphocytic infiltrate from "A0" to "A4"). Airway involvement can be seen as part of acute allograft rejection and is classified as "B grade" with a numerical grading scheme depending on the increasing severity of airway involvement from "B0" no airway inflammation, B1R low grade small airway inflammation, and B2R high grade small airway inflammation with "BX" indicating ungradable airway inflammation. A transbronchial biopsy with at least several pieces of alveolated lung parenchyma for evaluation can show no perivascular infiltrate (no rejection, grade A0); minimal rejection with a sparse perivascular infiltrate one or two cells thick, mild rejection (A1); an infiltrate that is usually just "cuffing" the vessels, usually more than several "lymphocytes thick" and visible at low power (A2); moderate rejection with lymphocytic infiltrate that also extends from around the vessels into the adjacent interstitium (A3); and severe rejection with perivascular infiltrates associated with lung injury with intra-alveolar fibrin and hyaline membrane formation (A4). Airway inflammation on transbronchial biopsy may show minimal or mild airway inflammation with rare mononuclear cells within bronchial or bronchiolar submucosa (B1R, encompassing previous grade of B1 and B2) with circumferential mononuclear cells within bronchial or bronchiolar submucosal eosinophils and few intraepithelial lymphocytes. Moderate to severe airway inflammation (B2R, encompassing previous grade of B3 and B4) consists of a dense mononuclear cell infiltrate containing many intraepithelial lymphocytes, epithelial cell apoptosis, and lymphocyte satellitosis. B2R high grade small airway infalmmation can also show features of epithelial detachment, fibrinopurulent exudate, and ulceration.

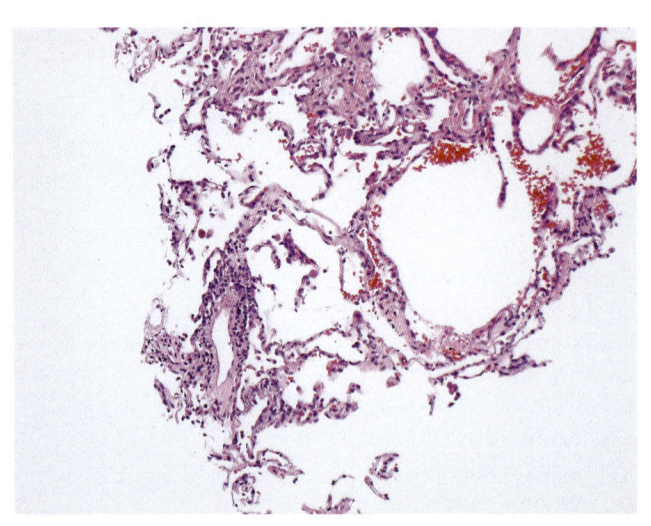

Figure 35.1: Medium power of transbronchial biopsy from lung transplant recipient shows minimal acute rejection (grade A1) with lymphocytes, about two lymphocytes thick cuffing a small blood vessel.

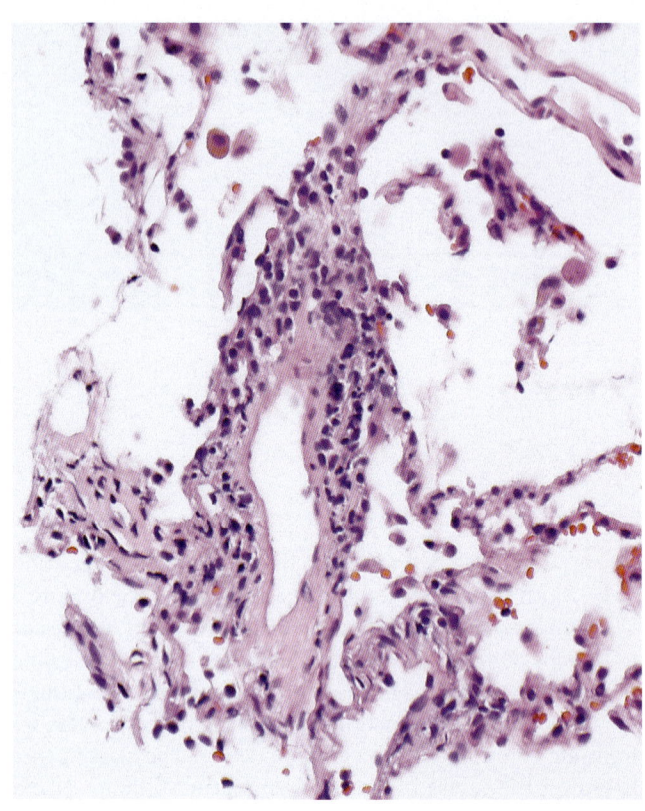

Figure 35.2: High power of the same transbronchial biopsy shows minimal acute rejection (grade A1) with lymphocytes, about two lymphocytes thick cuffing a small blood vessel.

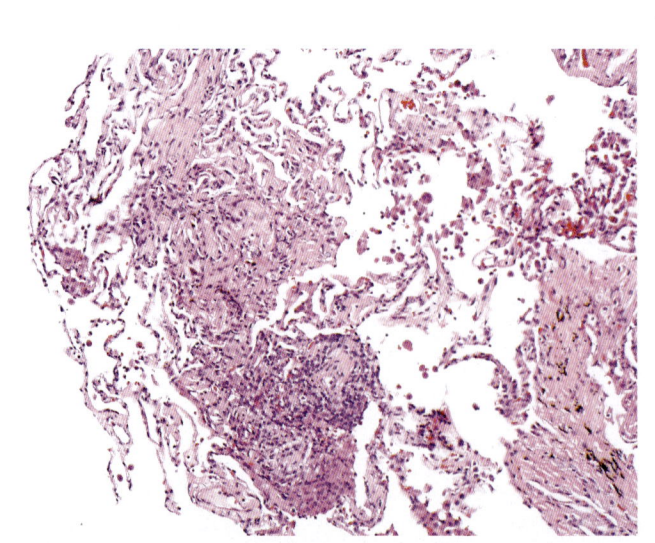

Figure 35.3: The perivascular lymphocytic infiltrates are readily seen cuffing a blood vessel in this low medium power of a transbronchial biopsy from a lung transplant recipient with mild acute rejection (grade A2).

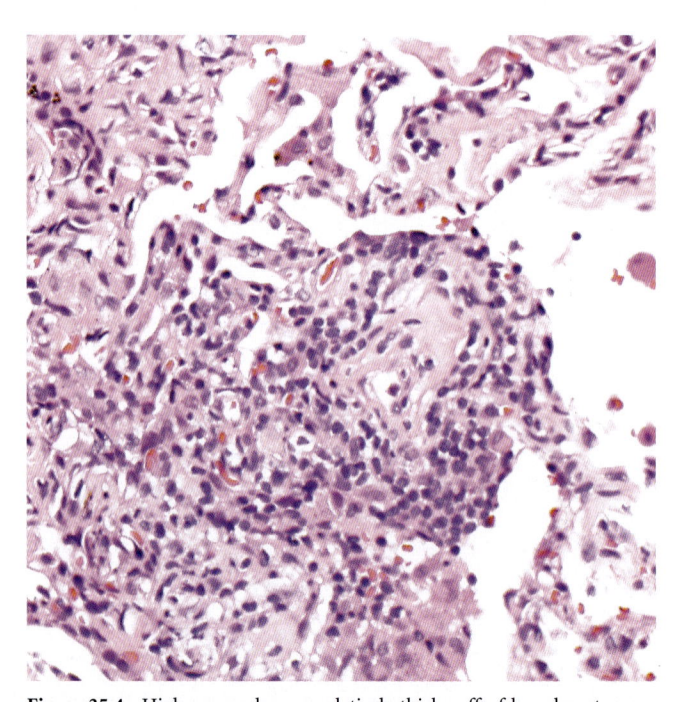

Figure 35.4: High power shows a relatively thick cuff of lymphocytes surrounding a blood vessel without extension into the adjacent interstitium in this transbronchial biopsy from a lung transplant recipient with mild acute rejection (grade A2).

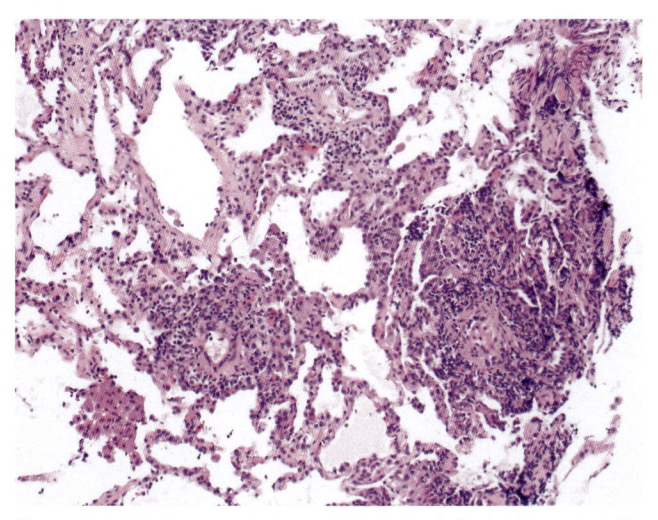

Figure 35.5: Medium power shows thick perivascular lymphocytic infiltrates extending into adjacent alveolar septa in a transbronchial biopsy from a lung transplant recipient with moderate acute rejection (grade A3).

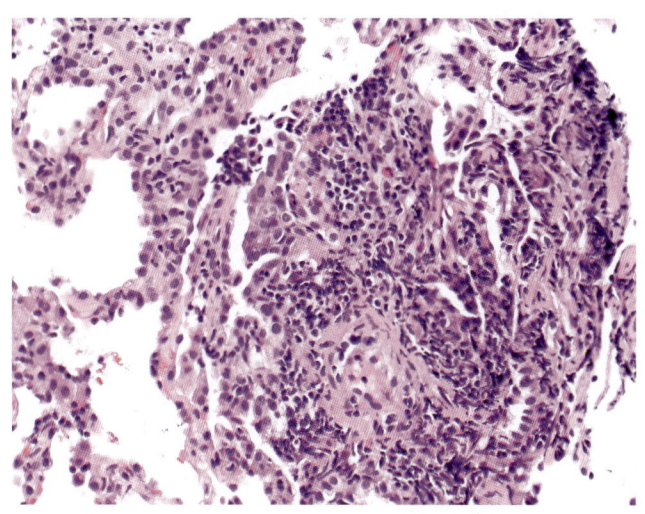

Figure 35.6: High power of the perivascular infiltrate of moderate acute rejection (grade A3) shows a predominantly lymphocytic infiltrate with some plasma cells and a few eosinophils.

Suggested Readings

Glanville AR. The role of bronchoscopic surveillance monitoring in the care of lung transplant recipients. *Semin Respir Crit Care Med* 2006;27:480–491.

Knoop C, Estenne M. Acute and chronic rejection after lung transplantation. *Semin Repir Crit Care Med* 2006;27:521–533.

Marboe CC. Pathology of lung transplantation. *Semin Diagn Pathol* 2007;24:188–198.

Stewart S, Winters GL, Fishbein MC, et al. Revision of the 1996 working formulation for the standardization of nomenclature in the diagnosis of lung rejection. *J Heart Lung Transplant* 2007; 26:1229–1242.

Other Transplant Associated Pathology

▶ Anna Sienko, MD
▶ Philip T. Cagle, MD

In addition to acute rejection, transbronchial biopsy is typically used for lung transplant recipients for diagnosis of opportunistic infections (cytomegalovirus, *Pneumocystis*, etc.), which are discussed in their respective separate chapters. Occasionally, acute rejection and infection may coexist in the same patient and both may be sampled in the same transbronchial biopsy. Some features traditionally associated with infection such as organizing pneumonia are now also thought to occasionally be features of acute rejection, further complicating interpretation of transbronchial biopsies. Correlation with the clinical findings may be very helpful in these situations.

In addition to acute rejection and infection, other histopathologic findings may be seen in transbronchial biopsies from lung transplant recipients. Chronic rejection is a transplant-associated pathology that is potentially diagnosable by transbronchial biopsy. Chronic rejection can be seen months to years posttransplant and is characterized by an obliterative bronchiolitis with inflammation of small airways with fibrosis resulting in complete luminal occlusion. The histopathologic diagnosis of chronic rejection requires sampling of a bronchiole by the bronchoscopist, which does not always occur with every biopsy. Clinicians may also make a diagnosis of bronchiolitis obliterans syndrome on a clinical basis. The finding of intra-alveolar macrophages is suggestive of small airways obstruction when a bronchiole is not sampled on the transbronchial biopsy.

Various other conditions can be potentially sampled on a transbronchial (or endobronchial) biopsy. Accelerated vascular arteriosclerosis is usually seen in long-term transplant patients who develop patchy arteriosclerosis of large and small vessels with narrowing of lumens due to fibrointimal and myointimal proliferation, concentric intimal sclerosis of veins, and arteriosclerotic plaque formation. Primary graft failure, which is usually seen within 3 days of transplant, is an acute lung injury syndrome resulting from ischemia-reperfusion injury and characterized by patchy or diffuse formation of hyaline membranes, interstitial edema, and organization (diffuse alveolar damage, or DAD). Anastomotic complications can be seen with necrosis of bronchial mucosa, submucosa, and cartilage. Thrombus formation, granulation tissue formation with mucosal ulceration, and fibrosis of submucosa can also be seen with anastomotic complications. Rarely hyperacute rejection can occur within minutes to hours posttransplant and is often fatal. Biopsy tissue shows edema, hyaline membrane formation, intra-alveolar hemorrhage, fibrin thrombi, and foci of necrosis of septa and bronchiolar mucosa.

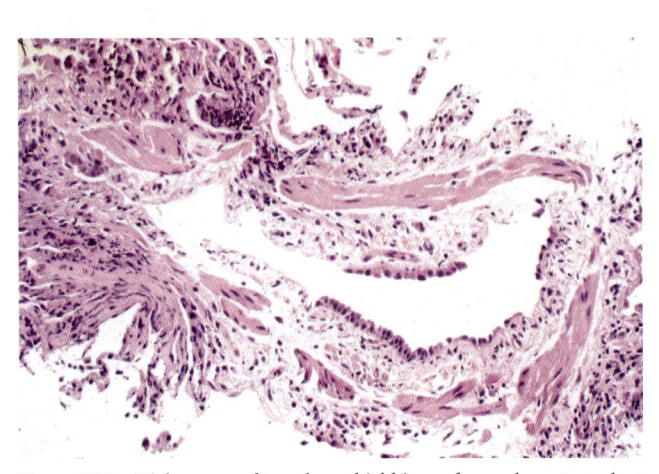

Figure 36.1: High power of transbronchial biopsy from a lung transplant recipient shows sampling of a bronchiole that has circumferential submucosal fibrosis. The submucosal fibrous tissue is immature with myxoid stroma. A diagnosis of obliterative bronchiolitis consistent with chronic rejection was made.

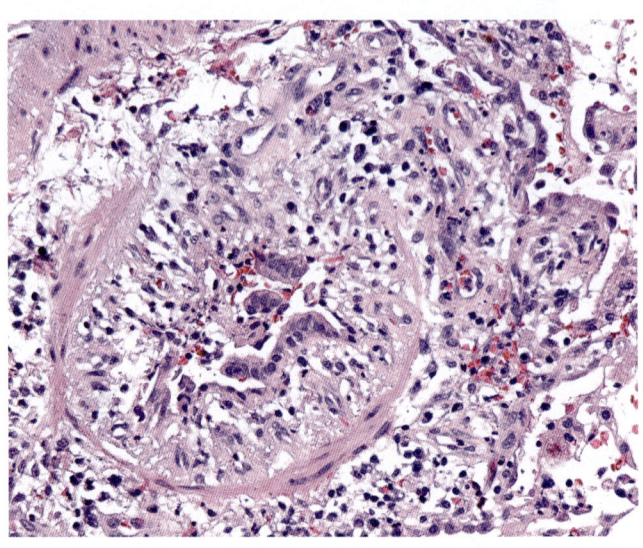

Figure 36.2: High power shows nearly complete obliteration of a bronchiolar lumen by immature submucosal fibrous tissue consistent with chronic rejection.

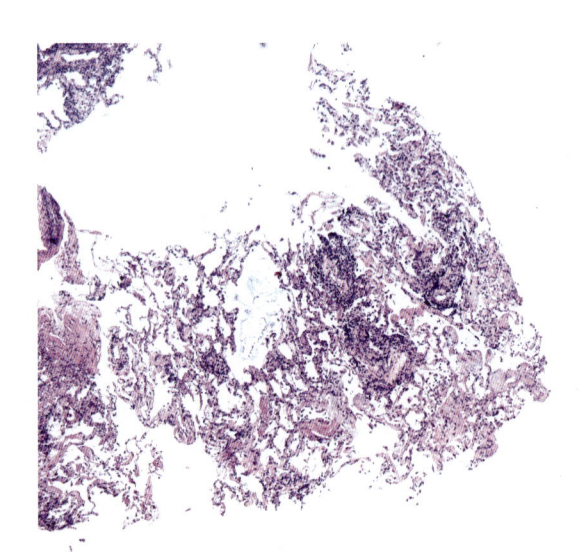

Figure 36.3: Low power of a transbronchial biopsy from a lung transplant recipient shows perivascular lymphocytic infiltrates with extension into adjacent alveolar septa consistent with grade 3 acute rejection. In addition, there are foci of intra-alveolar granulation tissue or organizing pneumonia. In this setting, the organizing pneumonia could be due to a simultaneous infection, an additional manifestation of acute rejection, or possibly some other etiology such as a drug reaction. Clinical correlation may be helpful in determining the most likely cause of the organizing pneumonia.

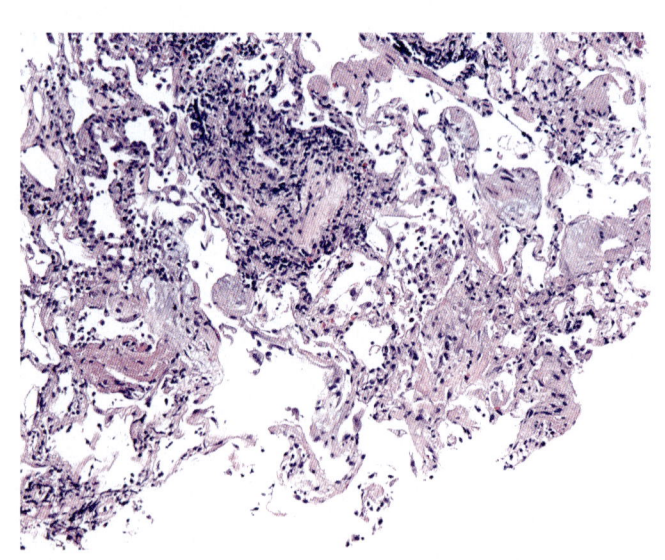

Figure 36.4: Higher power of the biopsy in Figure 36.3 shows the grade 3 acute rejection and adjacent foci of intra-alveolar granulation tissue with focal organizing fibrin.

Suggested Readings

Alalawi R, Whelan T, Bajwa RS, et al. Lung transplantation and interstitial lung disease. *Curr Opin Pulm Med* 2005;11:461–466.

Avery RK. Infections after lung transplantation. *Semin Respir Crit Care Med* 2006;27:544–551.

Corris PA. Lung transplantation. Bronchiolitis obliterans syndrome. *Chest Surg Clin N Am* 2003;13:543–557.

Frost AE. Bronchiolitis obliterans: the Achilles heel of lung transplantation. *Verh K Acad Geneeskd Belg* 2002;64:303–319; discussion 319–322.

Glanville AR. The role of bronchoscopic surveillance monitoring in the care of lung transplant recipients. *Semin Respir Crit Care Med* 2006;27:480–491.

Hummel M, Muller J, Dandel M, et al. Surveillance biopsies in heart and lung transplantation. *Transplant Proc* 2002;34:1860–1863.

Kubak BM. Fungal infection in lung transplantation. *Tranpl Infect Dis* 2002;4:S24–31.

Stewart S. Pulmonary infections in transplantation pathology. *Arch Pathol Lab Med* 2007;131:1219–1231.

Wahidi MM, Ernst A. The role of bronchoscopy in the management of lung transplantation recipients. *Respir Care Clin N Am* 2004;10:549–562.

Whelan TP, Hertz MI. Allograft rejection after lung transplantation. *Clin Chest Med* 2005;26:599–612, vi.

Nonneoplastic Large Airways Pathology

37

▸ Timothy C. Allen, MD, JD
▸ Jaishree Jagirdar, MD
▸ Keith M. Kerr, FRCPath

Endobronchial and transbronchial biopsy are used to diagnose neoplasms and infections involving the large airways, and these diseases were discussed in previous chapters. A few special nonneoplastic conditions of the large airways are mentioned here. Additional conditions involving the large airways are discussed in the pediatric disease chapters.

Asthma and Chronic Bronchitis

Asthma is a chronic inflammatory disorder involving both large and small airways associated with airway obstruction that is reversible either spontaneously or with treatment. Its incidence has increased over the last two decades. Asthma is diagnosed clinically, and traditionally, the surgical pathologist is not asked to diagnose asthma by examining tissue. However, characteristic histopathologic changes occur as a result of asthma. Therefore, the surgical pathologist will not receive a transbronchial biopsy for the specific purpose of diagnosing asthma but may encounter histopathologic changes due to asthma in a transbronchial biopsy performed for infection or other reasons. The pathologist should recognize the findings of asthma so they are not interpreted as some other type of pathologic process. On endobronchial or transbronchial biopsy, airway inflammation is the primary feature of asthma. Bronchial walls contain a mixed inflammatory infiltrate with a preponderance of eosinophils, hyperplastic bronchial and bronchiolar smooth muscle, basement membrane thickening, and goblet cell metaplasia within bronchial and bronchiolar epithelium. Transbronchial biopsy may show significant inflammation within surrounding alveolar septa.

Chronic bronchitis is clinically defined as persistent cough accompanied by sputum production lasting at least 3 months over at least 2 consecutive years, not attributable to another lung or heart condition. Chronic bronchitis, along with emphysema and obstructive bronchiolitis, are the three morphologic forms of chronic obstructive pulmonary disease (COPD), and they often present as a combination in individual patients. Mucus hypersecretion is a feature of the disease. The pathogenesis of chronic bronchitis involves chronic irritation by inhaled substances and microbiologic infections. The primary cause of chronic bronchitis is cigarette smoking.

As with asthma, chronic bronchitis is a clinical diagnosis, and the pathologist will not be asked to diagnose chronic bronchitis by examining tissue. However, similar to asthma, chronic bronchitis produces characteristic histopathologic changes, and these may be encountered on transbronchial biopsy performed for exacerbation of symptoms or to rule out infection or malignancy. Histologically, chronic bronchitis exhibits enlargement of mucus-secreting glands within the trachea and bronchi, increased inflammatory cells, specifically lymphocytes, and goblet cell metaplasia within bronchial and bronchiolar walls. Increased bronchial smooth muscle may arise in bronchial walls, and squamous metaplasia and dysplasia may be found in bronchial mucosa. The basement membrane thickness is within the normal range. Submucosal bronchial gland enlargement is an important feature of chronic bronchitis, and the Reid index assists in its evaluation. The Reid index, the calculated ratio of submucosal gland layer thickness to total airway wall thickness, from epithelium base to inner cartilage surface, is generally >0.5. The normal Reid index is 0.3.

Asthma and chronic bronchitis share many histologic features; however, the thickening of the basement membrane with asthma, and the normal range of its thickness with chronic bronchitis, is a key difference between these diseases histologically. Nonetheless, a study by Bourdin et al. found that routine analyses of endobronchial biopsy specimens, performed in the hope of discriminating between the two diseases in complicated cases such as smokers with asthma, do not appreciably assist in differentiating between these diseases.

Tracheobronchial Amyloidosis

Tracheobronchial amyloidosis, along with nodular amyloidosis (amyloid tumor) and diffuse alveolar-septal amyloidosis, is one of three patterns of respiratory tract involvement in this rare condition. The tracheobronchial form is generally limited to the submucosa of the trachea and major bronchi but may be found in smaller segmental airways. There may be diffuse thickening and nodularity of the airway mucosa or a more localized nodule or plaque that may obstruct an airway, mimicking a tumor at endoscopy.

Patients, mostly 60 to 70 years of age, are generally symptomatic with dyspnea and cough; hemoptysis is rarely reported. Most of these cases are localized primary amyloidosis, and although around 10% may show serum or urinary monoclonal proteins, associated lymphoproliferative disorders are uncommon.

Bronchial biopsies show an irregular deposition of amorphous, hyaline eosinophilic material in the connective tissues of the submucosa. This may show localized clumping with nodule formation. Deposition may be accentuated around blood vessels and bronchial glands, cuffing the latter in a ring of eosinophilic homogenous deposit. In general the submucosa is relatively paucicellular, but there may be lymphocytes, macrophages, plasma cells, and even multinucleated giant cells admixed with the amyloid. Osseous metaplasia may occur. The Congo Red stain is most useful for identifying the amyloid nature of the eosinophilic deposits, giving the amyloid protein a deep orange or reddish hue when viewed by ordinary light, and more specifically showing (apple-green) birefringence during polarizing microscopy.

Immunohistochemistry may be used as a supplement to diagnosis but is not necessary. Most tracheobronchial amyloid is AL-type protein, although some cases may demonstrate AA or ATTR (transthyretin) types.

Differential diagnosis includes light chain deposition disease, a carcinoid tumor stroma, basement membrane thickening in asthma or as a cross-cutting artifact, and tracheobronchopathia osteochondroplastica.

Relapsing Polychondritis

Relapsing polychondritis, a rare, chronic, systemic, immunologically mediated inflammatory disease involving the trachea and central bronchi, is characterized by recurrent widespread inflammatory lesions with progressive distortion of cartilaginous structures at these sites, ultimately causing their destruction. Other sites are frequently involved, including nose, glottis, external and middle ears, and joints. About a fourth of relapsing polychondritis patients also have another connective tissue disease. Patients generally present with painful joints, nose, or ears, and variable pulmonary expiratory and inspiratory obstruction is identified on pulmonary function testing. Impaired clearance of inflammatory debris from the airways and ineffective cough due to upper airway collapse cause bronchial obstruction. Infections, often mycobacterial or fungal, occur in up to a third of patients. Destruction and distortion of airways may ultimately cause bronchiectasis. Treatment revolves around maintaining adequate ventilation, and patients usually die due

Chapter 37 • Nonneoplastic Large Airways Pathology

to collapse of tracheal and bronchial rings after repeated bouts of inflammation, edema, destruction, and scarring of these structures. Patients with airway involvement are thought to have a worse prognosis, and early diagnosis of airway involvement is important because early aggressive treatment may delay or prevent irreversible cartilaginous destruction.

Microscopically, biopsy shows an inflammatory infiltrate of lymphocytes, plasma cells, and neutrophils within cartilage and pericartilaginous tissue. Granulation tissue, fibrosis, and cartilage destruction subsequently occur. Differential diagnosis includes other diseases for which cartilage destruction is a feature, such as granulomatous infections, bronchiectasis, and Wegener granulomatosis. Clinical history of disease involving other sites and history of recurrent disease are helpful in making an accurate diagnosis.

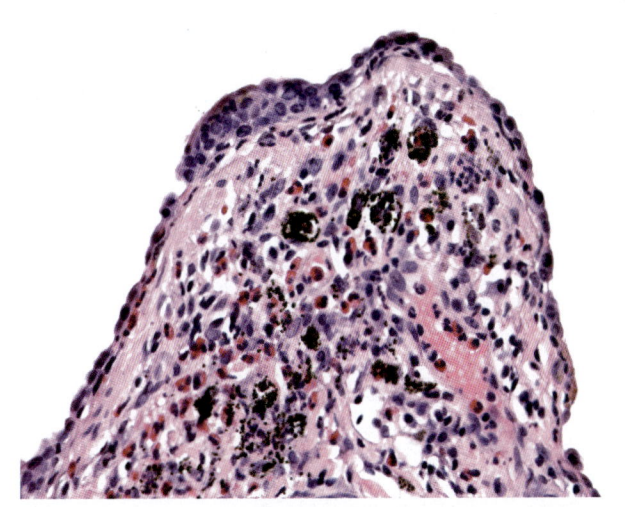

Figure 37.1: Transbronchial biopsy from a patient known to have asthma. The biopsy was not performed to diagnose asthma, but the bronchus shows submucosal infiltrates of eosinophils mixed with mononuclear cells, which is consistent with the patient's clinical history of asthma. The basement membrane is not noticeably thickened in this biopsy. The respiratory epithelium shows squamous metaplasia.

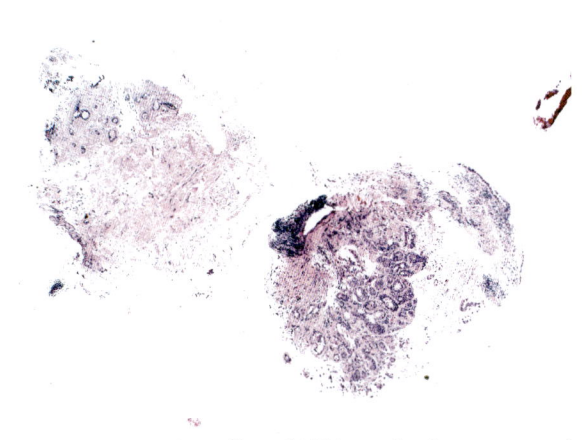

Figure 37.2: Low power view of bronchial biopsy showing two mucosal fragments from a patient with tracheobronchial amyloidosis.

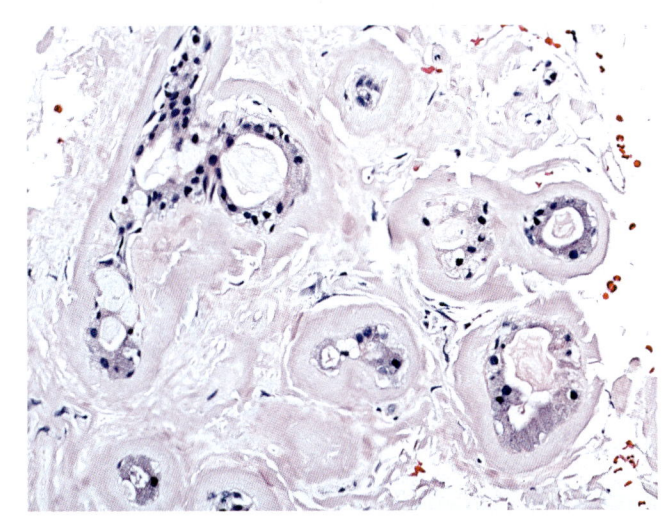

Figure 37.3: High power view of field at 10 o'clock in left-hand fragment in Figure 37.2. The amyloid deposits around the bronchial glands form an eosinophilic hyaline band around each acinus.

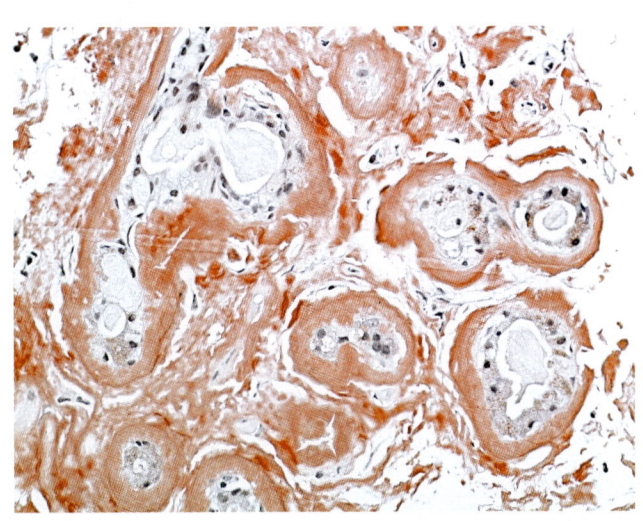

Figure 37.4: Congo Red stain shows deep orange/red staining of the amyloid deposits. Same field as Figure 37.3.

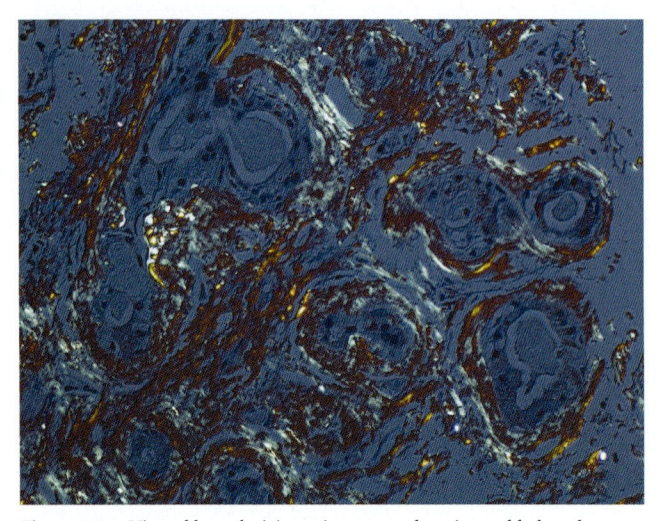

Figure 37.5: Viewed by polarizing microscopy, there is speckled apple-green birefringence in the amyloid deposits. Same field as Figure 37.4.

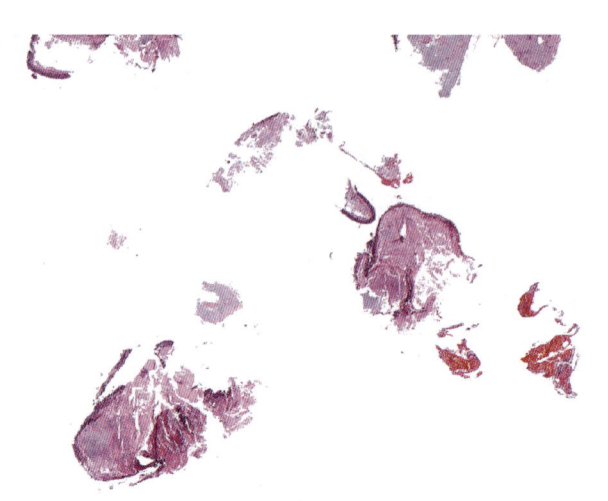

Figure 37.6: Low power of endobronchial biopsy from patient with relapsing polychondritis shows fragments with necrotic cartilage.

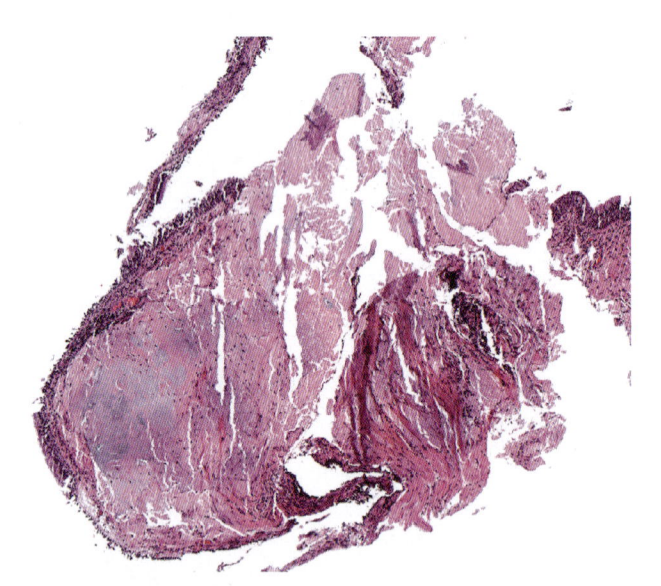

Figure 37.7: Medium power shows one of the endobronchial fragments with necrotic cartilage consistent with the diagnosis of relapsing polychondritis.

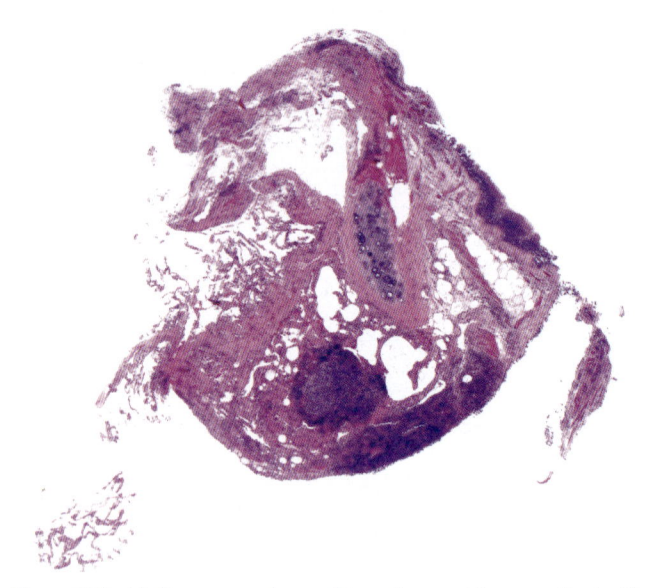

Figure 37.8: Medium power shows a biopsy fragment from a patient with relapsing polychondritis shows an inflammatory infiltrate and fibrosis.

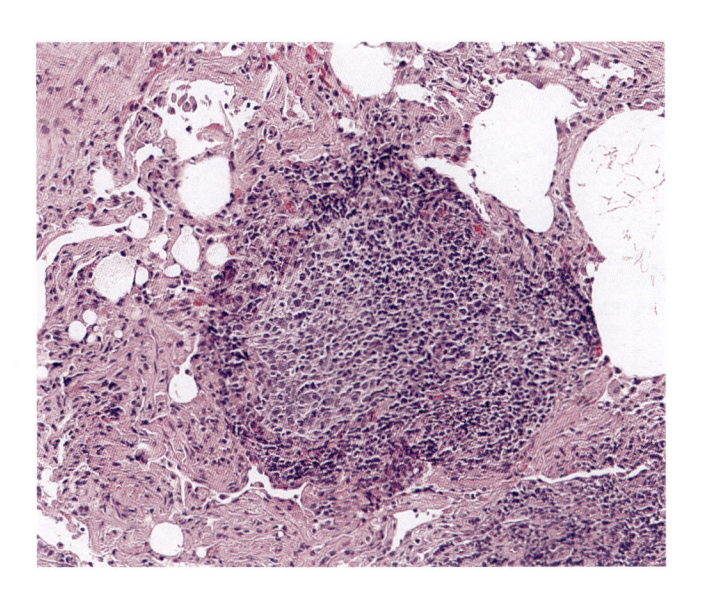

Figure 37.9: High power view of Figure 37.8 shows a lymphoid follicle and a mixed inflammatory cell infiltrate must prominent in the lower right.

Suggested Readings

Asthma and Chronic Bronchitis

Balzar S, Wenzel SE, Chu HW. Transbronchial biopsy as a tool to evaluate small airways in asthma. *Eur Respir J* 2002;20:254–259.

Bourdin A, Seer I, Flamme H, et al. Can endobronchial biopsy analysis be recommended to discriminate between asthma and COPD in routine practice? *Thorax* 2004;59: 488–493.

Hattotuwa K, Gamble EA, O'Shaughnessy T, et al. Safety of bronchoscopy, biopsy, and BAL in research patients with COPD. *Chest* 2002;122:1909–1912.

Laga AC, Allen T, Cagle PT. Asthma. In: Cagle PT, ed. *Color Atlas and Text of Pulmonary Pathology.* Philadelphia, Pa: Lippincott Williams & Wilkins; 2004.

Laga AC, Allen T, Cagle PT. Chronic bronchitis. In: Cagle PT, ed. *Color Atlas and Text of Pulmonary Pathology.* Philadelphia, Pa: Lippincott Williams & Wilkins; 2004.

Sutherland ER, Martin RJ, Bowler RP, et al. Physiologic correlations of distal lung inflammation in asthma. *J Allergy Clin Immunol* 2004;113:1046–1050.

Szilasi M, Donlinay T, Nemes Z, et al. Pathology of chronic obstructive pulmonary disease. *Pathol Oncol Res* 2006;12:52–60.

Tracheobronchial Amyloidosis

Berk JL, O'Regan A, Skinner M. Pulmonary and tracheobronchial amyloidosis. *Semin Respir Crit Care Med* 2002;23:155–165.

Cordier JF, Loire R, Brune J. Amyloidosis of the lower respiratory tract. Clinical and pathologic features in a series of 21 patients. *Chest* 1986;90:827–831.

Hui AN, Koss MN, Hochholzer L, et al. Amyloidosis presenting in the lower respiratory tract. Clinicopathologic, radiologic, immunohistochemical, and histochemical studies on 48 cases. *Arch Pathol Lab Med* 1986;110:212–218.

Pitz MW, Gibson IW, Johnston JB. Isolated pulmonary amyloidosis: Case report and review of the literature. *Am J Haematol* 2006;81:212–213.

Toyoda M, Ebihara Y, Kato H, et al. Tracheobronchial amyloidosis: histologic, immunohistochemical, ultrastructural and immunoelectron microscopic observations. *Hum Pathol* 1993;24:970–976.

Utz JP, Swensen SJ, Gertz MA. Pulmonary amyloidosis: the Mayo Clinic experience from 1980 to 1993. *Ann Intern Med* 1996;124:407–413.

Relapsing Polychondritis

Lee KS, Ernst A, Trentham DE, et al. Relapsing polychondritis: prevalence of expiratory CT airway abnormalities. *Radiology* 2006;240:565–573.

Lee-Chiong TL Jr. Pulmonary manifestations of ankylosing spondylitis and relapsing polychondritis. *Clin Chest Med* 1998;19:747–757.

Letko E, Zarirakis P, Baltatzis S, et al. Relapsing polychondritis: a clinical review. *Semin Arthritis Rheumatism* 2002;31:384–395.

Prince JS, Duhamel DR, Levin DL, et al. Nonneoplastic lesions of the tracheobronchial wall: radiologic findings with bronchoscopic correlation. *Radiographics* 2002;22: S215–230.

Role of Transbronchial and Endobronchial Biopsies in Children

▶ Megan K. Dishop, MD

Transbronchial and endobronchial biopsy have been performed in children and adolescents since the 1980s, with technical advances since 1995 allowing routine biopsy in infants and small children via a pediatric flexible bronchoscope. These biopsy procedures are now performed safely and routinely in pediatric lung transplant recipients for surveillance of rejection and other complications of transplantation. Outside of this clinical setting, however, transbronchial and endobronchial biopsies are performed infrequently in children and adolescents as compared with adults. In a 5-year experience at Texas Children's Hospital, a total of 358 biopsy procedures were performed at bronchoscopy, excluding biopsy of focal endobronchial lesions. Of these biopsies, 338 (94.4%) were performed in lung transplant recipients (57 patients) and only 20 (5.6%) were performed for other indications. The 20 biopsy procedures in non–lung transplant recipients included 11 transbronchial biopsy (TBB) only, 7 endobronchial biopsy (EBB) only, and 2 with both TBB and EBB. Indications included evaluation of infection, graft-versus-host disease and obliterative bronchiolitis in bone marrow transplant recipients, micronodular or suspected granulomatous disease (e.g., sarcoidosis, infection, hypersensitivity pneumonia), evaluation of mucus plugs and/or bronchiectasis, and, rarely, interstitial lung disease. A large series from the University of Florida included 38 pediatric TBBs from non–lung transplant patients over a 7-year period. These biopsies were considered diagnostic in 58%, contributory to diagnosis in 21%, and noncontributory to diagnosis in 21%. Adequacy and diagnostic yield were greater with use of the adult-size biopsy forceps compared with the pediatric equipment. In another study of the diagnostic evaluation of immunocompetent children with chronic interstitial lung disease, transbronchial biopsy was chosen as the first-line diagnostic procedure in 6 of 30 patients (20%) with lung biopsy. TBB using an adult bronchoscope yielded a specific diagnosis in three of six patients (50%; two sarcoidosis, one bronchiolitis obliterans), with subsequent diagnosis in the remaining three by open or thoracoscopic biopsy.

Although TBB may yield useful diagnostic information in selected circumstances, wedge biopsy by open or thoracoscopic procedure is generally preferred in the diagnosis of pediatric interstitial lung disease due to the importance of evaluating lung architecture and development, particularly in infants and young children. Evaluation of the pulmonary vasculature also necessitates wedge biopsy, for example, in children with vasculopathy secondary to congenital heart disease, lymphangiectasia, persistent pulmonary hypertension of the newborn, and idiopathic pulmonary hypertension in older children. Due to its greater diagnostic sensitivity, wedge biopsy may be chosen over transbronchial biopsy for diagnosis of entities with more subtle or focal diagnostic characteristics, for example, vasculitis in pulmonary hemorrhage syndromes, alveolar proteinosis and cholesterol clefts in genetic disorders of surfactant metabolism, and poorly formed granulomas in hypersensitivity pneumonitis. Hyperinflation in cystic fibrosis patients is also considered a relative contraindication to TBB due to the risk of pneumothorax, and wedge biopsy may be preferable in that clinical setting.

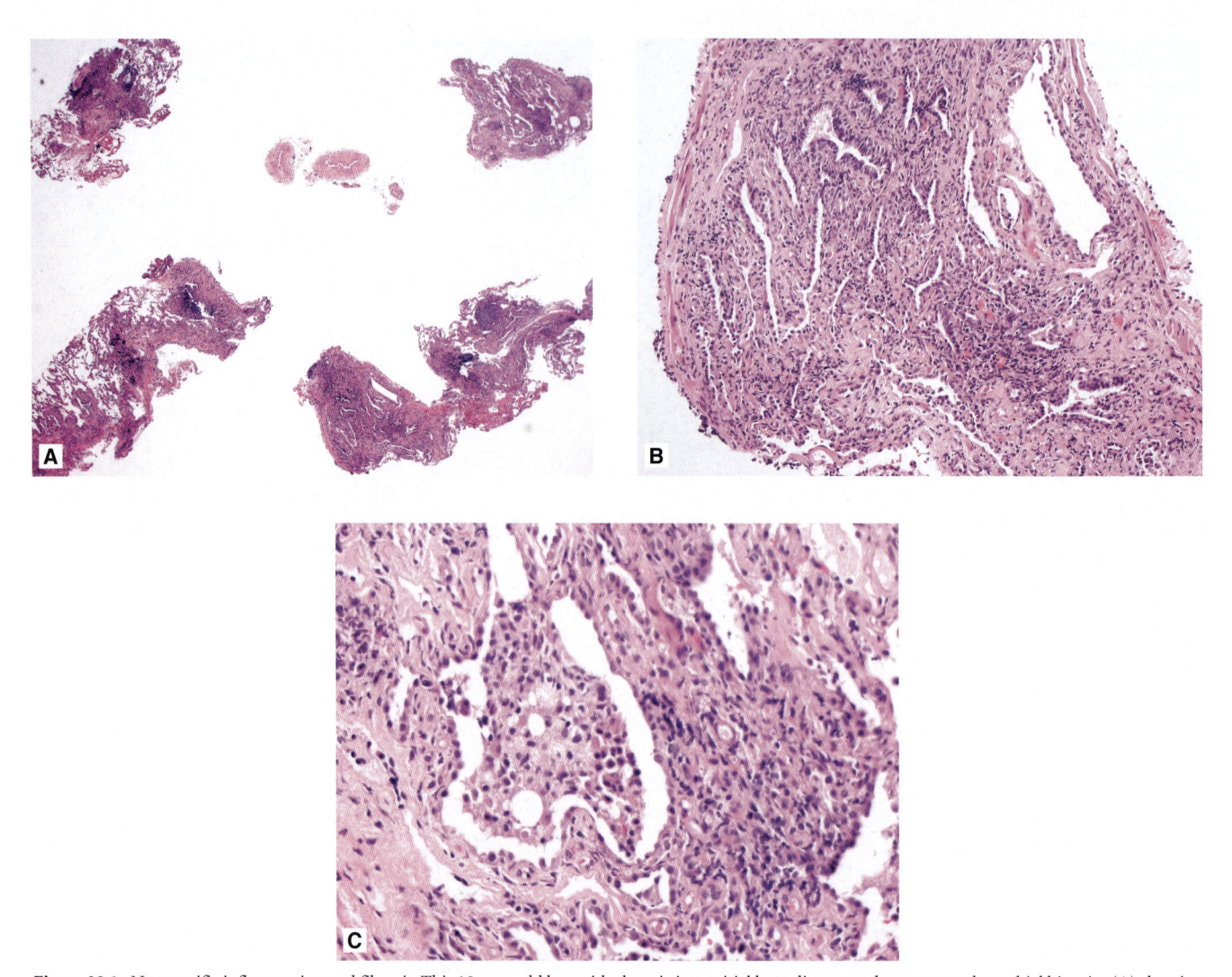

Figure 38.1: Nonspecific inflammation and fibrosis. This 10-year-old boy with chronic interstitial lung disease underwent transbronchial biopsies (A) showing patchy lymphocytic inflammation and mild fibrosis in the interstitium, as well as accumulation of foamy macrophages in some airspaces (B, C). Specific etiology remains undetermined.

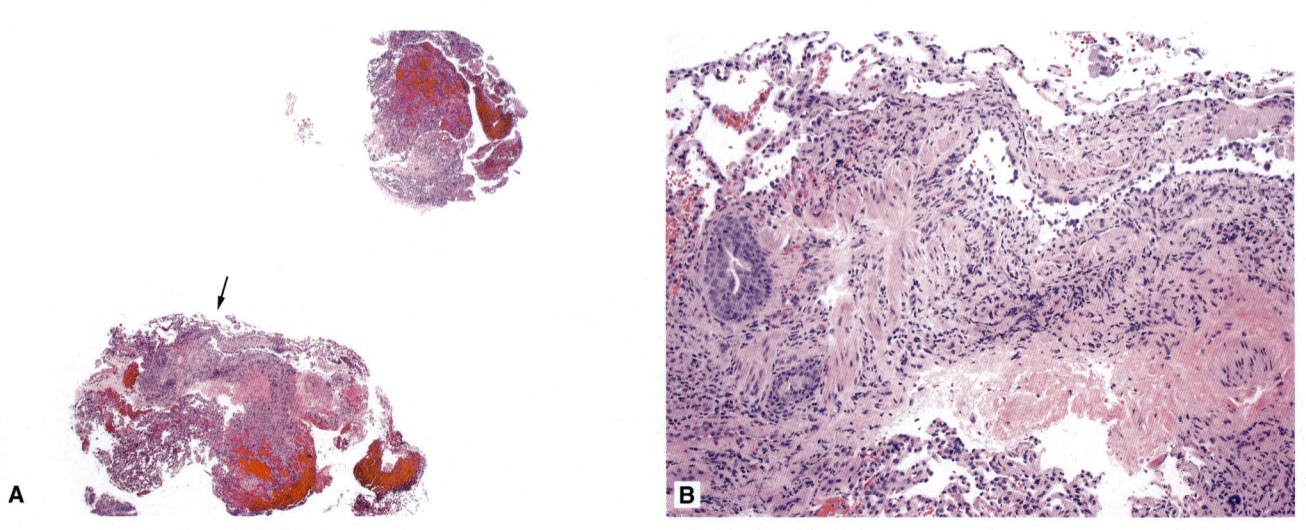

Figure 38.2: (*Continued*)

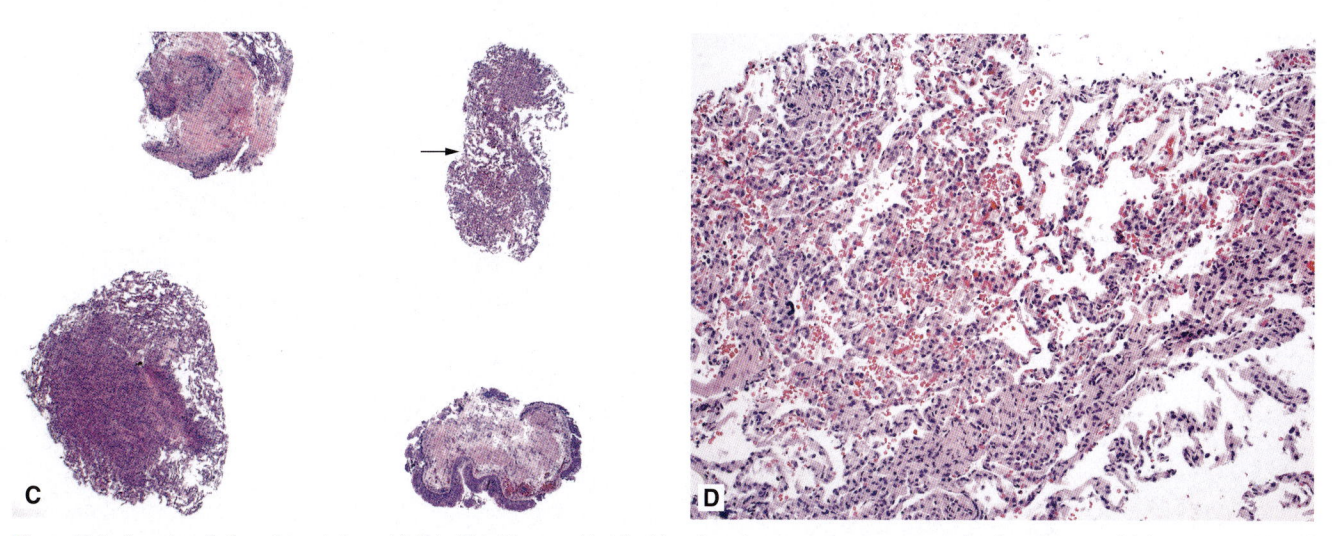

Figure 38.2: (*continued*) Lymphocytic bronchiolitis. This 13-year-old girl with asthmatic symptoms was suspected to have hypersensitivity pneumonitis and underwent transbronchial biopsy. Biopsy findings included focal airway injury and mild chronic inflammation (A, arrow, B) but no inflammation or granulomas in the alveolated parenchyma (C, arrow, D). She was later diagnosed with common variable immunodeficiency.

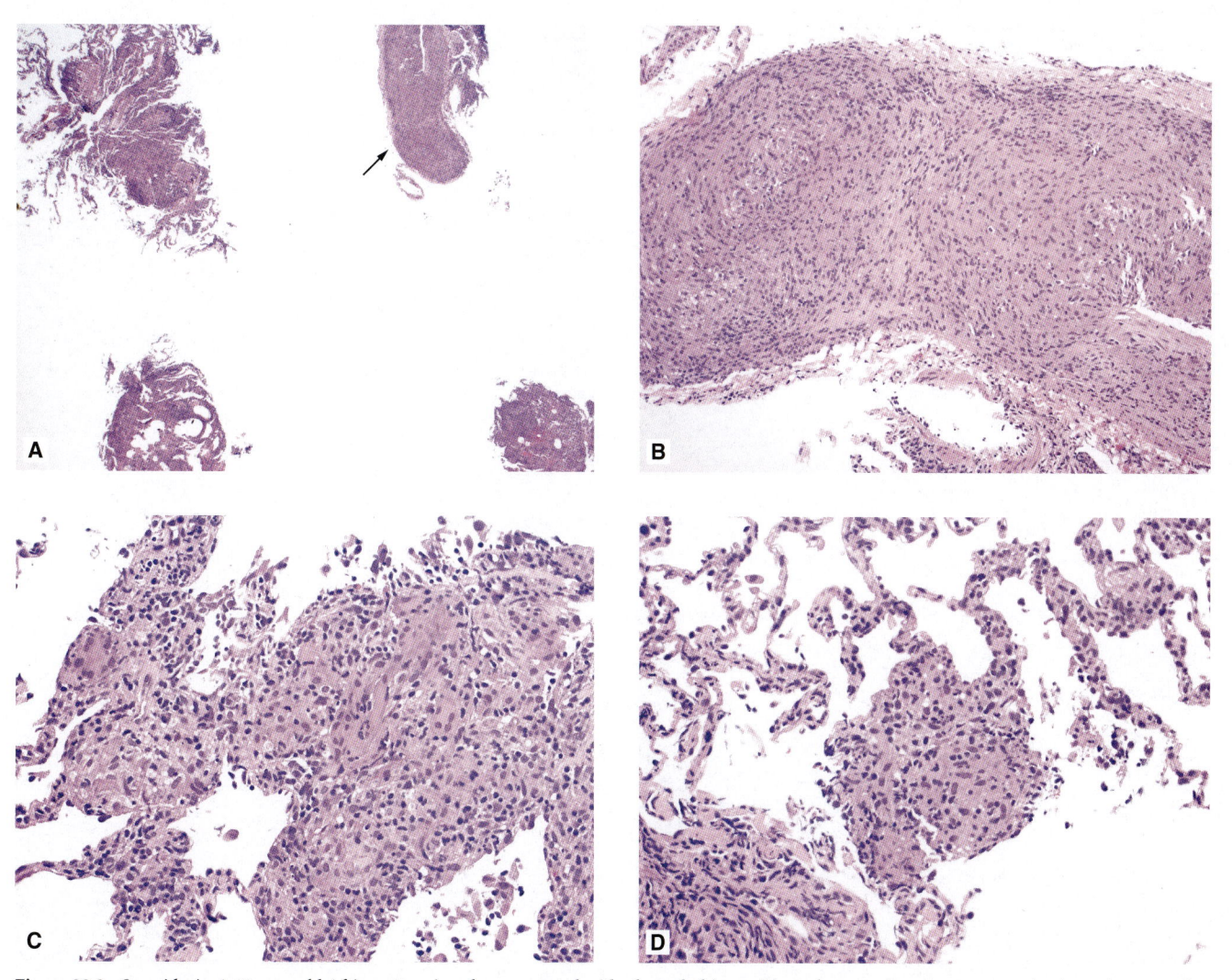

Figure 38.3: Sarcoidosis. A 12-year-old African American boy presented with photophobia, uveitis, and no respiratory symptoms. Angiotensin-converting enzyme was elevated, and he was found to have diffuse airway-centered interstitial lung disease on chest computed tomography, suggesting sarcoidosis. Transbronchial biopsy confirmed a region of noncaseating granulomatous inflammation in a vascular distribution adjacent to a bronchiole (A, arrow, B). Multiple small noncaseating granulomas were also present in the interstitium (C, D). No Schaumann bodies or asteroid bodies were seen.

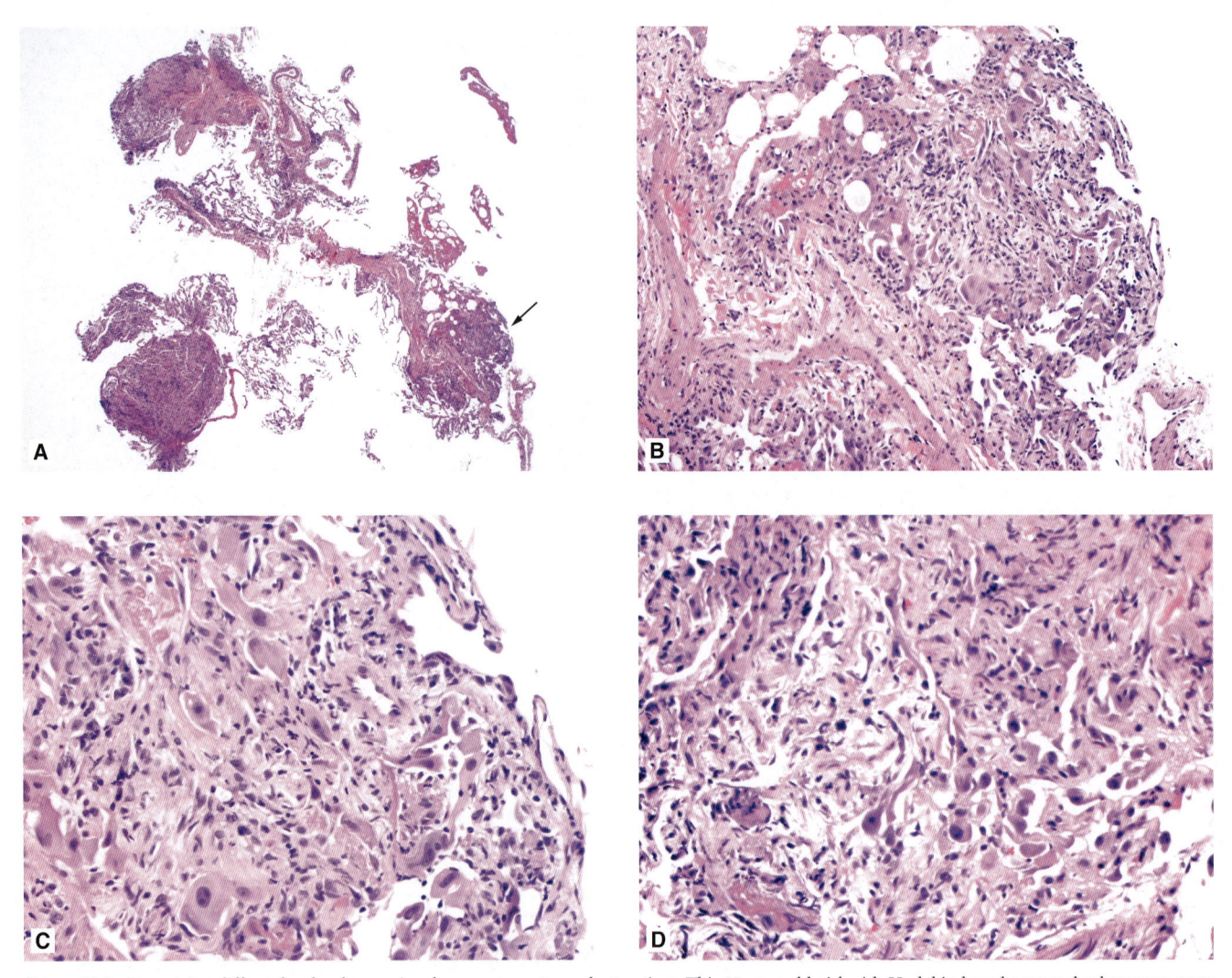

Figure 38.4: Organizing diffuse alveolar damage in a bone marrow transplant patient. This 15-year-old girl with Hodgkin lymphoma and subsequent acute lymphoblastic leukemia, status post bone marrow transplant, presented with pneumonia. Transbronchial biopsies demonstrated alveolar injury with reactive alveolar epithelial hyperplasia (A, arrow, B), focal hyaline membranes (C), and fibroblast proliferation indicating focal organization (D). Although no specific viral cytopathic effect was detected on biopsy, adenovirus was isolated from bronchoalveolar lavage culture.

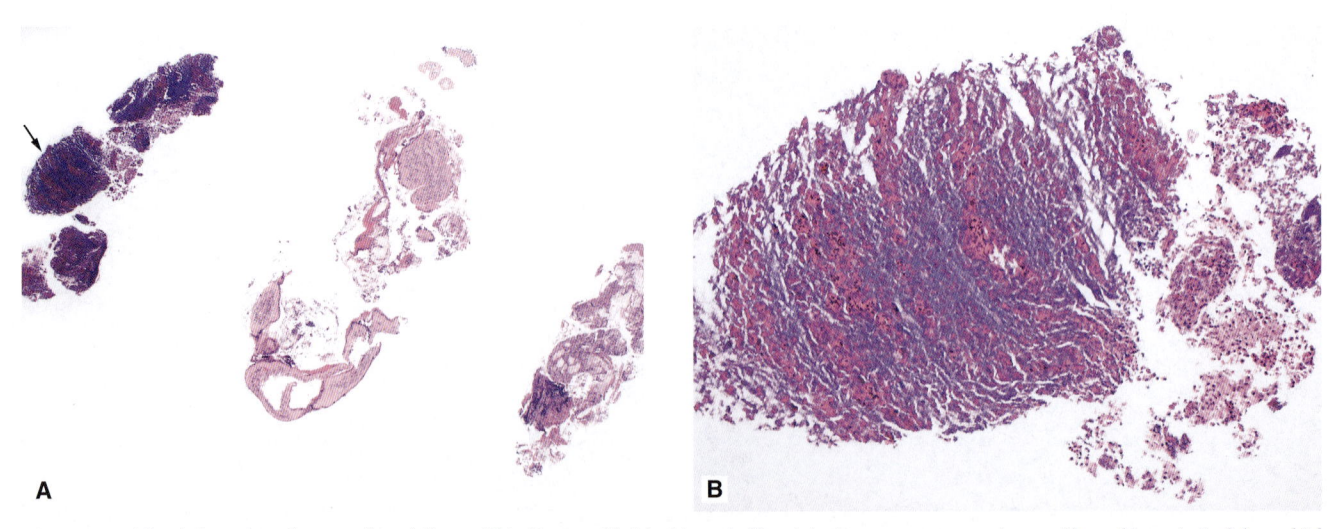

Figure 38.5: Allergic bronchopulmonary fungal disease. This 13-year-old girl with cystic fibrosis had recurrent mucus plugs and bronchiectasis. Endobronchial biopsies at the time of removal of a bronchial mucus plug demonstrated a dense aggregate of allergic mucin with typical laminar appearance (A, arrow, B), as well as bronchial mucosa with eosinophil infiltrates (*Continued*)

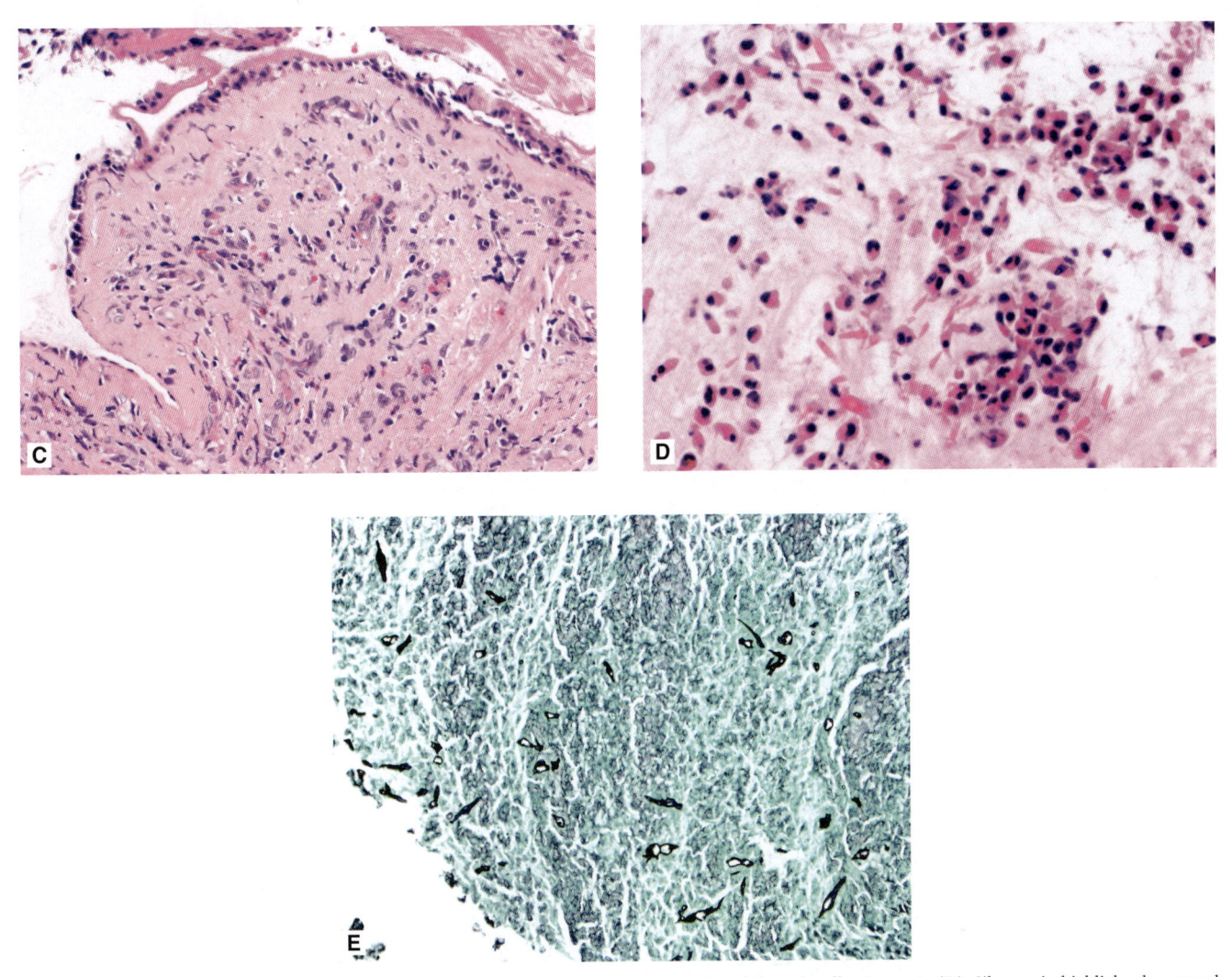

Figure 38.5: (*continued*) (C). Charcot-Leyden crystals were admixed with numerous eosinophils in the allergic mucin (D). Silver stain highlighted scattered fungal hyphae in the area of allergic mucin (E), consistent with *Aspergillus* isolated in culture. No invasive organisms were seen.

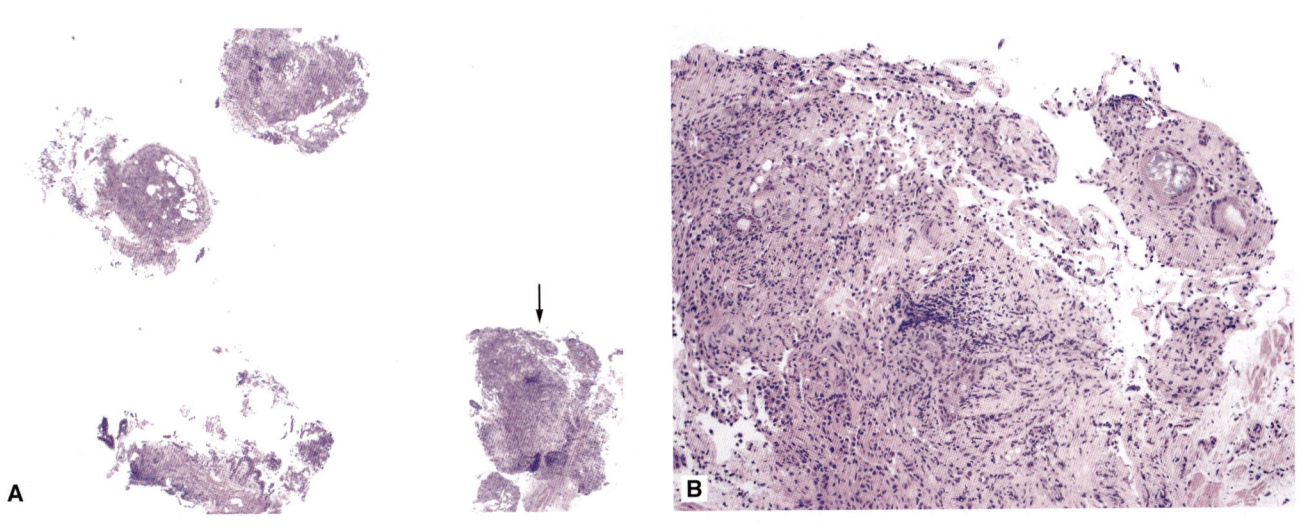

Figure 38.6: (*Continued*)

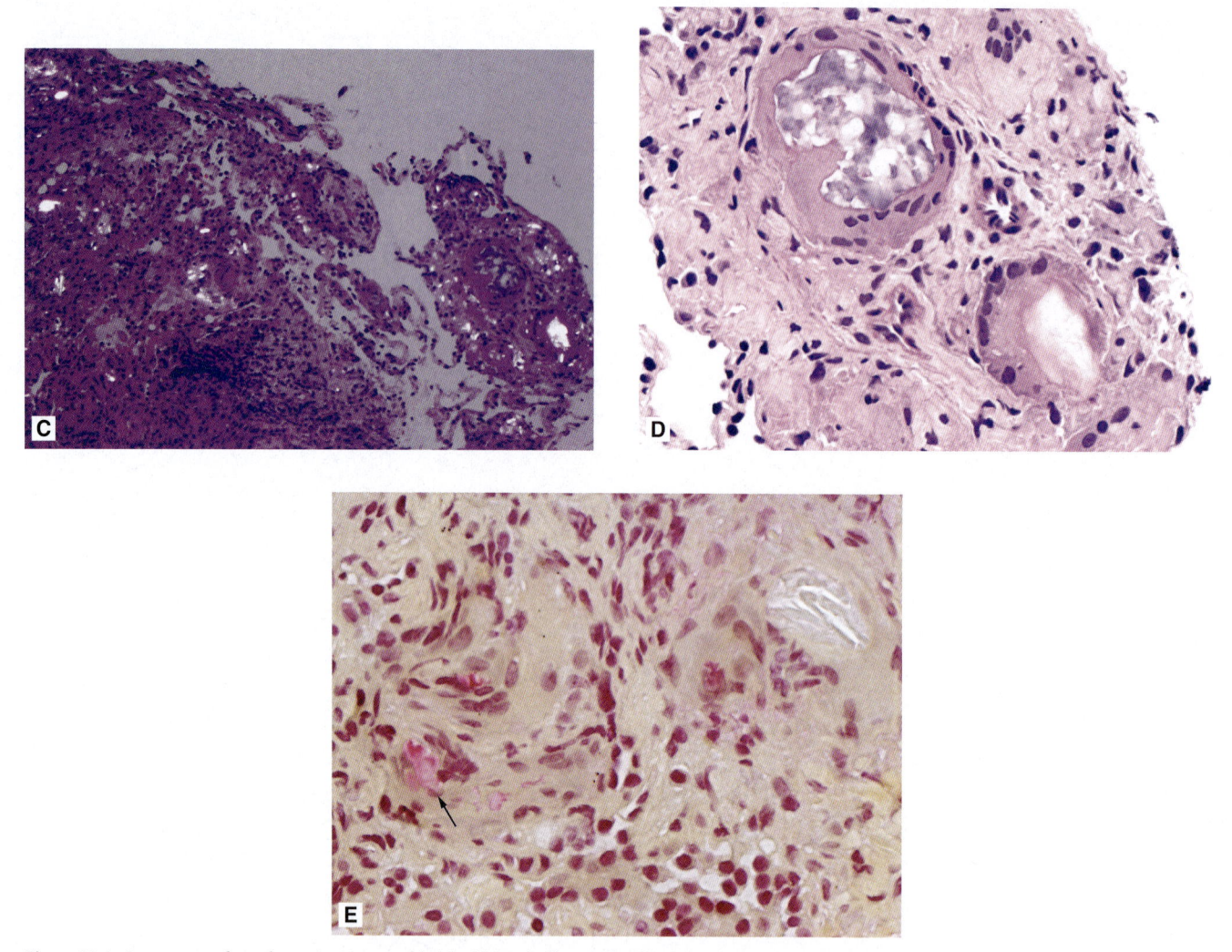

Figure 38.6: Intravenous drug abuse. An 18-year-old girl with cystic fibrosis, insulin-dependent diabetes mellitus, and a central line presented with declining pulmonary function tests and diffuse micronodular lung disease on chest computed tomography. Transbronchial biopsy showed patchy mild inflammation and multiple foreign body giant cells (A arrow, B). Some of the foreign material was demonstrable by polarizing microscopy (C). The giant cells contained two components: refractile pale yellow crystalline material (microcrystalline cellulose) (D, lower right) and more amorphous basophilic material forming "coral-like" branching patterns (crospovidone) (D, upper left). The crospovidone was also highlighted by mucicarmine stain (E, arrow) and periodic acid-Schiff stain (not shown). Microcrystalline cellulose and crospovidone are filler components of pharmaceutical tablets that form a foreign body giant cell reaction in the lungs when crushed and injected systemically.

Suggested Readings

Fan LL, Kozinetz CA, Wojtczak HA, et al. Diagnostic value of transbronchial, thoracoscopic, and open lung biopsy in immunocompetent children with chronic interstitial lung disease. *J Pediatr* 1997;131:565–569.

Kurland G, Noyes BE, Jaffe R, et al. Bronchoalveolar lavage and transbronchial biopsy in children following heart-lung and lung transplantation. *Chest* 1993;104:1043–1048.

Mullins D, Livne M, Mallory GB, et al. A new technique for transbronchial biopsy in infants and small children. *Pediatr Pulmonol* 1995;20:253–257.

Bronchial Masses in the Pediatric Population

▶ Megan K. Dishop, MD

Endobronchial biopsy is occasionally performed for diagnosis and/or excision of obstructive tracheal and endobronchial masses. Most bronchial lesions in children are benign, including predominantly nonneoplastic lesions, such as granulation tissue (sometimes related to foreign body aspiration), pyogenic granulomas, granulomatous infection, hamartomas, and juvenile-onset recurrent respiratory papillomatosis. Recurrent respiratory papillomatosis is typically caused by infection with human papillomavirus types 6 and 11 acquired during delivery, and it results in multiple recurrent squamous papillomas of the larynx, tracheobronchial tree, and, less commonly, the esophagus and pulmonary parenchyma. Frequent excisions are required for recurrent papillomas due to obstructive symptoms and rare occurrence of malignant progression.

Other endobronchial tumors include hemangiomas, myofibroblastic tumors, histiocytic lesions, bronchial neuroendocrine tumors (carcinoid tumor), adenoid cystic carcinoma, mucoepidermoid carcinoma, benign mucous gland adenoma, leiomyoma, and rarely metastatic tumors with an endobronchial component. Bronchogenic carcinoma has been reported in children but is exceptionally rare. Inflammatory myofibroblastic tumors account for approximately 20% of all primary lung tumors in children, most commonly forming intraparenchymal masses and only occasionally presenting as an endobronchial mass. Bronchial carcinoid tumors are the most common bronchial neoplasm in childhood, typically presenting in adolescents as endophytic polypoid masses with variable mural and extrabronchial extension. Although rare, carcinoid tumors account for approximately 80% of primary malignant lung tumors in children. They are considered low-grade malignancies with potential for local recurrence and distant metastasis.

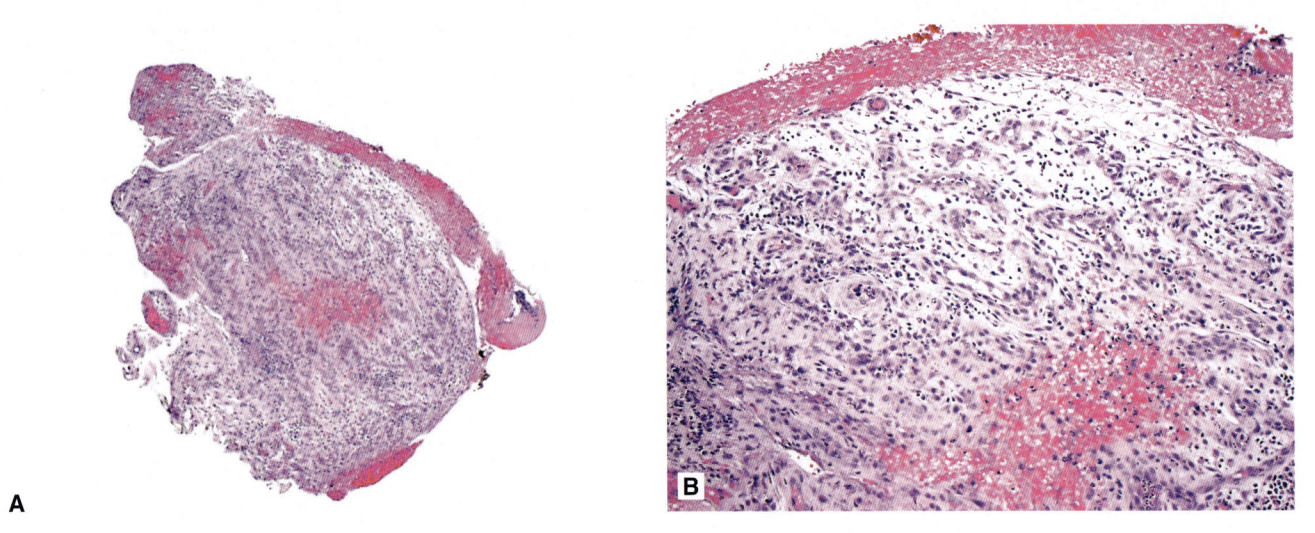

Figure 39.1: Endobronchial biopsy: granulation tissue. A 10-year-old boy presented with recurrent pneumonia and possible bronchial foreign body. Excisional biopsy of an endobronchial lesion (A) shows vascular proliferation in a myxoid inflammatory background, associated with surface hemorrhage (B), typical of granulation tissue.

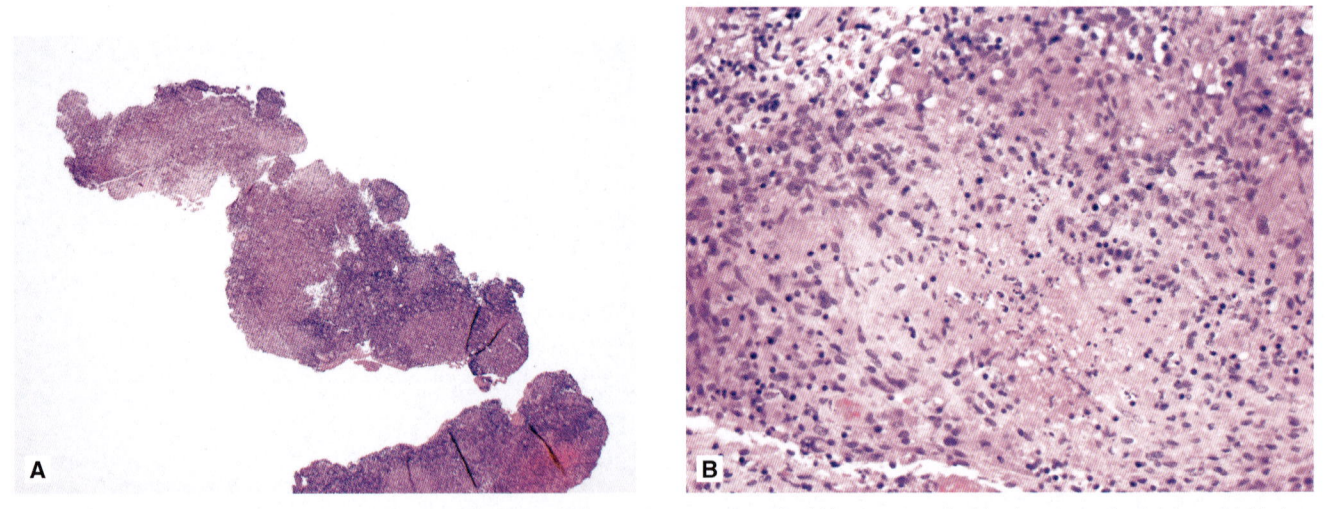

Figure 39.2: Endobronchial biopsy: necrotizing granulomatous inflammation. A 15-month-old boy presented with wheezing and a left bronchial lesion. Endobronchial biopsy (A) demonstrated chronic inflammation and epithelioid granulomas with focal central necrosis (B). Although no organisms were detected on special stains or culture, he was treated presumptively for mycobacterial infection.

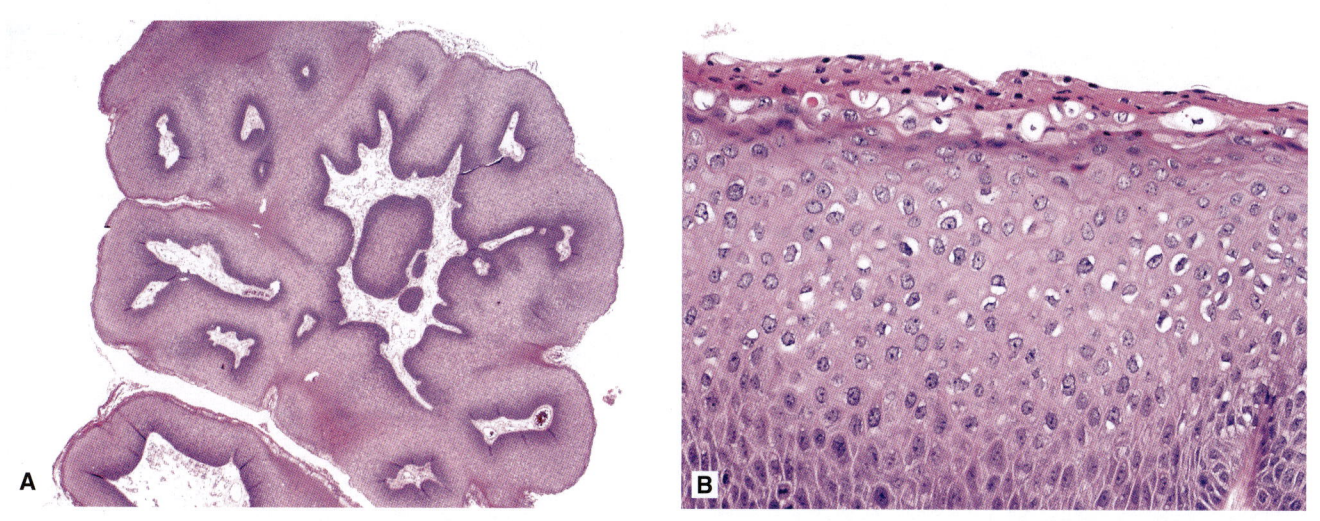

Chapter 39 • Bronchial Masses in the Pediatric Population

Figure 39.3: Endobronchial biopsy: juvenile-onset recurrent respiratory papillomatosis. A 5-year-old girl underwent multiple excisions of recurrent laryngeal and tracheobronchial squamous papillomas (A). Histologic features include focal parakeratosis and perinuclear halos typical of human papillomavirus cytopathic effect (B).

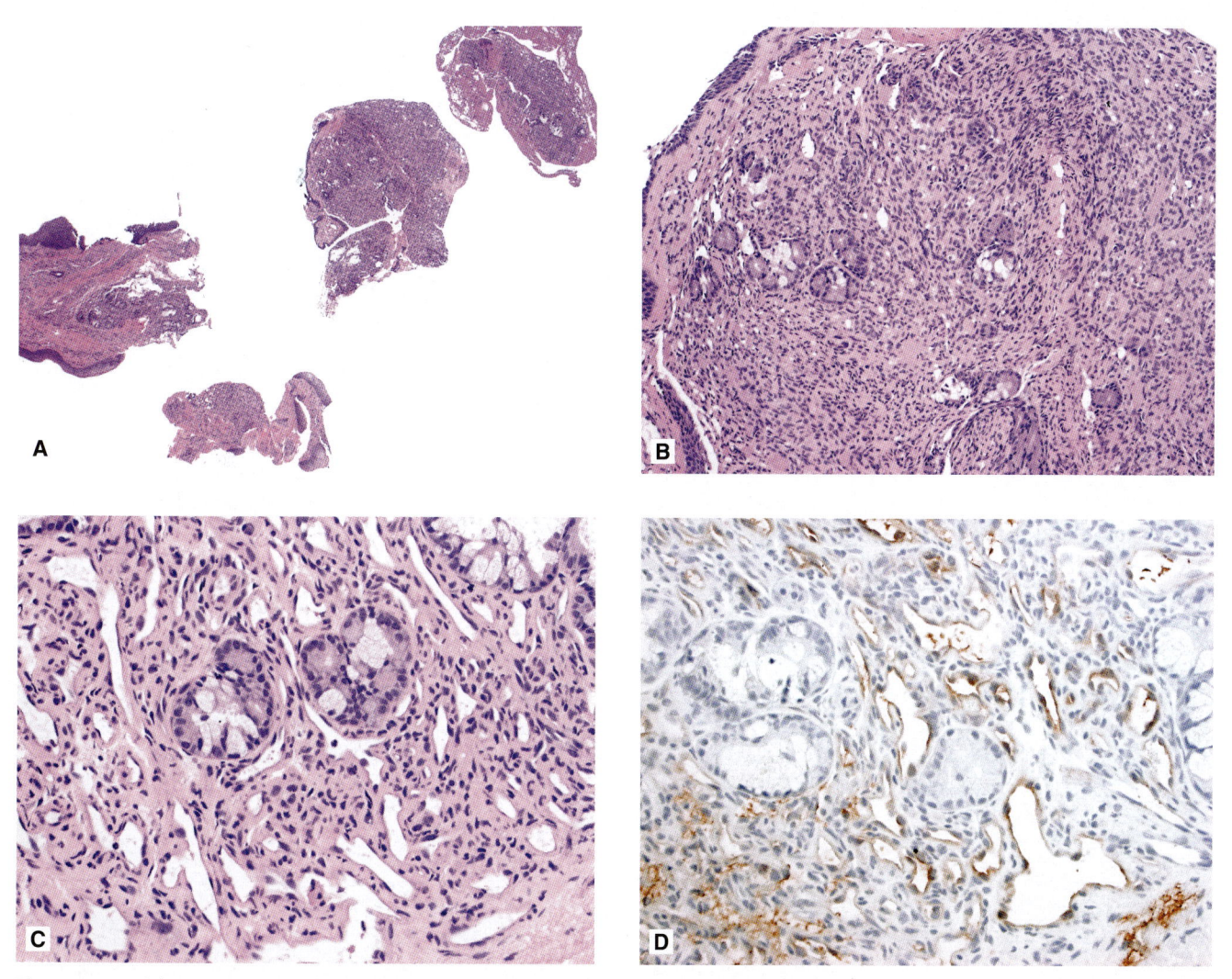

Figure 39.4: Endobronchial biopsy: infantile hemangioma. A 5-month-old infant girl with respiratory difficulty was found to have a 7-mm partially obstructive airway mass. Multiple biopsies (A) demonstrated a benign vascular proliferation of compact capillaries surrounding mucosal glands (B, C). Glut-1 immunohistochemistry demonstrates capillary endothelial staining (D), confirming the diagnosis of infantile hemangioma.

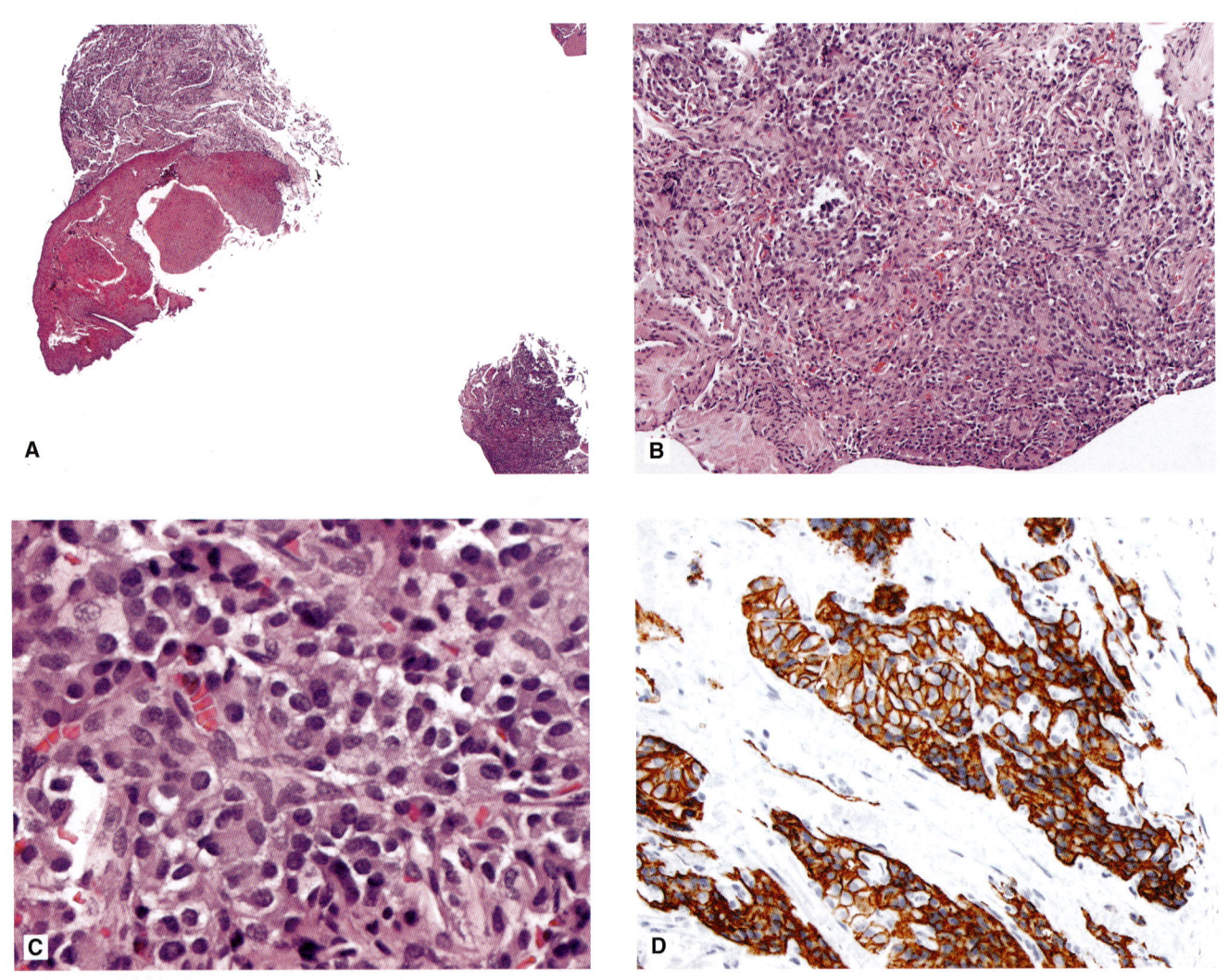

Figure 39.5: Endobronchial biopsy: carcinoid tumor. An 11-year-old boy was found to have a large partially obstructive right mainstem bronchus mass. Endobronchial biopsy showed a cellular subepithelial tumor (A) composed of round and polygonal cells with a rich vascular stromal network (B, C). Immunohistochemical evidence of neuroendocrine differentiation was demonstrated by positivity for CD56 (D), as well as chromogranin A and Cam 5.2.

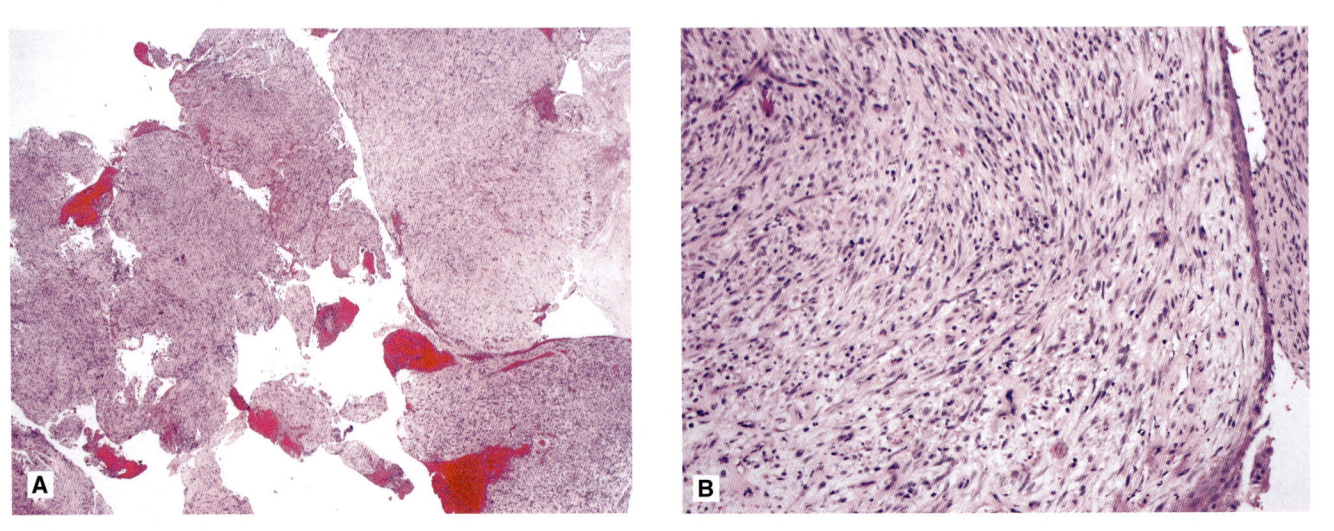

Figure 39.6: (*Continued*)

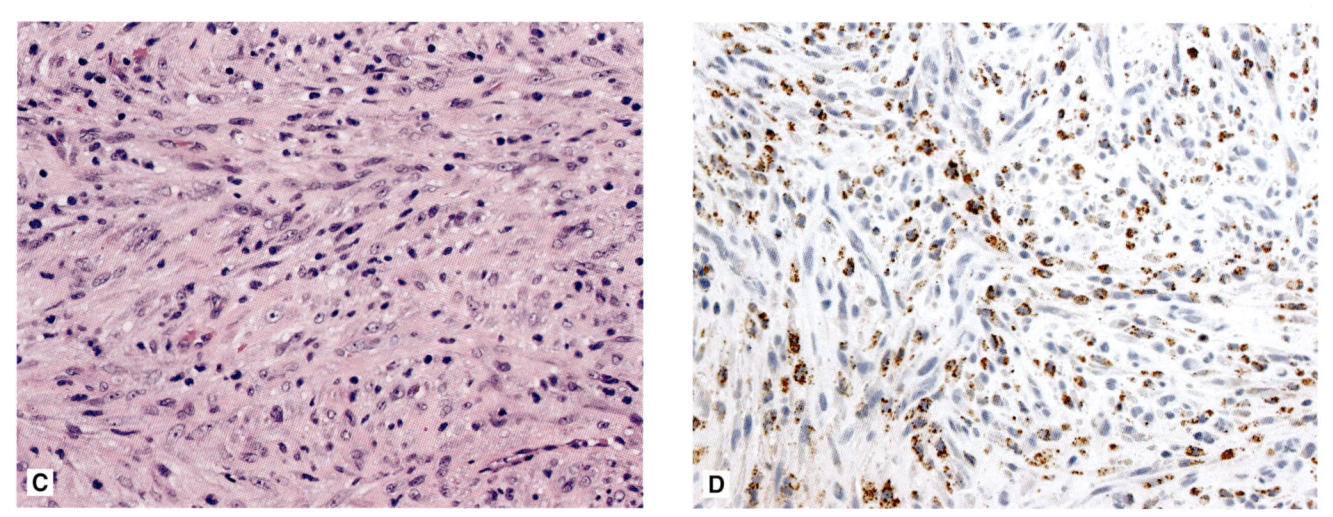

Chapter 39 • Bronchial Masses in the Pediatric Population

Figure 39.6: (*continued*) Endobronchial biopsy: inflammatory myofibroblastic tumor. A 4-year-old boy with decreased breath sounds on the right was found to have an obstructive right mainstem bronchus mass. Endobronchial biopsy demonstrated a proliferation of spindled and stellate myofibroblasts admixed with infiltrating lymphocytes (A–C). Immunohistochemistry was focally positive for smooth muscle actin and muscle specific actin, and diffusely positive for Alk-1 protein (D).

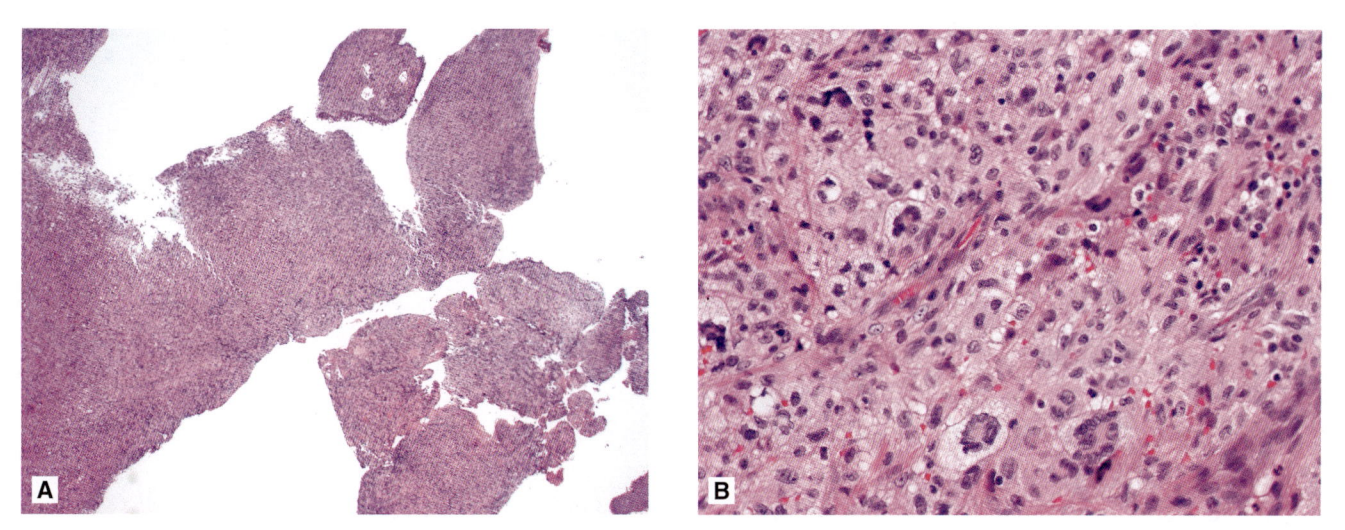

Figure 39.7: Endobronchial biopsy: juvenile xanthogranuloma. A 7-month-old infant boy presented with partial airway obstruction and no other systemic disease. Biopsy of a mass arising from the airway wall (A) showed a proliferation of histiocytes with abundant eosinophilic and foamy cytoplasm, occasionally forming Touton-type giant cells (B), typical of juvenile xanthogranuloma.

Suggested Readings

Al-Qahtani, Di Lorenzo M, Yazbeck S. Endobronchial tumors in children: Institutional experience and literature review. *J Pediatr Surg* 2003;38:733–736.

Curtis JM, Lacey D, Smyth R, et al. Endobronchial tumors in childhood. *Eur J Radiology* 1998;29:11–20.

Hartmann GE, Shochat SJ. Primary pulmonary neoplasms of childhood: a review. *Ann Thorac Surg* 1983;36:108–119.

Magid MS, Chen Y-T, Soslow RA, et al. Juvenile-onset recurrent respiratory papillomatosis involving the lung: a case report and review of the literature. *Ped Dev Pathol* 1998;1:157–163.

Souid AK, Ziemba MC, Dubansky AS, et al. Inflammatory myofibroblastic tumor in children. *Cancer* 1993;27:2042–2048.

Tracheobronchial Biopsy for Primary Ciliary Dyskinesia

▶ Megan K. Dishop, MD

Primary ciliary dyskinesia (PCD) is a rare disorder of immotile or abnormally motile cilia resulting in chronic recurrent respiratory infection, sinusitis, otitis media, and male infertility due to abnormal sperm motility. Incidence is approximately 1 in 20,000 individuals. Often familial, PCD demonstrates an autosomal recessive pattern of inheritance. Onset of symptoms is usually in childhood. Half of cases are associated with situs inversus (Kartagener syndrome), which may be a clue to diagnosis. Situs inversus results from abnormal ciliary motility in the embryonic node, which determines left-right asymmetry. Chronic headaches and hydrocephalus in some PCD patients are thought to result from impaired ciliary movement of the ventricular ependymal lining cells, and therefore abnormal cerebrospinal fluid flow. The major pulmonary complications of PCD result from impaired mucociliary clearance, leading to mucus stasis, chronic bronchitis, bronchiectasis, and chronic recurrent parenchymal infections. Histologic findings in the lung include mucus stasis, bronchiectasis, lymphocytic bronchitis and bronchiolitis, peri-airway fibrosis, and variable bronchopneumonia.

Biopsies of the tracheobronchial mucosa or nasal mucosa are often performed for screening of ciliary motility. Although there is no role for routine processing and light microscopy of tracheal or endobronchial biopsies in this setting, immediate direct wet mount preparations of brushings or biopsies are performed for evaluation of ciliary movement. The cilia are evaluated by assessing the presence or absence of coordinated movement, normally showing a rhythmic wavelike motion with each beat. Presence of squamous metaplasia or inflammation may cause secondary impairment or absence of ciliary movement, and detection of these features on direct microscopy may necessitate repeat biopsy at a different site or time. If the specimen is adequate and no ciliary movement is detected, ultrastructural examination is then performed to identify any structural abnormalities in the ciliary apparatus. The normal arrangement of microtubules in the ciliary axoneme includes 9 peripheral microtubule doublets interconnected by nexin links and 2 central individual microtubules (9 + 2 arrangement), which are connected to the peripheral doublets by radial spokes. Defects in any of these axonemal structures may occur, although the absence or truncation of outer and/or inner dynein arms is most frequently recognized in PCD patients.

Despite over 250 proteins in the normal cilium, mutations in only three genes encoding these proteins have been described to date, and unfortunately they account for a minority of cases. The known PCD genes encode intermediate and heavy chains of the outer dynein arms: DNAI1 (chromosome 9p13), DNAH5 (5p15), and DNAH11 (7p21).

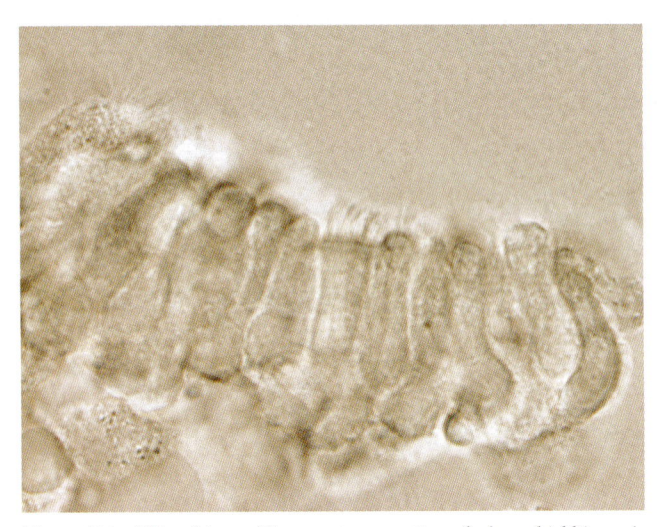

Figure 40.1: Ciliary biopsy. Direct wet preparation of a bronchial biopsy is evaluated by light microscopy to assess rhythmic and coordinated ciliary movement.

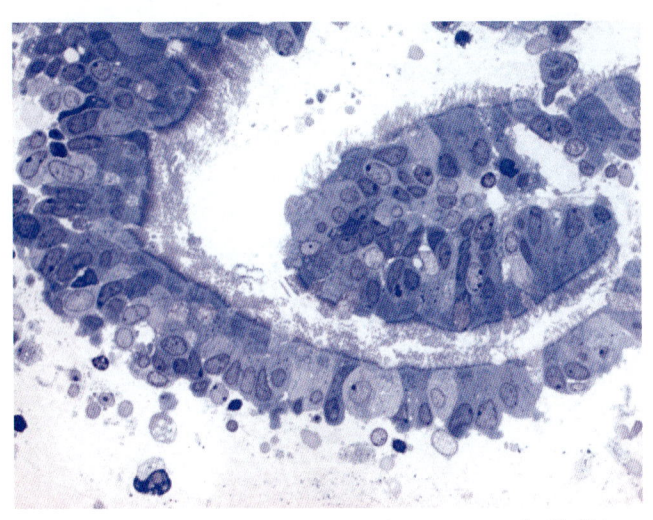

Figure 40.2: Ciliary biopsy. Thick section of epoxy resin-embedded biopsy material demonstrates ciliated columnar respiratory epithelium adequate for evaluation. Ultrastructural evaluation is performed on cilia oriented in cross section.

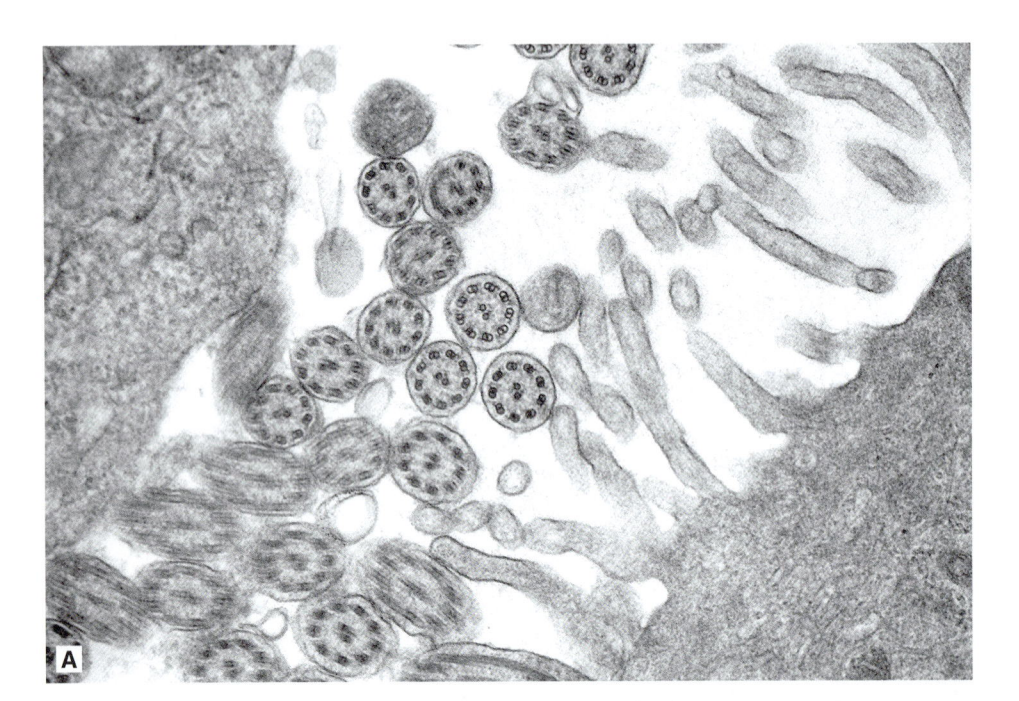

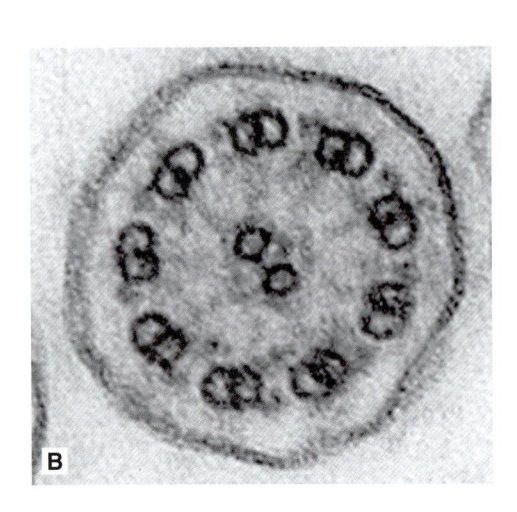

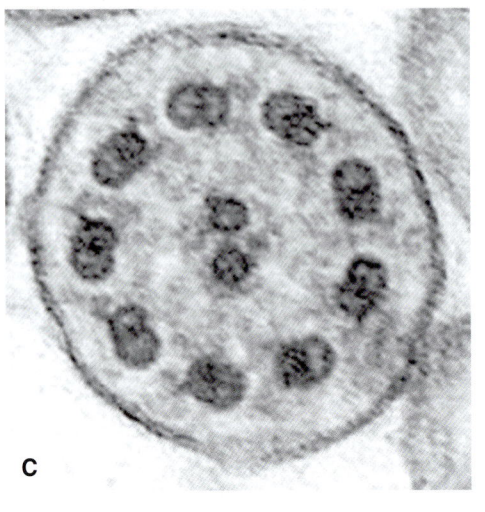

Figure 40.3: Ciliary biopsy. (A) Transmission electron microscopy demonstrates cilia oriented in cross section. (B) A normal ciliary axoneme shows 9 + 2 microtubular arrangement and well-visualized inner and outer dynein arms, including hooks of outer dynein arms. (C) This patient with immotile cilia has absent and truncated inner and outer dynein arms.

Suggested Readings

Carlen B, Stenram U. Primary ciliary dyskinesia: a review. *Ultrastruct Pathol* 2005;29:217–220.

Geremek M, Witt M. Primary ciliary dyskinesia: genes, candidate genes, and chromosomal regions. *J Appl Genet* 2004;45:347–361.

Holzmann D, Ott PM, Felix H. Diagnostic approach to primary ciliary dyskinesia: a review. *Eur J Pediatr* 2000;159:95–96.

MacCormick J, Robb I, Kovesi T, et al. Optimal biopsy techniques in the diagnosis of primary ciliary dyskinesia. *J Otolaryg* 2002;31:13–17.

Meeks M, Bush A. Primary ciliary dyskinesia (PCD). *Pediatr Pulmonol* 2000;29:307–316.

Roomans GM, Ivanovs A, Shebani EB, et al. Transmission electron microscopy in the diagnosis of primary ciliary dyskinesia. *Upsala J Med Sci* 2006;111:155–168.

Legal Aspects of Endobronchial and Transbronchial Biopsy

41

▶ Timothy C. Allen, MD, JD

Clinicians' medicolegal concerns about transbronchial and endobronchial biopsies generally arise from medical complications such as severe pneumothorax and severe bleeding. Pathologists also have to be cognizant of medicolegal consequences arising from the biopsies' diagnoses. Appropriate accessioning of the biopsy, gross examination, processing, and careful microscopic review are necessary as with any other surgical pathology specimen. For several issues specific to endobronchial and transbronchial biopsies, appropriate attention will help assure a correct diagnosis and allay medicolegal concerns as well.

The self-expectation or clinician pressure to render a diagnosis does not abrogate the pathologist's responsibility to identify artifacts, normal variations, nonspecific changes, and limited, nonrepresentative samples and therefore appropriately limit the diagnosis, even to the extent that no diagnosis is possible. Correlation with clinical and radiologic features helps avoid overinterpretation of the biopsy tissue.

Endobronchial and transbronchial biopsies are by definition specimens consisting of small fragments of tissue, often with associated blood. Specimen adequacy is a principal concern. Specimens labeled as endobronchial biopsies, for which the clinician may be primarily concerned with preneoplasia or another endobronchial process, may contain underlying lung parenchymal tissue in which focal or subtle pathologic changes are present. If an endobronchial biopsy contains little or no intact mucosa due to mucosal sloughing or crush or other artifact, the specimen is not representative of the patient's airway mucosa and bronchial wall and is unsatisfactory for the determination of preneoplasia. Such a finding should be noted in the microscopic description or diagnosis, and no opinion regarding preneoplasia in the specimen should be rendered.

Specimens labeled as transbronchial biopsies should contain enough lung parenchymal tissue without crush or other artifactual changes so that a reliable diagnosis may be rendered. If lung parenchyma is not representative of the patient due to the amount of lung parenchyma present or is otherwise suboptimal for diagnosis due to artifactual changes, processing or staining issues, or other factors, it should be noted in the microscopic description or diagnosis, and no opinion regarding a parenchymal process should be rendered.

With posttransplant transbronchial biopsies performed for evaluation of infection and rejection, the updated International Society for Heart and Lung Transplantation classification system indicates that at least five pieces of alveolar parenchyma are necessary to render a reliable diagnosis; and further that three hematoxylin and eosin (H&E) stained slides from three levels in the block, as well as a trichrome stain or other stain for connective tissue, be reviewed.

Certain interstitial lung diseases such as organizing pneumonia and diffuse alveolar damage are diagnosable with transbronchial biopsy. Various interstitial lung diseases such as usual interstitial pneumonia, fibrotic variant of nonspecific interstitial pneumonia, and asbestosis, among other diseases, are characterized by mature fibrosis. These diseases have a variety of prognoses and treatments but share similar histologic features. The necessity of evaluating the extent and distribution of fibrosis or other parenchymal lesions, the temporal heterogeneity or homogeneity of the disease process, and the focal nature of some features preclude the reliable diagnosis of these diseases by transbronchial biopsy. Although the transbronchial biopsy has a role in the diagnosis and management of these diseases as discussed in individual chapters, these particular fibrotic interstitial lung diseases cannot generally be diagnosed reliably on a histologic basis without a surgical lung biopsy specimen, at least a wedge biopsy.

Pathologists may feel pressured to render a diagnosis of a fibrotic interstitial lung disease on transbronchial biopsy, but extreme caution should be used to give an accurate and not overly broad diagnosis based on the tissue present in the transbronchial biopsy. Diagnosing a transbronchial biopsy simply as "interstitial lung fibrosis" is meaningless and may be dangerously overbroad because the term may be taken by clinicians as synonymous with usual interstitial pneumonia.

Suggested Readings

Cagle PT. Endobronchial and transbronchial biopsies. In: Cagle PT, ed. *Diagnostic Pulmonary Pathology*. New York: Marcel Dekker; 2000.

Frost AE. Transbronchial biopsies: clinical perspective. In: Cagle PT, ed. *Diagnostic Pulmonary Pathology*. New York: Marcel Dekker; 2000.

Stewart S, Fishbein MC, Snell GI, et al. Revision of the 1995 working formulation for the standardization of nomenclature in the diagnosis of lung rejection. *J Heart Lung Transplant* 2007;26:1229–1242.

Index

Note: Page numbers followed by "*f*" refer to illustrations; page numbers followed by "*t*" refer to tables.

AAH. *See* Atypical adenomatous hyperplasia
Acanthamoeba, 66
ACE. *See* Angiotensin-converting enzyme
Acetylsalicylic acid, 106*t*
Acid-fast bacillus, 59, 60*f*
Acquired immunodeficiency syndrome. *See* AIDS
Actin, 121
Acute allograft rejection, 131, 132*f*, 133*f*
Acute bacterial pneumonia, 52*f*, 86*f*
Acute bronchiolitis, 55
Acute fibrinous and organizing pneumonia, 77, 78*f*
Acute interstitial pneumonia (Hamman-Rich syndrome), 68*t*, 115–116
Acute transplant rejection, 131, 132*f*, 133*f*
Adenocarcinoma(s), 23
    cells, 14*f*
    classifications of, 9
    clear cell, 8*f*, 9
    differentiated, 12*f*–13*f*
    fetal, 8*f*
    invasive, 8*f*, 31*f*
    location of, 8
    lung, 29–30
    mucinous (colloid), 8*f*
    papillary, 13*f*–14*f*
    patterns of, 15*f*
    pulmonary, 16*f*
    Signet-ring cell, 8*f*
    types of, 8*f*
    variants of, 8*f*
    WHO classifications of, 7–8, 8*t*
Adenoid cystic carcinomas, 10, 18*f*–19*f*
Adenoma(s)
    mucous gland, 43
    pleomorphic, 43, 44*f*–45*f*
Adenosquamous carcinomas, 9–10
Adenovirus, 47, 48*f*, 48*t*, 49*f*
AFB. *See* Autofluorescence bronchoscopy
AIDS (acquired immunodeficiency syndrome), 49*f*, 60*f*
Airway(s)
    involvement of, 131
    mucosa, 48*f*
    pathology, neoplastic large, 139–141, 141*f*, 142*f*, 143*f*
Alveolar lipoproteinosis, 93, 94*f*
Alveoli, 15*f*
Amiodarone, 68*t*, 74*t*, 91, 105
Amphotericin B, 106*t*
ANCA. *See* Antineutrophil cytoplasmic antibody
Angiotensin-converting enzyme (ACE), 109
Antibiotics, 106*t*
Anticoagulants, 84*t*, 106*t*
Antimicrobials, 51

Antineutrophil cytoplasmic antibody (ANCA), 109
Aspergillus, 62*t*
Aspiration, 68*t*, 83
    of barium/charcoal, 79
    of particulate gastric contents, 79
    pneumonia, 79, 80*f*
Asthma, 139–140, 141*f*
Atelectasis, 79
Atypia, 7
    marked, 37*f*
    mild, 11*f*
Atypical adenomatous hyperplasia (AAH), 35
Autofluorescence bronchoscopy (AFB), 35
Azathioprine, 106*t*

BAC. *See* Bronchioloalveolar carcinoma
Balamuthia, 66
Barium, 79
Basaloid carcinomas, 17*f*
Biopsy(ies). *See also* Endobronchial biopsies; Tracheobronchial biopsies; Transbronchial biopsies
    bronchial, 22, 25*f*, 39
    endoscopic, 9
    lung, 15*f*
        endobronchial, 97
        wedge, 1, 121, 145
    open, 65
    procedures, 7
        bleeding during, 3
    tissue, 7
Bladders, 29
Blastomyces, 62*t*
Bleeding
    during biopsy procedures, 3
    minor, 1
    significant, 1
Bleomycin, 74*t*, 106*t*
Blood, 106*t*
    cells, red, 65, 85*f*
    vessels, 6*f*, 96*f*
Blue bodies, 3
BOOP. *See* Bronchiolitis obliterans organizing pneumonia
Bowel diseases. *See* Crohn's disease; Inflammatory bowel diseases
Bradyzoites, 65
Breasts, 29, 30, 30*f*, 31*f*
Bronchial cartilages, 5*f*
Bronchial glands, 2*f*
Bronchial walls, 2*f*
    collapse of, 3
    inflammation of, 49*f*
Bronchiectasis, 61, 101
Bronchiolitis, 101, 146*f*–147*f*

Bronchiolitis obliterans organizing pneumonia
    (BOOP), 73
Bronchioloalveolar carcinoma (BAC)
    detection of, 9
    patterns, 9
Bronchitis, 101
    chronic, 139–140
Bronchus, 6f, 18f–19f
Burns, 68t
Busulfan, 106t

Calcium oxalate crystals, 3
Calcospherites. *See* Psammoma bodies
Cancer(s). *See also specific types of cancers*
    colorectal, 29–30, 31f, 32f
    metastatic, sites of, 29
Candida, 62t
Capillaritis, 83, 101
Carbol fuchsin, 59
Carcinoembryonic antigen (CEA), 30
Carcinoma(s), 3. *See also specific types of carcinomas*
    adenoid cystic, 10, 18f–19f
    adenosquamous, 9–10
    basaloid, 17f
    breast, 30, 30f, 31f
    invasive, 15f–16f
    lung, 31f
        diagnosis of, 7
        mixed-type, 9–10
        types of, 7
    mucoepidermoid, 10
    other, 8f
    pleomorphic, 17f–18f
    renal cell, 30, 33f
    salivary-type, 10
    sarcomatoid, 8f, 9, 18f–19f
    undifferentiated, 17f
Carcinoma in situ (CIS), 7–8
    definition of, 35
    lesions, 35, 37f
CEA. *See* Carcinoembryonic antigen
Cell(s). *See also* Langerhans cells; Large cell carcinomas;
        Squamous cell carcinomas; Squamous
        cell papillomas
    adenocarcinoma, 14f
    carcinomas, renal, 30, 33f
    Clara, 9, 13f–14f
    clear, 8f, 9
    cuboidal, 5f
    epithelial, 4f, 45f
        crushed "infiltrating," 10f
    giant, 98f, 125
    inflammatory, 17f–18f
    large lymphoma B-, 39, 41f
    lung carcinomas, small, 3, 7
    lymphoma, T-, 39
    mesothelial, 5f
    mononuclear, 80f
    necrosis, alveolar epithelial, 79
    neuroendocrine tumors
        large, 21–22, 22t, 26f
        small, 21–22, 22t, 23f–25f
    papillomas, squamous cell, 43, 44f
    plasma dyscrasia, 40
    pleomorphism of, 17f–18f
    red blood, 65, 85f
    Signet-ring adenocarcinoma, 8f
    spindle, 23
    tumor, 7, 18f
        infiltration of, 21
        power of, 26f
        types, 8
Charcoal, 79
Charcot-Leyden crystals, 3, 89, 149f
Chemicals, 84t
Chemotherapy, 68t
Chest radiographs, 83, 127
Children
    bronchial masses in, 151, 152f, 153f, 154f, 155f
    transbronchial biopsies and, 145, 146f, 147f, 148f,
        149f, 150f
Chlorambucil, 106t
Cholesterol clefts, 3, 80f, 93
Chromatin, 11f, 22, 24f
Chromogranin, 22, 25f, 27f
Chronic bronchitis, 139–140
Churg-Strauss syndrome, 83, 85f, 109
Cilia, 157
CIS. *See* Carcinoma in situ
Clara cells, 9, 13f–14f
Coal, 112f
Cocaine, 84t
Coccidiosis, 62t
Collagen, 21
    deposition of, 67
    vascular diseases, 67, 68t
        diagnosis of, 102, 102f, 103f
        manifestations of, 101
Colon, 29, 32f
Colorectal cancers, 29–30, 31f, 32f
Computed tomography, 83
Confluent sarcoid, 95
Congestion, 79
Connective tissue diseases, 84t
COP. *See* Cryptogenic organizing pneumonia
Cornstarch, 125, 126f
Cresyl violet, 57
Crohn's disease, 109, 110f
Crospovidone, 125
Crush artifact(s), 3, 4f
    presence of, 21, 23
    substantial, 7
Cryptococcus, 62t
Cryptogenic organizing pneumonia (COP), 73, 74t, 75f,
        115–116
Crystal(s)
    calcium oxalate, 3
    Charcot-Leyden, 3, 69, 149f
Cyclophosphamides, 106t
Cystic fibrosis, 149f–150f
Cysts, 65–66, 66f
Cytarabine, 106t
Cytokeratins, 10f, 22
    express, 25f, 33f
Cytology, samples of, 1
Cytomegalovirus, 47, 48t, 49f
Cytoplasm(s), 8, 27f, 59
    eosinophilic, 12f, 32f
    presence of, 21, 22
Cytoxan, 102f

DAD. *See* Diffuse alveolar damage
Dermatomyositis, 68t, 83, 101
Desmin, 121
Desquamative interstitial pneumonia (DIP), 115, 127
Diabetes mellitus, insulin-dependent, 149f–150f

Index

Diffuse alveolar damage (DAD), 83, 84t, 135, 148f, 161
    causes of, 67, 68t
    infections and, 68t
    phases of, 67, 69f
Diffuse idiopathic pulmonary neuroendocrine cell hyperplasia (DIPNECH), 35
DIP. *See* Desquamative interstitial pneumonia
DIPNECH. *See* Diffuse idiopathic pulmonary neuroendocrine cell hyperplasia
Drug(s), 67, 68t
    abuse, intravenous, 125, 126f, 149f–150f
    causing lung diseases, 106t
    for organizing pneumonia, 74t
    pulmonary hemorrhage and, 84t
    reactions, 103f, 105, 106t, 107f
Dusts, inorganic, 111
Dyscrasia, plasma cell, 40
Dysplasia. *See also* specific types of dysplasia
    moderate, 36f
    severe, 37f
Dystrophic ossification, 3

EGFR. *See* Epidermal growth factor receptor
EGFR-targeted tyrosine kinase inhibitors (Erlotinib, Gefitinib), 9
Ehrlichia chaffeensis, 65
Ehrlichia ewingii, 65
Endobronchial biopsy(ies)
    high power of, 2f
    legal aspects of, 161–162
    low power of, 2f
    overview of, 1
Enzyme immunoassay testing, 55
Eosinophils, 73, 89, 90f
Epidermal growth factor receptor (EGFR), 9
Epithelium, 36f
    metaplastic squamous, 10f–11f
    respiratory, 10f, 17f, 36f
    squamous
        atypical, 7, 37f
        stratified, 44f
Epstein-Barr virus, 39
Erlotinib. *See* EGFR-targeted tyrosine kinase inhibitors
Escherichia coli, 51
Estrogen receptors, 121

Fat, 81
Ferruginous bodies, 3
Fibrin, 3, 67, 86f, 87f, 127
Fibrinolytic agents, 106t
Fibroblasts, 67, 75f, 86f
Fibrosis, 61, 101
    cystic, 149f–150f
    interpretation of, 6f
    parenchymal, 5f
    pulmonary, 102f
    septal, 79, 80f
Fleas, 65
Forceps, transbronchial biopsy, 3
Fungus. *See also* specific types of fungus
    diseases, types of, 62t, 148f–149f
    etiologies of, 61, 62f

Gastrointestinal tracts, 29, 32f
Gaucher disease, 91
Gefitinib. *See* EGFR-targeted tyrosine kinase inhibitors
Genes, PCD, 157
Genitourinary tracts, 29
Giemsa stains, 65
Gland(s), 43
    bronchial, 2f
    submucosal, 15f
GMS. *See* Gomori methenamine silver
Gold, 74t, 106t
Gomori methenamine silver (GMS), 57, 58f, 59, 61, 93
Goodpasture syndrome, 68t, 83
Gram stains, 59
    negative, 51, 65
    positive, 51
Granulomas, 65–66, 73, 95, 97, 109
    noncaseating, 147f
    pyogenic, 151
Grocott silver stain, 61

Haemophilus influenzae, 51
Hamartomas, chondroid, 43, 45f
Hamman-Rich syndrome. *See* Acute interstitial pneumonia
H&E. *See* Hematoxylin and eosin
Headaches, 157
Heart failure, 71
Heat, 68t
Hemangiomas, 151, 153f
Hematologic disorders, 68t
Hematolymphoid malignancies, 39–40, 39f, 40f
Hematoxylin and eosin (H&E), 4, 33f
    examination of, 29, 73
    standard, 22
Hemorrhage(s)
    fresh procedural, 4f
    intra-alveolar
        causes of, 84t
        etiologies of, 83–84, 85f, 86f, 87f
    localized, 84t
    pulmonary, 67
        causes of, 84t
        drugs and, 84t
    variable, 67
Henoch-Schönlein purpura, 84t
Heroin, 106t
Herpes simplex, 47, 48t, 49f, 50f
Histiocytes, 55, 59, 60f, 90f, 97
Histoplasma, 62t
HIV (human immunodeficiency virus), 83
Hodgkin lymphomas, 39
Human immunodeficiency virus. *See* HIV
Hyaline, 67
Hydrocephalus, 157
Hypereosinophilic syndromes, 89, 90f
Hyperplasia, 35
    atypical adenomatous, 35
    diffuse idiopathic pulmonary neuroendocrine cell, 35
    type II pneumocyte, 67, 91
Hypersensitivity pneumonitis, 73, 97, 98f, 99f

Idiopathic pulmonary fibrosis (IPF), 115
Idiopathic pulmonary hemosiderosis, 83
Immunofluorescence techniques, 65
Immunohistochemistry, 22, 25f, 31f, 140
    CK20+/CK7-/CDX2+/MUC2+, 30, 32f
Immunostaining, 10f
Immunostain(s), 49f, 57, 65
    calretinin, 5f
    panel of, 40
Immunosuppressive therapies, 102f
Infection(s), 83, 84t, 93, 139
    diffuse alveolar damage and, 68t
    granulomatous, 151, 152f

Infection(s) (Cont.)
  organizing, 74t
  other, 65–66, 66f
Inflammation, 7, 93, 109
  of bronchial walls, 49f
  chronic, 12f, 80f
Inflammatory bowel diseases, 109, 110f. See also Crohn's disease
Influenza, 47, 48t. See also Viruses
Inhalants, 67, 68t, 74t
Inhalation
  injuries, 68t
  of inorganic dusts, 111
Insulin-dependent diabetes mellitus, 149f–150f
Interstitium, 56f, 67, 89
Intra-alveolar hemorrhage
  causes of, 84t
  etiologies of, 83–84, 85f, 86f, 87f
IPF. See Idiopathic pulmonary fibrosis
Iron, 83, 112f

Juvenile xanthogranulomas, 151, 153f
Juvenile-onset recurrent respiratory papillomatosis, 151, 153f

Kartagener syndrome. See Situs inversus
Keratin, 11f
Kidneys, 29
Klebsiella pneumoniae, 51

Langerhans cell(s)
  giant, 59, 60f, 95
  histiocytosis, 127–128, 128f, 129f
Large cell carcinoma(s), 8f
  diagnosis of, 9
  neuroendocrine, 8f
  with rhabdoid phenotype, 8f
Leishmania donovani, 66
Lesion(s)
  CIS, 35, 37f
  focal endobronchial, 1
  mixed, 43
  preinvasive
    diagnosis of, 35, 36f, 37f
    recognized, 35
  SD, 35
Leukemia, 40
LIP. See Lymphocytic interstitial pneumonia
Lipoma(s)
  endobronchial, 45f
  relationships of, 43
Liver, 29
L-tryptophan, 106t
Lung(s), 39–40, 101. See also specific types of lung diseases
  biopsies, 15f
    endobronchial, 97
    wedge, 1, 121, 145
  diseases, 1
    drugs causing, 106t
    interstitial, 146f, 161
  metastases, 29–30
  transplant recipients, 131, 132f, 133f
  tumors
    heterogeneous, 9–10
    WHO classifications of, 9
Lung carcinoma(s), 31f. See also specific types of lung carcinomas
  diagnosis of, 7
  mixed-type, 9–10
  types of, 7

Lung parenchyma, 49f
  alveolar septa of, 2f
  collapsed, 3, 5f
  compression of, 3, 4f
  invasion of, 8
Lymph nodes, 95
Lymphangioleiomyomatosis, 121, 122f
Lymphocytes, 3, 4f, 55, 97
Lymphocytic bronchiolitis, 146f–147f
Lymphocytic interstitial pneumonia (LIP), 115, 117f
Lymphoma(s). See also specific types of lymphomas
  large
    anaplastic, 40f
    B-cell, 39, 41f
  systemic, 40
  T-cell, 39

MAC. See *Mycobacterium avium-intracellulare* complex
Macrophages, 90f, 117f, 118f
  foamy, 75f, 80f
  hemosiderin-laden, 3, 83
  location of, 56f
  pigmented, 112f, 113f
  scattered, 93
MALT lymphoma. See Mucosa-associated lymphoid tissue
Melanoma(s)
  identification of, 30
  metastatic, 32f, 33f
Melphalan, 106t
Mesenchymomas, 43
Metabolic disorders, 68t
Metaplasia, squamous, 40f, 43
Methadone, 106t
Methotrexate, 106t, 107f
Microcrystalline cellulose, 125
Micromyces, 62t
Milk, 79
Mitomycin, 106t
Mitral stenosis, 83
Morbidity, 1, 51
Morrhuate sodium, 106t
Mortality, 1, 51
Mucin
  extracellular, 8–9
  presence of, 8, 15f
  stains, 71
Mucoepidermoid carcinomas, 10
Mucosa(s), 135, 157
  airway, 48f
  bronchial, 2f, 7, 8, 21
    fragments of, 24f–25f, 40f
    infiltration of, 25f
Mucosa-associated lymphoid tissue (MALT lymphoma), characteristics of, 39
Mycobacteria, 59, 60f
Mycobacterium avium-intracellulare complex (MAC), 59, 60f
Mycobacterium kansasii, 59
Mycobacterium scrofulaceum, 59
Mycobacterium tuberculosis, 59, 60f
Mycobacterium xenopi, 59
Mycoplasma pneumoniae, 55, 56f

Naloxone, 106t
Narcotics, 68t
Necrosis, 50f, 135
  alveolar epithelial cell, 79
  coagulative, 21, 26f
  dirty, 29–30

Neoplasm(s), 139
    adjacent to, 4
    benign, occurrence of, 43
    hematologic, 39–40
    primary pulmonary, 39
    vascular spread of, 4*f*
Niemann-Pick disease, 91
Neuroendocrine marker(s)
    CD45, 22, 25*f*
    CD56, 22, 25*f*
    NSE, 25*f*
    PGP9.5, 25*f*
Neuroendocrine tumor(s), 30
    carcinoid, 21, 22*f*, 23, 27*f*
    categories/WHO classifications of, 21–23, 22*t*
    large cell, 21–22, 22*t*, 26*f*
    small cell, 21–22, 22*t*, 23*f*–25*f*
Neutrophils, 40*f*, 55, 56*f*
NSIP. *See* Nonspecific interstitial pneumonia
Nitrofurantoin, 68*t*, 106*t*
Nitrosureas, 106*t*
Non-Hodgkin lymphomas, primary pulmonary, 39
Non-small cell carcinoma(s), 7
    cases of, 15*f*–16*f*, 17*f*
    invasive, 11*f*–12*f*
Nonspecific interstitial pneumonia (NSIP), 115–116, 117*f*
Nonsteroidal anti-inflammatory agents, 106*t*
Nuclear molding, 23*f*–24*f*
Nuclei, 21, 41*f*
Nucleoli
    indistinct, 24*f*
    prominent, 21–22, 41*f*

Pancreas, 29
Papilloma(s). *See also specific types of papillomas*
    glandular, 43
    squamous cell, 43, 44*f*
Papillomatosis, juvenile-onset recurrent respiratory, 151, 153*f*
Parainfluenza, 47, 48*t*
Paraquat, 84*t*
Parasites, 65
PAS. *See* Periodic acid-Schiff stains
PCD. *See* Primary ciliary dyskinesia
Penicillamine, 68*t*, 84*t*, 106*t*
Periodic acid-Schiff stains (PAS), 71
    Alcian blue, 3, 14*f*, 33*f*
    uses of, 59, 61, 93
Phaeohyphomycosis, 62*t*
Pleomorphic carcinomas, 17*f*–18*f*
Pleomorphism(s)
    of cells, 17*f*–18*f*
    cellular, 23
    nuclear, 13*f*, 15*f*, 23
Pleura, 3, 5*f*
Pneumoconioses, 111, 112*f*
Pneumocystis jiroveci, 57, 58*f*
Pneumocytes, 4
Pneumonia(s). *See also specific types of pneumonia*
    acute bacterial, 52*f*, 86*f*
    aspiration, 79, 80*f*
    bacterial, 51
    broncho, 51
    community-acquired, 55
    eosinophilic, 89, 90*f*
    "golden," 91
    herpes, 49*f*
    interstitial, 1, 80*f*, 98*f*
        idiopathic, 115–116, 117*f*, 118*f*

    lipid, 91, 92*f*
        exogenous, 79
    lipoid, 79, 91, 92*f*
    lobar, 51
    organizing, 73, 74*f*, 74*t*, 75*f*, 98*f*, 103*f*, 161
        acute fibrinous and, 77, 78*f*
    pneumocystis, 57, 58*f*
    postobstructive, 91, 92*f*
    types of, 51, 52*f*
Pneumothorax, 1, 127, 145
Polyangiitis, microscopic, 68*t*
Polyarteritis
    microscopic, 83, 109
    nodosa, 68*t*
Polychondritis, relapsing, 140–141, 142*f*, 143*f*
Polymyositis, 68*t*, 83, 101
Prednisone, 102*f*
Primary ciliary dyskinesia (PCD), 157, 158*f*
Primary pulmonary neoplasms, 39
Primary pulmonary non-Hodgkin lymphomas, 39
Procarbazine, 106*t*
Progesterone receptors, 121
Progressive systemic sclerosis, 101
Propoxyphene, 106*t*
Prostatic acid phosphatase. *See* PSA
Protamine, 106*t*
PSA (prostatic acid phosphatase), 20
Psammoma bodies (calcospherites), 3
Pseudomonas, 51, 52*f*
Pulmonary adenocarcinomas, 16*f*
Pulmonary alveolar proteinosis, 93, 94*f*
Pulmonary edema, 71, 72*f*, 93
Pulmonary eosinophilia, 89, 90*f*
Pulmonary fibrosis, 102*f*
Pulmonary hemorrhage, 67, 68*t*
    causes of, 84*t*
    drugs and, 84*t*
Pulmonary hypertension, 83, 101
Pulmonary leishmaniasis, 66
Pulmonary vasculitis, 67

Radiation, 68*t*, 74*t*
Rapamycin. *See* Sirolimus
RBILD. *See* Respiratory bronchiolitis-associated interstitial lung disease
Renal cell carcinomas, 30, 33*f*
Respiratory bronchiolitis-associated interstitial lung disease (RBILD), 115, 128
Rheumatoid arthritis, 68*t*, 83, 101, 103*f*
Rickettsia rickettsii, 65
Rickettsia typhi, 65
Rickettsiae, 65
Rocky Mountain spotted fever, 65

Salicylates, 106*t*
Salivary-type carcinomas, 10
Sarcoidosis, 95, 96*f*, 147*f*
Sarcomas, metastatic, 29
Sarcomatoid carcinomas, 8*f*, 9, 18*f*–19*f*
Schaumann bodies, 3, 147*f*
Scleroderma, 68*t*, 83, 102*f*
SD. *See* Squamous dysplasia
Serologic testing, 55
Shock, 67, 68*t*
Signet-ring cell adenocarcinomas, 8*f*
Silica, 112*f*
Sirolimus (rapamycin), 107*t*
Situs inversus (Kartagener syndrome), 157
Sjögren syndrome, 101

Small cell lung carcinoma(s), 3, 7
Smokers
    cigarette, 127–128, 128f, 129f
    pigment, 115–116, 117f, 118f
Specimens, 161
Spores, 61
Sporotrichosis, 62t
Squamous cell carcinoma(s), 7–8, 30
    basaloid, 8f, 9
    clear cell, 8f
    diagnosis of, 11f
    papillary, 8f
    small cell, 8f
    variants of, 8f
Squamous cell papillomas, 43, 44f
Squamous dysplasia (SD), 7
    angiogenic, 36f
    definition of, 35
    lesions, 35
Squamous epithelium
    atypical, 7, 37f
    metaplastic, 10f–11f
    stratified, 44f
Squamous metaplasia, 40f, 43
Stain(s). *See also* Periodic acid-Schiff stains
    Giemsa, 65
    Gram, 59
        negative, 51, 65
        positive, 51
    Grocott silver, 61
    iron, 4
    mucin, 71
    special, 107f
    toluidine blue, 57
Staphylococcus aureus, 51
Steroids, 89
Stomach, 29
Streptococcus pneumoniae, 51
Streptokinases, 84t
Stroma, 12f, 45f
    chondroid, 43
    fibrovascular, 44f, 45f
    little, 23
    myxoid, 73, 75f
    subepithelial, 16f
Strongyloides, 65
Sulfasalazine, 106t
Sulfonamides, 106t
Surgery, 1
Synaptophysin, 22, 25f, 26f
Systemic lupus erythematosus, 68t, 86f, 101

Tachyzoites, 66f
Talc, 106t, 125, 126t
Testis, 29
Texas Children's Hospital, 145
Thoracoscopy, 1
Thyroid transcription factor-1 (TTF-1), 14f, 22–23, 30
Ticks, 65
Tissue(s)
    biopsies, 7
    compression, 3
    diseases, connective, 84t
Tocainide, 106t
Toluidine blue stains, 57
Toxic shock syndrome, 68t
Toxins, 67
Toxoplasma gondii, 65

Tracheobronchial amyloidosis, 140, 141f
Tracheobronchial biopsy(ies), 157, 158f
Transbronchial biopsy(ies), 8, 43
    basis for, 1
    children and, 145, 146f, 147f, 148f, 149f, 150f
    deep, 3
    forceps, 3
    high power of, 2f, 5f
    legal aspects of, 161–162
    low power of, 4f, 5f, 6f
    material, 22
    overview of, 1
Transplant associated pathology, 135, 136f. *See also*
        Acute transplant rejection; Lungs
Trimellitic anhydride, 84t
Trophozoites, 57, 65–66, 66f
TTF-1. *See* Thyroid transcription factor-1
Tuberculosis, 59
Tumor(s). *See also specific types of tumors*
    cells, 7, 18f
        infiltration of, 21
        power of, 26f
    crushed, 25f
    endobronchial, 32f, 151, 153f, 154f, 155f
    high-grade malignant, 26f
    inflammatory myofibroblastic, 151, 153f
    neuroendocrine
        carcinoid, 21, 22t, 23, 27f
        categories/WHO classifications of, 21–23, 22t
        large cell, 21–22, 22t, 26f
        small cell, 21–22, 22t, 23f–25f
    papillary, 13f–14f
    WHO classifications of, 7–8, 8t
Typhus, 65

UIP. *See* Usual interstitial pneumonia
United States (U.S.), 65
University of Florida, 145
U.S. *See* United States
Usual interstitial pneumonia (UIP), 115–116, 117f, 118f

Vacuole(s)
    intracellular, 12f
    mucin, 13f, 32f
Valvular heart diseases, 71
Vasculitis, 84t
    capillaritis, 83
    pulmonary, 67
    sarcoid, 95
Vinblastine, 106t
Virus(es). *See also* Influenza; *specific types of viruses*
    measles, 47, 48t
    respiratory syncytial, 47, 48t
    types of, 47, 48t

Wegener granulomatosis, 68t, 83, 109
WHO. *See* World Health Organization
World Health Organization (WHO)
    adenocarcinoma classifications of, 7–8, 8t
    definitions, 9
    lung tumor classifications of, 9
    neuroendocrine tumor classifications of,
            21–23, 22t
    tumor classifications of, 7–8, 8t

Xanthogranulomas, juvenile, 151, 153f

Yeast, 61